The Career Advisor Series offers three healthcare career directories to cover the whole spectrum of jobs in this crucial and fast-growing field:

Healthcare Career Directory—Nurses and Physicians covers:

Critical Care Nurse

Long-Term Care Nurse

Neurologist

Nurse Practitioner

Oncology Nurse

Pathologist

Pediatrician

Psychiatrist

Specialty Nurse

Surgeon

Traveling Nurse

Therapists and Allied Health Professionals Career Directory is

designed to cover licensed health workers, other than physicians, nurses, and public health professionals, who provide one-on-one services to patients, including:

Athletic Trainer

Audiologist

Chiropractor

Dental Hygienist

Dietician

Massage Therapist

Medical Assistant

Occupational Therapist

Pharmacist

Physical Therapist

Physician Assistant

Recreational Therapist

Respiratory Therapist

Speech-Language Pathologist

Sports Medicine Specialist

Surgical Physician Assistant

Medical Technologists and Technicians Career Directory is designed to cover

the more technical healthcare careers, including:

Cardiac and Pulmonary Rehabilitation Specialist

Cytotechnologist

Correctional Healthcare Administrator

Electroneurodiagnostic Technologist

Emergency Medical Technician

Health Information Manager

Health Sciences Librarian

Health Services Administrator

Histotechnologist

Infection Control Specialist/Epidemiologist

Laboratory Medical Personnel

Medical Illustrator

Nuclear Medicine Technologist

Ophthalmic Allied Health Professional

Optometric Technician

Radiologic Technologist

Surgical Technologist

THERAPISTS AND ALLIED HEALTH PROFESSIONALS

CAREER DIRECTORY

Gale Research Inc. proudly presents the first edition of the *Therapists and Allied Health Professionals Career Directory*. The hallmark of this volume, part of Gale's Career Advisor Series, is the essays by active professionals. Here, industry insiders describe opportunities and challenges in all segments of the allied health professions, including:

- Occupational therapy
- Speech-language pathology/audiology
- Physical therapy
- Sports medicine
- Athletic training
- Recreational therapy
- Massage therapy/bodywork
- Respiratory therapy

- Physician assistantship
- Surgical physician assistantship
- Medical assistantship
- Chiropractic healthcare
- Dental hygiene
- Pharmacy
- Dietetics/nutrition

In fully up-to-date articles, they describe:

- What to expect on the job
- Typical career paths
- What they look for in an applicant
- How their specialty is unique

Provides Excellent Job Hunting Resources

Once this "Advice from the Pro's" has given you a feel for allied health careers, the *Directory* offers even more help with your job search strategy:

- **The Job Search Process** includes essays on determining career objectives, resume preparation, networking, writing effective cover letters, and interviewing. With worksheets and sample resumes and letters. **FEATURES:** Resumes are targeted to the realities of allied health professions.

- **Job Opportunities Databank** provides details on hundreds of organizations that hire at entry-level. **FEATURES:** In addition to the entry-level information, entries also include information on all-important internship opportunities.

- **Career Resources** identifies sources of help-wanted ads, professional associations, employment agencies and search firms, career guides, professional and trade periodicals, and basic reference guides and handbooks. **FEATURES:** Resource listings include detailed descriptions to help you select the publications and organizations that will best meet your needs.

Master Index Puts Information at Your Fingertips

This edition is thoroughly indexed, with access to essays and directory sections both by subject and by organization name, publication title, or service name.

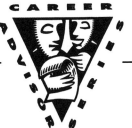

CAREER ADVISOR SERIES

ISSN 1070-7263

THERAPISTS AND ALLIED HEALTH PROFESSIONALS

CAREER DIRECTORY

A Practical, One-Stop Guide to Getting a Job as an Allied Health Specialist

1ST EDITION

Bradley J. Morgan and Joseph M. Palmisano, Editors

Diane M. Sawinski, Associate Editor

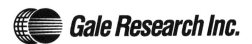

Gale Research Inc.

DETROIT • WASHINGTON, D.C. • LONDON

Editors: Bradley J. Morgan and Joseph M. Palmisano
Associate Editors: Joyce Jakubiak and Diane M. Sawinski
Assistant Editor: Wendy H. Mason
Aided by: Mary Alampi, Susan E. Edgar, Susan P. Hutton,
Peggy Kneffel Daniels, Katherine H. Nemeh, Lou Ann J. Shelton,
and Devra M. Sladics
Senior Editor: Linda S. Hubbard

Research Manager: Victoria B. Cariappa
Research Supervisor: Gary J. Oudersluys
Research Associate: Tracie A. Wade
Research Assistants: Andreia L. Earley, Charles A. Jewell,
Colin C. McDonald, Michele L. McRobert, Michele P. Pica,
Phyllis Shepherd, and Barbara Thornton

Production Manager: Mary Beth Trimper
Production Assistant: Shanna Philpott Heilveil

Technical Design Services Manager: Art Chartow
Art Director: Cindy Baldwin
Graphic Designer: Mary Krzewinski

Supervisor of Systems and Programming: Theresa Rocklin
Programmer: Timothy Richardson

Data Entry Supervisor: Benita L. Spight
Data Entry Group Leader: Gwendolyn S. Tucker
Data Entry Associates: Beverly Jendrowski and Fredrick L. Penn Jr.

Some data were included from *Ward's Business Directory,* copyrighted by Information Access Company.

ISBN 0-8103-9155-4
ISSN 1070-7263

Printed in the United States of America

Published simultaneously in the United Kingdom
by Gale Research International Limited
(An affiliated company of Gale Research Inc.)

The trademark **ITP** is used under license.

Contents

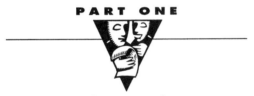

PART ONE

Advice from the Pro's

1 Occupational Therapy—A Great Bet in Today's Career Game

Marian Kavanagh Scheinholtz, M.S., OTR/L, Clinical Education
Program Coordinator, Dept. of Rehabilitation Medicine, National
Institutes of Health, and Howard Holland, APR, Public Relations Dept.,
The American Occupational Therapy Association, Inc.

*Examines how to begin a personally and financially rewarding career in the growing
field of occupational therapy.* **1**

**2 Speech-Language Pathology and Audiology:
Careers That Make a Difference**

Patricia A. Cole, Ph.D., Director, Membership and Career Development,
American Speech-Language-Hearing Association

*Explores the preparation needed to land a job helping others communicate—a career
in speech-language pathology and audiology.* **5**

**3 Medical Social Work in a Physical Therapy Clinic:
A Unique Opportunity**

Jennie Petrovich, MSW, Greater Lansing Rehabilitation Agency

*Ironing out personal problems with the help of a medical social worker allows
patients to more easily direct their energy into physical rehabilitation.* **15**

v

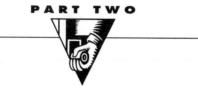

The Job Search Process

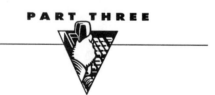

Job Opportunities Databank

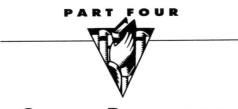

Acknowledgments

The editors would like to thank all the pro's who took the time out of their busy schedules to share their first-hand knowledge and enthusiasm with the next generation of job-seekers. A special thanks to Kathleen M. Daniels, Assistant Director of the Career Planning and Placement Office at the University of Detroit Mercy, who provided much needed help with the job search section.

Thanks are also owed to the human resources personnel at the companies listed in this volume and to the public relations staffs of the associations who provided excellent suggestions for new essays. Joseph Donovan of the College of Allied Health Sciences at Thomas Jefferson University deserves special mention.

Introduction

"Corporate America has developed a deep, and perhaps abiding, reluctance to hire."

—*Business Week*, February 22, 1993

As the above quote indicates, getting and keeping a job these days can be a demanding proposition. Despite an economy that is finally recovering from the latest recession, many firms are still downsizing and are reluctant to increase staff levels.

What this means is that the job search is an increasingly competitive process. To beat the competition, job seekers need information. By utilizing the *Therapists and Allied Health Professionals Career Directory*, job seekers gain all the information they need to make the best possible decisions during their job search. The *Directory* is a comprehensive, one-stop resource that includes:

- Essays by industry professionals that provide practical advice not found in any other career resource
- Job search guidance designed to help you get in the door in allied health
- Job and internship listings from leading hospitals, healthcare facilities, and pharmaceutical companies in the United States
- Information on additional career resources to further the job hunt
- A Master Index to facilitate easy access to the *Directory*

The *Directory* is organized into four parts that correspond to the steps of a typical job search—identifying your area of interest, refining your presentation, targeting agencies, and researching your prospects.

Advice from the Pro's: An Invaluable Tool

Instead of offering "one-size-fits-all" advice or government statistics on what the working world is like, the *Therapists and Allied Health Professionals Career Directory* goes into the field for first-hand reports from experienced professionals working in all segments of allied health. This "Advice from the Pro's" is offered by people who know what it's like to land that first job and turn it into a rich and rewarding career.

Learn about:

- the various opportunities available for dieticians from Pam Michael of the American Dietetic Association, the leading association for dieticians in the United States.
- the increasing importance of physician assistants from Lisa Mustone Alexander, director of the physician assistant program at the George Washington University Medical Center.
- the rewards of working as a physical therapist or athletic trainer in sports medicine rehabilitation from Janet Ventimiglia, manager of the Center for Athletic Medicine, Henry Ford Hospital.
- and 10 other areas of specialization, including:

Occupational therapy	Surgical physician assistantship
Speech language pathology/audiology	Medical assistantship
Recreational therapy	Chiropractic healthcare
Massage therapy/bodywork	Dental hygiene
Respiratory therapy	Pharmacy

The essays cover the most important things a job applicant needs to know, including:

- What college courses and other background offer the best preparation
- Specific skills that are needed
- What organizations look for in an applicant
- Typical career paths
- Salary information

The Job Search Process: Making Sense of It All

What is the first thing a new job-hunter should do?

What different types of resumes exist and what should they look like?

What questions are off-limits in an interview?

These important questions are among the dozens that go through every person's mind when he or she begins to look for a job. Part Two of the *Therapists and Allied Health Professionals Career Directory*, **The Job Search Process**, answers these questions and more. It is divided into five chapters that cover all the basics of how to aggressively pursue a job:

- **Getting Started: Self-Evaluation and Career Objectives.** How to evaluate personal strengths and weaknesses and set goals.
- **Targeting Companies and Networking for Success.** How to identify the organizations you would like to work for and how to build a network of contacts.
- **Preparing Your Resume.** What to include, what not to include, and what style to use. Includes samples of the three basic resume types and worksheets to help you organize your information.
- **Writing Better Letters.** What letters should be written throughout the search process and how to make them more effective. Includes samples.
- **Questions for You, Questions for Them.** How to handle an interview and get the job.

Job Opportunities Databank: Finding the Job You Want

Once you're ready to start sending out those first resumes, how do you know where to start? The **Job Opportunities Databank**, Part Three of the *Directory*, includes listings for nearly 350 hospitals, rehabilitation centers, intermediate and long-term care facilities, and pharmaceutical companies in the United States that offer entry-level jobs in allied health. These listings provide detailed contact information and data on the organizations' business activities, hiring practices, benefits, and application procedures—everything you need to know to approach potential employers. And since internships play an increasingly important role in the career research and employment process, information on the internship opportunities offered by the organizations listed is also included.

For further information on the arrangement and content of the **Job Opportunities Databank**, consult "How to Use the Job Opportunities Databank" immediately following this introduction.

Career Resources: A Guide to Organizations and Publications in the Field

Need to do more research on the specialty you've chosen or the organizations you'll be interviewing with? Part Four of the *Directory*, **Career Resources**, includes information on the following:

- Sources of help-wanted ads
- Professional associations
- Employment agencies and search firms
- Career guides
- Professional and trade periodicals
- Basic reference guides and handbooks

Listings contain contact information and descriptions of each publication's content and each organization's membership, purposes, and activities, helping you to pinpoint the resources you need for your own specific job search.

For additional information on the arrangement and content of **Career Resources**, consult "How to Locate Career Resources" following this introduction.

Master Index Speeds Access to Resources

A Master Index leads you to the information contained in all four sections of the *Directory* by citing all subjects, organizations, publications, and services listed throughout in a single alphabetic sequence. The index also includes inversions on significant keywords appearing in cited organization, publication, and service names. For example, the "National Athletic Trainers' Association" would also be listed in the index under "Athletic Trainers' Association; National." Citations in the index refer to page numbers.

Information Keeps Pace with the Changing Job Market

This first edition of the *Therapists and Allied Health Professionals Career Directory* contains essays in the Advice from the Pro's section by leading professionals in the allied health field on subjects of particular interest to today's job seekers. All employers listed in the **Job Opportunities Databank** were contacted by telephone or facsimile to obtain current information, and **Career Resources** listings were obtained from selected material in other databases compiled by Gale Research Inc.

Comments and Suggestions Welcome

The staff of the *Therapists and Allied Health Professionals Career Directory* appreciates learning of any corrections or additions that will make this book as complete and useful as possible. Comments or suggestions for future essay topics or other improvements are also welcome, as are suggestions for careers that could be covered in new volumes of the Career Advisor Series. Please contact:

Career Advisor Series
Gale Research Inc.
835 Penobscot Bldg.
Detroit, MI 48226-4094
Phone: 800-347-GALE
Fax: (313)961-6815

Bradley J. Morgan
Joseph M. Palmisano

How to Use the
Job Opportunities Databank

The **Job Opportunities Databank** comprises two sections:
Entry-Level Job and Internship Listings
Additional Companies

Entry-Level Job and Internship Listings

Provides listings for nearly 350 general medical and surgical hospitals, rehabilitation centers, intermediate and long-term care facilities, and pharmaceutical companies in the United States. Entries in the **Job Opportunities Databank** are arranged alphabetically by organization name. When available, entries include:

- **Organization name.**
- **Address and telephone number.** A mailing address and telephone number are provided in every entry.
- **Fax and toll-free telephone number.** These are provided when known.
- **Business description.** Outlines the organization's business activities.
- **Corporate officers.** Lists the names of executive officers, with titles.
- **Number of employees.** Includes the most recently provided figure for total number of employees. Other employee-specific information may be provided as well.
- **Average entry-level hiring.** Includes the number of entry-level employees the organization typically hires in an average year. Many organizations have listed "Unknown" or "0" for their average number of entry-level jobs. Because of current economic conditions, many organizations could not estimate their projected entry-level hires for the coming years. However, because these firms have offered entry-level positions in the past and because their needs may change, we have listed them in this edition.
- **Opportunities.** Describes the entry-level positions that the organization typically offers, as well as the education and other requirements needed for those positions.

- **Benefits**. Lists the insurance, time off, retirement and financial plans, activities, and programs provided by the organization, if known.
- **Human resources contacts**. Lists the names of personnel-related staff, with titles.
- **Application procedure**. Describes specific application instructions, when provided by the organization.

Many entries also include information on available internship programs. Internship information provided includes:

- **Contact name**. Lists the names of officers or personnel-related contact who are responsible for the internship program.
- **Type**. Indicates the type of internship, including time period and whether it is paid, unpaid, or for college credit. Also indicates if an organization does not offer any internships.
- **Number available**. Number of internships that the organization typically offers.
- **Number of applications received**. Total number of applications received in a typical year.
- **Application procedures and deadline**. Describes specific application instructions and the deadline for submitting applications.
- **Decision date**. Final date when internship placement decisions are made.
- **Duties**. Lists the typical duties that an intern can expect to perform at the organization.
- **Qualifications**. Lists the criteria a prospective applicant must meet to be considered for an internship with the organization.

Additional Companies

Covers those organizations that elected to provide only their name, address, and telephone number for inclusion in the *Directory*. Entries are arranged alphabetically by organization name.

How to Locate
Career Resources

The **Career Resources** chapter contains six categories of information sources, each of which is arranged alphabetically by resource or organization name. The categories include:

▼ Sources of Help-Wanted Ads

- **Covers:** Professional journals, industry periodicals, association newsletters, placement bulletins, and online services that include employment ads or business opportunities. Includes sources that focus specifically on allied health professions, as well as general periodical sources such as the *National Business Employment Weekly*.
- **Entries include:** The resource's title; name, address, and telephone number of its publisher; frequency; subscription rate; description of contents; toll-free and additional telephone numbers; and facsimile numbers.
- **Sources:** *Job Hunter's Sourcebook* (published by Gale Research Inc.) and original research.

▼ Professional Associations

- **Covers:** Trade and professional associations that offer career-related information and services.
- **Entries include:** Association name, address, and telephone number; membership; purpose and objectives; publications; toll-free or additional telephone numbers; and facsimile numbers. In some cases, the publications mentioned in these entries are described in greater detail as separate entries cited in the Sources of Help Wanted Ads, Career Guides, Professional and Trade Periodicals, and Basic Reference Guides and Handbooks categories.
- **Sources:** *Encyclopedia of Associations* (published by Gale Research Inc.) and original research.

▼ Employment Agencies and Search Firms

- **Covers:** Firms used by organizations to recruit candidates for positions and, at times, by individuals to pursue openings. Employment agencies are generally geared towards filling openings at entry- to mid-level in the local job market, while executive search firms are paid by the hiring organization to recruit professional and managerial candidates, usually for higher-level openings. Also covers temporary employment agencies because they can be a method of identifying and obtaining regular employment. Includes firms that focus specifically on allied health professions, as well as some larger general organizations.

- **Entries include:** The organization's name, address, and telephone number; whether it's an employment agency, executive search firm, or temporary agency; descriptive information, as appropriate; toll-free and additional telephone numbers; and facsimile number.
- **Sources:** *Job Hunter's Sourcebook.*

▼ Career Guides

- **Covers:** Books, kits, pamphlets, brochures, videocassettes, films, online services, and other materials that describe the job-hunting process in general or that provide guidance and insight into the job-hunting process in allied health.
- **Entries include:** The resource's title; name, address, and telephone number of its publisher or distributor; name of the editor or author; publication date or frequency; description of contents; arrangement; indexes; toll-free or additional telephone numbers; and facsimile numbers.
- **Sources:** *Professional Careers Sourcebook* and *Vocational Careers Sourcebook* (published by Gale Research Inc.) and original research.

▼ Professional and Trade Periodicals

- **Covers:** Newsletters, magazines, newspapers, trade journals, and other serials that offer information to allied health professionals.
- **Entries include:** The resource's title; the name, address, and telephone number of the publisher; the editor's name; frequency; description of contents; toll-free and additional telephone numbers; and facsimile numbers. Publication titles appear in italics.
- **Sources:** *Gale Directory of Publications* and *Broadcast Media* and *Newsletters in Print* (published by Gale Research Inc.) and original research.

▼ Basic Reference Guides and Handbooks

- **Covers:** Manuals, directories, dictionaries, encyclopedias, films and videocassettes, and other published reference material used by professionals working in allied health.
- **Entries include:** The resource's title; name, address, and telephone number of the publisher or distributor; the editor's or author's name; publication date or frequency; description of contents; toll-free and additional telephone numbers; and facsimile numbers. Publication titles are rendered in italics.
- **Sources:** *Professional Careers Sourcebook, Vocational Careers Sourcebook,* and original research.

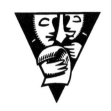

ADVICE
FROM THE
PRO'S

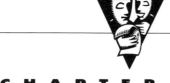

Occupational Therapy—
A Great Bet in Today's Career Game

**Marian Kavanagh Scheinholtz, M.S., O.T.R./L.,
Clinical Education Program Coordinator, Dept. of Rehabilitation
Medicine, National Institutes of Health, and
Howard Holland, APR,
Public Relations Dept., The American Occupational Therapy
Association, Inc.**

Where can you invest two to four years in a college degree that offers the entree to an amazing variety of career options beginning with your first job and continuing throughout your work life? What field offers you the opportunity to choose from among jobs working with newborn infants, school children, teens, or the elderly? What field offers positions in hospitals, schools, nursing homes, and industry throughout the continental U.S. and abroad? Where will you find employability, job mobility, good salaries, and benefits with an eight-to-five or even part-time work week? Where can you move up and move ahead without returning to school, find plenty of management opportunities, or enjoy a wide open field for your services as a consultant or business owner?

The answer is occupational therapy! What is it that people do in this wonderful career and why the funny name? The term *occupational therapy* accounts for a certain amount of the confusion, although the profession itself has been around the healthcare scene for more than 70 years. Simply stated, occupational therapy is treatment based on the idea that most people who are sick or have a physical or mental disability can still do many things for themselves. In almost every case, they are a lot better off for doing so! It isn't hard to understand that people who are active or *occupied* with carrying out their daily activities are more independent and productive and get better faster. The key to applying this concept as therapy is the contribution of trained professionals who can determine just how much and what kind of activity is beneficial to a particular individual at each step along the way.

People are most often introduced to occupational therapy when they are having difficulty functioning effectively in one or more aspects of life because of developmental, physical, or mental problems. If you have seen the movie *Dad*, starring Tom Hanks, you have seen an excellent capsule version of the concept of occupational therapy applied to meeting the needs of an older person. When his wife is suddenly hospitalized, an elderly gentleman finds he is totally helpless in carrying out the simplest of daily tasks. When his routine is broken down into steps listed on reminder cards, he finds that he can indeed prepare a simple meal, wash a load of laundry, and prepare a shopping list.

But not only elderly people benefit from occupational therapy. People with many different kinds of health problems also need specialized help in performing life's many tasks. Four-year-old Kelly was born with cerebral palsy. Occupational therapy was part of his life right from the start. An occupational therapist worked with him in the hospital nursery and taught his parents how they could stimulate his development at home. During his first two years, an occupational therapist visited his home twice a week to update his activity program and to give his mother hints on how she could encourage his self-sufficiency. At the age of three, Kelly was enrolled in a special nursery school for children with disabilities in the county school system. Here, occupational therapists consult regularly with classroom teachers on how children with disabilities should sit or be positioned, and adapt toys and learning materials for their special needs. Because Kelly has poor hand function, the occupational therapist has adapted a number of battery-powered toys with switches that he can enjoy.

Connie, a supermarket employee was injured in a fall on the job. The physician who treated her back injury referred her to an occupational therapist. The therapist advised Connie on resuming her household routine and completing tasks such as cleaning, laundry, and child care without causing pain or damage to her back. After evaluating her physical capabilities, the therapist provided several adaptive devices, such as an aid to help her put on her stockings. When Connie was ready to return to her job, the occupational therapist visited her work place and showed her how she could rearrange her work area and reposition some of the equipment for greater safety and less fatigue.

Oliver, in his mid-30's, has schizophrenia. Due to the frequent recurrence of his symptoms over the past 13 years, his ability to function independently has deteriorated. Recently, Oliver began taking a new medication that significantly improved his symptoms, but he still has many difficulties living in the community. He lacks skills to interact appropriately in work and social situations. He is unable to manage his money. He has trouble structuring his time and though he is able to get jobs, he loses them after a few days. Oliver was treated by an occupational therapist who used cooking and computer activities to help him improve his concentration and problem-solving abilities. She guided him to develop a structured daily schedule and to plan his spending. With his therapist, Oliver developed realistic goals for returning to work and began to initiate activities related to those goals.

Employment Benefits

Because of the many kinds of people with whom they work and the individual challenges faced by each patient, the occupational therapy profession attracts people who enjoy using creativity and problem-solving skills. Those who are employed in the field enjoy a high degree of autonomy and self-direction in their daily work that contributes to high career satisfaction. In fact, most of those who choose occupational therapy careers stay in some aspect of the profession throughout their work lives. The field is ideal for the career re-entry individual or older learner who will find maturity and life experience to be welcomed assets in the education process as well as in professional life.

Employment Opportunities

Employers nationwide are anxiously seeking candidates to fill the growing number of positions available in occupational therapy. The American Occupational Therapy Association estimates that there is currently a 25 percent shortage in the field at a time when the U.S. Bureau of Labor Statistics is predicting a 55 percent increase in available positions by the year 2005. This rapid growth is due to a greater awareness of the value of occupational therapy in preparing people to function independently in the mainstream of life as well as to an increasing survival rate of individuals who are affected by serious illness and injury.

Entry into the field is available at both technical and professional levels. You can become an occupational therapy assistant by completing a two-year associate degree program at one of more than 80 colleges and universities throughout the country. To enter the field as an occupational therapist, you may enroll in a four-year baccalaureate degree program or if you already have a bachelor's degree, you could be eligible for what is termed an *entry-level master's degree*. (To receive a free list of programs located throughout the United States, contact: The American Occupational Therapy Association, Public Relations Department, 1383 Piccard Drive, Rockville, MD 20850, or call their toll-free CareerLine, 1-800-366-9799.)

Top Companies in Hiring/Promoting People with Disabilities

Ranked by percentage of disabled employees at each company.
1. IBM, with 15.6%
2. Federal government, 10.0%
3. AT & T, 6.4%
4. McDonald's, 5.1%
5. State government, 3.8%
6. Marriott, 3.3%
7. General Electric, 2.6%
8. E. I. du Pont de Nemours, 2.3%
9. General Motors Corp., 2.0%
9. Boeing, 2.0%
11. Hewlett-Packard, 1.5%
11. Sears, Roebuck & Co., 1.5%

Source: *HR Magazine*

Entry into the field at either the technical or professional level is very competitive. Candidates often have excellent grade point averages and volunteer experience in a healthcare facility where they have been able to observe occupational therapy practitioners at work.

Occupational therapy jobs abound in both major metropolitan areas and in smaller, rural communities. Specialized regional facilities, such as a rehabilitation hospital, may employ as many as 50 therapists at any one time, while a nursing home might contract with one therapist operating a private practice to treat individual patients on an as-needed basis. Overall, 32 percent of occupational therapists work in general, psychiatric, and pediatric hospitals, 19 percent in public and private schools, and 12 percent in rehabilitation hospitals or centers. Others work in colleges and universities, home health agencies, skilled nursing homes, and private practice. Among occupational therapy assistants, 26 percent work in hospitals, 21 percent in skilled nursing homes and intermediate care facilities, and 17 percent in public and private schools. Other occupational therapy assistants work in community mental health centers, rehabilitation hospitals, residential care facilities, day care programs, and community agencies.

Direct patient treatment is only one of many career opportunities in occupational therapy. With experience comes eligibility for a variety of positions in healthcare management, as well as heading an occupational therapy department.

Salaries

In 1992, half of all new therapists earned an average of $32,400 in their first position and received between three and four job offers. Salaries in high-paying areas such as Washington, DC, are often substantially higher. Benefits include sign-on bonuses, tuition reimbursement for the costs of basic education and funds for continuing education or advanced degrees, as well as health and medical insurance, paid vacation, and child care. Occupational therapy assistant salaries averaged $21,200 nationally with higher cost areas offering salaries substantially higher.

The Future in Occupational Therapy

Occupational therapy practitioners, like all healthcare professionals, face a challenging future in light of the pressures on the healthcare system and impending healthcare reform. But regardless of changes in the environment, occupational therapists and certified assistants—together with all allied health professionals—can look forward to a continued role in helping meet the nation's healthcare needs.

▼

MARIAN KAVANAGH SCHEINHOLTZ is clinical education program coordinator for the Department of Rehabilitation Medicine at the National Institutes of Health, Bethesda, MD. She holds a bachelor of science degree from the University of Pittsburgh and a master's degree in occupational therapy from Virginia Commonwealth University.

HOWARD HOLLAND, a graduate of Furman University and the Duke University Divinity School, is an accredited member of the Public Relations Society of America. He works at the American Occupational Therapy Association's national office in Rockville, MD, in the public relations department.

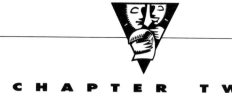

Speech-Language Pathology and Audiology: Careers That Make a Difference

Patricia A. Cole, Ph.D.,
Director, Membership and Career Development,
American Speech-Language-Hearing Association

Surprisingly, a large segment of the American population is not familiar with the professions of speech-language pathology and audiology. The professions represent the discipline of communication sciences and disorders. I will start by stating that there is a great deal of flexibility after one enters the professions. You can be almost anything you want to be—clinical service provider, researcher, professor/teacher, scientist, entrepreneur, or administrator. The careers are rewarding by virtue of the impact they have in helping individuals restore or enhance their communication skills.

The Practice of the Professions

Speech-Language Pathologists

Speech-language pathologists assess, evaluate, diagnose, and treat speech and language disorders in infants and toddlers, preschool and school-age children, and adults. They provide guidance and assistance for communication and development disorders and related areas; they conduct research in human communication and its disorders. The range of services provided by speech-language pathologists include:

- **Screening** to identify individuals who require further speech-language evaluation to determine the presence or absence of a communication disorder;

- **Preventing, evaluating, assessing** and **interpreting,** and **diagnosing** communication disorders;

- **Planning, directing,** and **conducting** rehabilitative and counseling programs to treat disorders;

- **Assessing, selecting, developing,** and **determining** the need for augmentative communication systems (sign language, gesture systems, communication boards, electronic devices, mechanical devices, and other computer assisted devices);

- **Providing elective services** to nonstandard English speakers who do not have a communication disorder;

- **Enhancing speech-language proficiency** and **communication effectiveness** such as accent reduction; and

- **Screening** of hearing and other factors for the purpose of speech-language evaluation and/or the initial identification of individuals with other communication disorders.

Audiologists

Audiologists identify, assess, and treat individuals of all ages with hearing handicaps. They are involved in preventing and detecting hearing problems and the management of existing communication disorders. The specific services provided by qualified audiologists include:

- **Screening** and **identifying** persons who require further evaluation to determine the presence or absence of a hearing problem;

- **Preventing, evaluating, assessing** and **interpreting,** and **diagnosing** communication disorders related to peripheral and central auditory system dysfunctions;

- **Planning** and **directing** habilitative and aural rehabilitation and counseling programs to treat peripheral and central auditory disorders and hearing problems that include, but are not limited to, selecting, fitting, and dispensing of:
    - a. auditory prosthesis, hearing aid, or assistive listening and alerting devices and providing orientation/training in their use;
    - b. counseling, guidance, and auditory training;
    - c. speech reading training; and
    - d. language habilitation.

- **Facilitating** the conservation of auditory system function, and **developing** and **implementing** environmental and occupational hearing conservation programs; and

- **Screening** for speech-language and other factors affecting communication function for the purposes of audiologic evaluation and/or initial identification of individuals with other communication disorders.

Speech-language pathologists and audiologists also engage in the following:

- Planning for discharge/termination and ensuring that the patient/client's family understands the communication abilities and program;

- Monitoring the effectiveness of treatment rendered to improve the communication skills of the patients/clients served; and

- Counseling and consulting with the clients/patients, their families, and others involved in the patients'/clients' life (e.g., teachers, employers, etc.).

They may teach and engage in basic and applied research associated with human communication and its disorders. Finally, they may serve as administrators or managers of programs and services in and/or related to communication disorders or maintain private consulting agencies or private practices.

Professional Practice Credentials

Currently, to practice the profession of speech-language pathology and/or audiology, one must hold a master's or doctoral degree, and preferably—though not required—the American Speech-Language-Hearing Association's Certificate of Clinical Competence (CCC) and a state license, where applicable. Individuals who desire to work in school-based settings may have to obtain state education agency certification. Presently, there are 43 states that regulate the practice of speech-language pathology and audiology.

All institutions and/or agencies accredited by the ASHA Educational Standards Board (ESB) and Professional Services Board (PSB) require speech-language pathologists and audiologists to hold the ASHA CCC. Also, effective January 1, 1994, to qualify for the ASHA National Certification, all graduate course work and clinical practicum must have been initiated and completed at an ASHA ESB accredited institution. Agencies or institutions that accept medicare and are regulated by the Healthcare Financing Administration required speech-language pathologists to be licensed by the state, eligible for the ASHA CCC, or be in the process of obtaining certification. Practitioners engaged in private practice usually hold master's or doctoral degrees and have the ASHA national certification and a state license.

To obtain the ASHA National Certification in speech-language pathology and/or audiology, one must hold a master's or doctoral degree, which includes completion of academic and clinicalpracticum requirements, passage of the National Examinations in Speech-Language Pathology and Audiology (NESPA), and completion of a Clinical Fellowship (CF).

The Clinical Fellowship is similar to the residency requirement that physicians must complete. It is a paid, professional experience. However, the clinical fellow is supervised by an individual who holds the American Speech-Language-Hearing Association's (ASHA) Certificate of Clinical Competence. A total of 36 supervisory activities that include direct observation of diagnostic treatment procedures and other professional activities are required of the clinical supervisor. The clinical fellow selects the employment setting based on its appropriateness in meeting the necessary clinical fellowship requirements. The clinical fellow and supervisor must complete the ASHA mandatory Clinical Fellowship Registration Agreement.

Also, as stated earlier, education agency certification and/or state licensure are needed for employment, depending upon the setting. While in graduate school, one should contact the state education department and state licensure board for specific requirements of each state in which s/he desires to practice. Usually, most graduate schools, especially those accredited by ASHA, prepare students to meet the state education and licensure credentials.

It is further recommended that students take the NESPA during their last semester of graduate course work. Some educational programs have included the standardized tests as part of their requirements for completing the master's degree. The NESPA are the area specialty tests of the National Teachers Examinations (NTE) programs administered by Educational Testing Services (ETS). The examinations are administered nationwide three times a year. A number of institutions and associations have begun to implement preparation courses for the NESPA.

Preparation for the Professions

To prepare for a career in speech-language pathology and audiology, it is recommended that one obtains a background strong in pre-science/health, mathematics, liberal arts, and a stalwart foundation in oral and written communication beginning at the high school level and continuing through graduate school. Students should concentrate on maintaining a "B" average or above in order to be eligible to enter a program of study in or related to communication disorders. Presently, with the steadfast competition and entry requirements for college, it is imperative that individuals establish a good pre-college and undergraduate academic track record.

Top 10 Job Markets

Ranked by: Total new jobs by 1995.
1. Washington, DC, with 118,200 new jobs
2. Anaheim, CA, 108,800
3. Atlanta, GA, 104,600
4. Phoenix, AZ, 92,000
5. San Diego, CA, 77,100
6. Tampa-St. Petersburg, 76,300
7. Orlando, FL, 70,300
8. Dallas, TX, 69,300
9. Riverside, CA, 67,700
10. Minneapolis-St. Paul, 64,700

Source: *Money*

It is recommended that students at the high school level consider courses in biology, physiology, physics, and mathematics. Also, a number of high schools offer courses in the social sciences, such as psychology and sociology. It is recommended, therefore, that courses of this nature be taken during the pre-college years as well. Moreover, students should enhance their reading and standardized test-taking skills during this period and establish good note taking and studying habits. If at all available, attendance at a summer pre-college program or volunteering at a facility that provides speech-language and hearing services would be an excellent and rewarding experience.

As one matriculates to the pre-professional and formative years of preparation, it is strongly urged to attend a college or university that provides undergraduate training in the professions. It is not, however, *mandatory* that the students' bachelor degrees be in communications sciences and disorders, although some programs have this *preference*. Over the last several years, larger numbers of individuals have changed careers and entered the professions of speech-language pathology and audiology. If one does not have an undergraduate degree in communication sciences and disorders, prerequisite courses are required. The number and specific course offerings vary. Each college or university establishes its own guidelines, so it is recommended that career changers contact the school of interest to obtain information on the requirements.

Nonetheless, it is absolutely necessary that a very rigorous liberal arts and sciences emphasis be sought. Because of the intimate relationship that the discipline of communication sciences and disorders has with other disciplines, courses such as linguistics, anatomy and physiology, psychology, counseling, physical science, biology, and statistics should be taken. In addition, students should focus on required and additional course work to enhance their analytical oral and written communication skills.

Finally, a word of caution to the traditional undergraduate student—don't allow the extraneous distractors, such as partying, to interfere in the pursuit of obtaining the degree which is absolutely *necessary* for entry into a graduate program. However, a balanced, well-rounded undergraduate experience should be obtained. Moreover, a "B" average cumulative GPA is mandatory for eligibility into the majority of graduate schools in the United States and necessary for receiving fellowship and scholarship awards.

In general, graduate programs require that individuals obtain the minimum requirements for entry into the professions. Some variation does occur, however. All programs in communication sciences and disorders should cover the following basic content areas:

1. Fundamental studies of the processes of normal speech and hearing, including anatomy and physiology, acoustics, and the psychological aspects of human communication.

2. The nature and management of disorders of speech, language, and hearing.

3. The measurement and evaluation of speech production, language abilities, and auditory processes.

4. The management procedures, such as principles in remedial methods used in habilitation and rehabilitation for children and adults with various communication disorders.

5. Research methodology in the study of disorders of communication.

All graduate programs provide students the opportunity to receive supervised clinical practicum experiences. Under the current ASHA standard, a minimum of 350 clinical hours is accrued in the various communication disorders categories (e.g., language, voice, fluency, stuttering disorders, articulation, phonological disorders, and hearing disorders) upon completion of most programs. Students usually have the opportunity to obtain clinical experience at one or more external practicum placement sights, such as hospitals, rehabilitation centers, public/private schools, or agencies.

Communication sciences and disorders programs that are accredited by the American Speech-Language-Hearing Association (ASHA) must comply with prescribed academic course work and practicum requirements necessary for obtaining the CCC in speech- language pathology and audiology and the ASHA Code of Ethics. New standards for the CCC were adopted in 1988, and became effective January 1, 1993 for certification applicants. Moreover, effective January 1, 1994, only graduate course work and clinical practicum from an ASHA ESB accredited program will be accepted.

Selecting a College/University

It is highly recommended that students select a college/university that will provide them with the essential criteria for entry into the professions and ultimately, the work force. There are presently 299 programs, in communication sciences and disorders (283 at the bachelor's level, 232 at the master's level, and 59 at the doctoral level). Of the master's level programs, 199 are accredited by the ASHA Educational Standards Board (ESB). Accreditation is voluntary for all educational programs that offer master's degrees in speech-language pathology and audiology. Also, ASHA's Professional Services Board accredits clinical facilities, including college/university clinics, where students obtain clinical practicum experiences. For a listing of programs in communication sciences and disorders, contact the American Speech-Language-Hearing Association.

Securing financial assistance to attend both undergraduate and graduate school is critical for most individuals. Today, the majority of students enrolled in post-secondary schools receive financial aid in some form. There are a number of sources available for students considering a major in speech-language pathology and audiology. To obtain federal funding, students must be a U.S. citizen or meet non-citizen eligibility requirements.

Employment Opportunities

Because speech-language pathology and audiology are such diverse disciplines, one has the opportunity to choose from a variety of employment settings. Speech-language pathologists provide professional services in the following work environments:

- public and private schools
- rehabilitation centers
- community clinics
- private practice offices
- state and local health departments
- state and federal government agencies
- home care
- centers for the developmentally disabled
- research laboratories
- hospitals
- nursing care facilities
- colleges and universities
- adult day care centers

Audiologists are employed in similar facilities:

- hospitals
- private practice offices
- college and university clinics
- public and private schools
- state and federal government agencies
- long-term care and home health facilities
- health department and community centers
- research laboratories

Salaries

The income for speech-language pathologists and audiologists vary depending upon their employment setting and geographic location. According to a 1992 ASHA survey, the median salary for speech-language pathologists was $34,000; audiologists earned $35,782. Individuals who were certified in both areas earned an average income of $44,300. Salaries were found to be higher in the Northeastern and Western parts of the country and lower in the Midwestern and Southern regions. Also, individuals employed in private practice and administrative/managerial capacities obtained higher incomes. Fringe benefits for the professions are excellent.

In the Future

The job outlook for the professions is outstanding. According to the 1991-92 *Occupational Outlook Handbook,* employment of speech-language pathologists and audiologists is expected to increase faster than the average for all occupations through the year 2000. The healthcare employment setting is expected to have the fastest growth, due to the increase in the number of persons age 75 and over and the rise of baby boomers to middle age, who are more susceptible to neurological disorders which may have accompanying speech, language, and hearing problems. The demand will also increase for educational institutions as a result of federal mandates such as the Americans with Disabilities Act and public laws that stipulate speech-language and hearing services to all individuals with disabilities. Finally, it is projected that private practice opportunities will boost due to the use of contractual services that are currently in use by hospitals, schools, and nursing homes.

The future of the audiology and speech-language pathology professions appears excellent. Federal law, dictating that children with disabilities will receive free and appropriate public education, means that school districts are hiring or contracting with more audiologists and speech-language pathologists. Greater awareness of the importance of early identification and diagnosis of hearing disorders in infants and toddlers, the aging of the U.S. population, a growing number of young adults suffering hearing loss, and the concern over prevention of occupationally induced hearing loss combine to paint a bright picture for future employment opportunities for audiologists.

The future of the speech-language pathology profession appears excellent as well. More frequent recognition of problems in preschool- and school-age children by teachers and parents, combined with the increased number of older citizens, has created a growing need for speech and language services. There are shortages of qualified personnel in some areas of the country, especially in inner city, rural, and less populated areas.

Moreover, there is a serious demand for multicultural persons who are bilingual. Presently, more than five million racial-ethnic multicultural individuals have a speech, language, or hearing disorder, and approximately 41.3 million American children and adults have a speech, language, or hearing disorder. In addition, job opportunities in medically related areas are expected to grow at an above average rate. Although competition for positions in some areas is keen, the potential for private practice and contract work is increasing rapidly.

All persons with communication disabilities deserve to have caring, committed, and dedicated individuals to provide appropriate professional services. Wouldn't you like to enter a career that helps people communicate? The rewards are abundant!

▼

DR. PATRICIA A. COLE is the director of the Membership and Career Development Division at the American Speech-Language-Hearing Association (ASHA). Her responsibilities include recruiting and retaining undergraduate and graduate students into the National Student Speech Language Hearing Association (NSSLHA), recruiting international affiliates and graduating master's degree candidates; designing, implementing, and marketing career information and development programs for high school and college students; making professional presentations; providing technical information; and conducting individual career consultations. She also supervises activities related to member benefits and member operations, the ASHA Convention Placement Center, the Employment Referral Service, and the National Student Speech Language Hearing Association.

Before assuming her current role, Dr. Cole was an assistant professor and clinical supervisor at Howard University, Washington, DC. She was also co-principal investigator of two federally funded research grants. In addition, she chaired the recruitment committee and served as a career advisor and consultant for the School of Communications Education Advisory Center. Dr. Cole served on the Executive Board of the National Student Speech Language Hearing Association in the capacity of consultant-at-large and advisor for multicultural concerns. She was advisor to the Howard University chapter of the NSSLHA and student liaison advisor for the District of Columbia Speech-Language-Hearing Association (DCSHA). She also served on the DCSHA Executive Board. Prior to her appointment at Howard, Dr. Cole was a practicing speech-language pathologist for the Montgomery County and the Vicksburg, MS, public school systems.

Dr. Cole received her Ph.D. from Howard University in communications sciences. Her major area of concentration was speech-language pathology, with a research focus in language-learning disabilities. Dr. Cole's master's degree and clinical training were completed at the University of Mississippi, and she received her bachelor's degree from Tougaloo College, Tougaloo, MS.

Dr. Cole is a certified member of ASHA and a member of the American Society of Association Executives. She also holds membership in other learned societies.

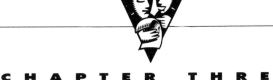

Medical Social Work in a Physical Therapy Clinic: A Unique Opportunity

Jennie Petrovich, M.S.W.,
Greater Lansing Rehabilitation Agency

Social work is an exciting profession, in part because of the wide range of work settings from which to choose. Contrary to popular belief, all social workers are not connected to the welfare system. There are job opportunities in education, industry, politics, healthcare, and numerous other settings in the public and private sector. Selecting a specific career path within the field was a difficult decision for me, but I knew that I wanted to be able to utilize as many of my skills as possible. My current position as a medical social worker in a private physical therapy clinic allows me to do just that. I am pleased to have discovered this unique and challenging career.

The Social Work/Physical Therapy Connection

In order for a physical therapy clinic to be registered as a rehabilitation facility, the U.S. Department of Health and Human Services requires that one of the following be on staff: a psychologist, a vocational specialist, or a professional social worker. This adjunct service must be available to patients free of charge while they are involved in therapy. The extent to which these services are provided varies greatly among agencies. Some meet the requirement by hiring the social worker on a contractual or part-time basis to simply refer patients to community resources if problems are identified. Other clinics hire full-time social workers who are available to assess patients' needs and actually provide the appropriate interventions.

A social worker in this setting, in very simple terms, is there to assist patients and physical therapists (P.T.'s) in any way possible to make the rehabilitation process go smoothly and efficiently. People generally enter a physical therapy clinic because they are faced with an injury or disability that is impacting their daily functioning to some degree. The problem could stem from any number of sources, including auto accidents, work injuries, diseases, or athletic injuries, to name a few. The person may be unable to work, participate in usual recreational activities, maintain their homes, enjoy a sex life, or even dress themselves.

Being unable to perform everyday activities that most of us take for granted can lead to a variety of emotional reactions, including anger, depression, frustration, and interpersonal difficulties. Financial concerns also tend to be prominent, as the person may be faced with temporary or permanent unemployment, legal battles, healthcare costs, and an unsure future. If left unattended, the combination of these factors can be overwhelming and interfere with their ability to put the necessary effort into physical therapy, thus prolonging an already difficult situation. Social workers are uniquely qualified to provide the range of intervention necessary to help patients make the most of the rehabilitation process and move ahead with their lives.

The Delivery of Services

Not all patients are in *need* of—or *want*—social work services. They are able to request the services at any point during treatment, but people are often hesitant to ask for help, and/or believe that *nothing* can help (which is why simply referring them to community resources can be ineffective). To reach more patients, an intake form is generally used, which screens for the presence of the difficulties I have mentioned. If these factors are noted, either on the form, or by the attending staff, the social worker meets with the patient to further assess the situation, explain the scope of services, and intervene as appropriate.

A typical day at the clinic begins with examining new intake forms to identify patients in need of services. The clinic treatment schedule must then be reviewed so that a plan can be made as to who will be seen on that day. Physical therapy patients tend to be scheduled at very short notice, which makes it difficult to plan one's day ahead of time. New patients must be fit in as soon as possible among those already receiving services.

Physical Rehab Starts from Within

I commonly see patients with marital and/or parenting difficulties, grief reactions, substance abuse issues, as well as histories of child abuse, sexual abuse, and highly dysfunctional families of origin. Helping patients to organize their personal issues provides them an increased feeling of control and frees them to channel their energy into physical rehabilitation.

The type of services provided, as well as the length and frequency of sessions, can vary greatly among patients. Common services provided include community resource allocation, advocacy, serving as a liaison between various professionals, educating the patient about topics such as stress management and the psychosocial aspects of a particular physical condition, crisis intervention, and various forms of counseling. The counseling may involve allowing isolated patients to ventilate their concerns and fears, helping them to problem-solve solutions to new life problems, teaching cognitive/behavioral techniques for managing chronic pain, and supporting their self-esteem as they are faced with the inability to carry out their usual roles.

For some people, brief psychotherapy is appropriate. Injury and illness can leave people feeling emotionally vulnerable, exacerbating any pre-existing problems. As their old wounds come to the surface, the patients can become easily overwhelmed, increasingly tense, and less likely to benefit from physical therapy. Given that some patients are not involved in physical therapy for an extended period of time, they may be referred elsewhere for long-term psychotherapy, if appropriate.

Working with patients' families can also be helpful, as they highly impact and are impacted *by* the situation. A common example would be that of an older couple comprised of one healthy spouse and one who has had a stroke. Not only must the stroke victim struggle with the loss of functioning, but the spouse must contend with a partner who may be very different from the one they had known. They may be thrust into and frightened by a range of new responsibilities, resentful of not having the retirement they had planned, and sad or frustrated that their spouse can no longer communicate with them clearly. Family members can be helped to grieve their losses, plan for the future, and achieve a balance between caring for their loved one and attending to their own needs.

Another possible area of service is group work. The type of group is limited only by one's creativity. Groups designed to teach patients to manage chronic pain have been found to be quite successful. My agency has also sponsored programs for parents of handicapped children and people who have experienced back injuries. On occasion, our social work staff has been contracted by businesses and community groups to make presentations on stress management, time management, and coping with pain. These experiences have been very rewarding and serve as good public relations and income for the clinic.

Education

To work in this setting as a social worker, there is a minimum requirement of a B.A. in social work from a college accredited by the Council on Social Work Education, plus one year experience in a healthcare setting. Job options will be quite limited if you do not continue your education beyond this point. Employers (in all settings) are increasingly requiring candidates to hold a master's degree in social work (M.S.W.). The graduate program generally involves two years of full-time education that includes internships. Some universities offer an accelerated, 12- to 15-month program for those who have an undergraduate degree in social work.

The undergraduate training tends to be quite broad-based, and specific courses in medical social work may not be offered at this level; however, electives can generally be found in a variety of departments that would provide useful background. Courses on substance abuse, grief, and race and gender issues would be beneficial. Volunteer work may not be required, but I feel that it is invaluable and should be sought out in the first two years of college. Social work is an incredibly broad field, and this exposure can help a student to focus their academic and vocational goals. It also looks good on a resume. Senior year of study does include an internship and you may be able to request or seek out a placement in a medical setting.

Graduate study for clinical social work involves more in-depth exploration of human behavior, mental disorders, and methods of intervention. Depending on individual interests, it may involve training in psychotherapy with children, adults, families, couples, and/or groups. Electives may be chosen related to special settings, including medical social work. I also did an independent study to further my knowledge in this area. In conjunction with the classroom work, an ongoing internship provides an opportunity to utilize the skills learned. Look for a placement that provides exposure to health issues, a variety of clients and concerns, and brief therapy techniques.

Finding a Job That Suits You

Investigate various health agencies in your area (and others) to get a sense of typical hiring requirements; they often vary among cities and rural areas, and in different parts of the country. Finding entry-level positions in medical social work can be quite difficult. Nursing homes, the public health department, and home health agencies are good places to start looking. Hospitals may be a possibility, but they generally look for more experience. Any job in which you work with persons with handicaps would be useful, such as vocational rehabilitation or community mental health centers. You might also get involved with organizations such as the Arthritis Foundation and the Multiple Sclerosis Society to expand your experience and knowledge base. In addition, participating in the local chapter of the National Association of Social Workers (NASW) can provide useful contacts.

Obtaining a job in a physical therapy clinic may require you to promote yourself and your profession quite heavily. I am fortunate to work in a clinic whose administration recognizes that the social worker is an integral part of the rehabilitation process, and not simply a licensure requirement. All organizations are not this enlightened. Be aware of the fact that basic social work services in a physical therapy/rehabilitation facility do not generate revenue—an important consideration in private clinics. You may need to help other professionals to understand your role and how you can be an asset to the company. Don't expect this to happen overnight, but if you are tactful, enthusiastic, and consider the economics of the situation, you may be able to win them over.

Salaries within the profession and *this* specialty can vary greatly depending on the agency and the location. The NASW has recommended minimum salaries of $20,000 per year for a person with a B.S.W. and $25,000 for one with an M.S.W. Recently, I have seen a range of M.S.W. starting salaries between $23,000 and $27,000, with medical social work jobs tending to be at the higher end of the scale.

The career ladder for this specialty can be somewhat limited; however, there are numerous opportunities for program development and professional growth. The paperwork is minimal, compared to many social work jobs, and the extent to which you are busy with patients tends to run hot and cold. Days with slow patient loads provide time to enrich the level of services by developing educational programs, supportive groups, and other methods of assisting patients as well as the company.

The position can be quite isolating because you do not work with other social workers. Our agency does have another social worker who also provides my clinical supervision, but smaller clinics may only have one social worker on staff. Be aware that you may need social work supervision in order to earn more advanced certifications within the profession. In some cases, it is possible to hire this supervision independently. Contact the local NASW for guidance in this regard.

A social worker in this setting must be able to work with other professionals assertively, cooperatively, and respectfully. Good organizational skills and a willingness to be flexible are also imperative, as the schedule for the day can change quickly. Given the level of independence on the job, a person must be highly motivated, reliable, and demonstrate sound judgement.

Helping people to successfully overcome major life hurdles can be a very challenging, rewarding experience. It requires an ability to face a barrage of intense emotions, such as anger and grief. Without letting it become intertwined with one's own issues, I continually strive to keep my work life and home life separate, which allows me to approach patients with the energy and compassion needed to serve them effectively. The job remains interesting because of the ongoing variety. There are few settings that involve working with such a wide range of people in regard to age, income level, and functioning level, and allows the opportunity to truly address the needs of the *whole person.*

Looking to the Future

It is difficult to speculate the extent to which changes in the nation's healthcare system will impact the medical social work profession. Hopefully, it will be recognized that social workers can facilitate greater efficiency in the delivery of services and the prevention of additional, costly problems. I am optimistic that social workers will have an increasingly prominent role in a variety of medical settings, including physical therapy clinics. Together with other medical professionals, social workers can make a difference in improving patients' quality of life and paving the way for a healthier future.

▼

JENNIE PETROVICH earned her bachelor of arts degree at Michigan State University, where she had a dual major in social work and psychology. She later returned to M.S.U. to complete her master's degree in social work, and is now certified as a social worker in the state of Michigan. In addition to the field of healthcare, Ms. Petrovich's experience includes work with chronically mentally ill adults, injured/handicapped workers, and the families of troubled adolescents. She currently lives in Mason, MI, and is employed by Greater Lansing Rehabilitation Agency.

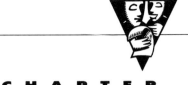

Physical Therapists as Sports Medicine Specialists—A New Choice

Janet Ventimiglia, P.T.,
Manager, Center for Athletic Medicine, Henry Ford Hospital

G iven the increasing popularity of maintaining an active lifestyle—step aerobics, "wall climbing", triathalons, or just plain walking two blocks to the corner store—the risk of injury has also increased. Once the physician is seen and a diagnosis of the injury is made, the patient used to be left to his or her *own* devices where exercise and rehabilitation were concerned. But more and more frequently, these patients are being referred to specialists in sports medicine rehabilitation—physical therapists and/or athletic trainers with specialized training in rehabilitation of surgical and nonsurgical injuries of the *athlete*.

Career Preparation

To pursue a degree in physical therapy (P.T.) requires a strong background in the sciences. The core curriculum in all programs is basically the same: physics, chemistry, anatomy, physiology, and neurology. In addition to these, include those sciences directly involved in the study of human motion: kinesiology, biomechanics, and exercise physiology. Most programs take applications after the completion of the sophomore year and the basic college curriculum: English, biology, clinical psychology, and general humanities. Some programs accept students directly into the P.T. program upon entering as a freshman based solely on high school GPA and SAT/ACT scores. Once the student is in the program, an area of interest will generally become apparent: neuro or cardiac rehabilitation, pediatrics, orthopedics, sports, etc.

A career in **sports medicine** can involve any number of healthcare specialists: not only physical therapists, but also physicians, psychiatrists, and athletic trainers. If, as a physical therapist, you wish to specialize in sports medicine, there are several avenues you can pursue. First, once the core curriculum is completed in the pursuit of a B.S. in P.T. or an M.S. in P.T. (a lot of programs have become mandatory master's programs), an *advanced clinical specialist certification* can be pursued through the

American Board of Physical Therapy Specialties. This involves a great deal of independent study and the passage of clinical competencies in patient care, administration, educational services, and research. Another option would be to attain a master's degree in exercise physiology, kinesiology, or biomechanics through a university setting—all of these subspecialties are directly applicable to the science of physical therapy and research.

A newer, more innovative approach is found through a *fellowship* program offered through HEALTH SOUTH, located in Birmingham, AL. In this program, physical therapists spend six weeks rotating through each of three sport rehabilitation sites, observing surgery, working in patient care, and getting more experience in the acute, *on the field* care of athletes. This enables them to gain the necessary credentials and hours of training necessary to sit for their national certification exam and become an **athletic trainer** (P.T., A.T.C.).

Getting Started in Sports Medicine

By far, the simplest way to pursue a career in sports medicine is to begin work in a specialty clinic catering to athletic medicine injury evaluation and follow-up rehabilitation. Some clinics prefer new employees to first get a broader background of experience (pediatrics, neurology, or cardiology) before specializing, but others will hire new grads simply because of their interest in athletic medicine.

My workplace, the Center for Athletic Medicine, is a progressive orthopedic rehabilitation facility specializing in the evaluation and treatment of sport injuries. The staff rehabilitates the Detroit area professional athletic teams, as well as the area high school and weekend athletes. The physical therapists are highly skilled in bringing an injured athlete from the point of injury to full return of sport ability. They have a close working relationship with the orthopedic surgeons and exchange ideas and suggestions freely. As part of the overall Bone and Joint Center at Henry Ford Health System, they play an integral part in producing revenue and contributing to an overall highly regarded service.

As a new graduate, primary responsibilities lie strictly in providing patient care and applying the basic sciences in functional rehabilitation. Education is emphasized at all levels of experience and participation in national continuing education courses is highly encouraged. As experience increases, so too does a trend toward expertise in particular areas—not only joint-specific but in the areas of mobilization, soft tissue manipulation, the treatment of the back and cervical spine in the athlete, etc. In conjunction with an increase in experience, promotion into managerial positions is possible. These differ from clinic to clinic, but range from being the coordinator of student programs (arranging clinical internships for university students), supervisor of rehabilitation (overseeing day-to-day operations involving the P.T.'s in the clinic), or supervisor of external programs (organizing community involvement, high school athletic trainer coverage, and other areas).

How Much Will I Make?

Because of the high demand for physical therapists and the increasingly shorter supply, salaries in the field remain highly competitive. Those with specialized training command a higher salary. For example, if you already have a degree in athletic training (A.T.C.), have completed a B.S. or M.S. in physical therapy, and have passed the state licensing exam (P.T., A.T.C.), your starting salary would be approximately five to eight percent higher than someone with just a P.T. degree.

The starting salary for a new graduate in an urban setting can range from $36,000 to $42,000 annually, with yearly reviews and increases. Some institutions do regional salary surveys so that the hospital remains competitive in that particular market and then adjusts salaries accordingly. A private, suburban-based clinic will generally offer a higher salary. But the educational opportunities in a large urban teaching hospital more than compensate for the difference.

A Hot Career

Overall, a therapist specializing in athletic medicine is highly marketable, can work in a private clinic or teaching hospital, or own their own clinic. They would have opportunities to treat the *elite* athletes or *weekend warriors* and be challenged daily to keep up with the latest advances in medicine and physical rehabilitation.

Those P.T.'s with adequate financial backing can open their own practice, accept physician referrals (currently, we cannot diagnose or self-refer), and become a highly independent business person with a comparably high salary. With reimbursement rates from insurance companies constantly changing, much research must be done to make sure this type of endeavor is sound.

Qualifications

The candidates we look to hire must have a definite interest in orthopedics and want to work with a population that is highly motivated, ranging in age from adolescents to active senior citizens, with a wide variety of orthopedic injuries. They must be extremely personable, given the large number of patients they would treat per day (14-20), and have a high desire to continue learning. Experienced P.T.'s are very marketable and great strides have been made to make salaries commensurate with experience.

JANET VENTIMIGLIA, P.T., received her B.S. in physical therapy from Marquette University in Milwaukee, WI. She did her clinical internships at Billings Hospital in Chicago, IL and at Hessler Rehabilitation Institute in West Orange, NJ. She has been at Henry Ford Hospital since 1980, and has been manager of rehabilitation at the Center for Athletic Medicine since 1984. The medical staff currently works with the Detroit Lions, Tigers, and Red Wings, as well as the Detroit Rockers, Turbos, and Drive. They treat a wide variety of surgical and non-surgical injuries in the athletic population, and average over 14,000 patient visits a year.

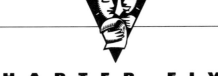

CHAPTER FIVE

Athletic Trainers: Premier Professionals in Athletic Healthcare

Danny T. Foster, M.A., A.T.C.,
Director, Athletic Training Education Program and
Associate Director, Department of Athletic Training Services,
University of Iowa

An **athletic trainer** is a highly qualified allied healthcare professional educated and experienced in the management of healthcare problems associated with sports participation. In cooperation with physicians and other allied health personnel, the athletic trainer functions as an integral member of the athletic healthcare team in secondary schools, colleges and universities, sports medicine clinics, professional sports programs, and other athletic healthcare settings. The athletic trainer works with medical personnel, athletic administrators, coaches, and parents in the development and coordination of efficient and responsive athletic healthcare delivery systems.

A certified athletic trainer is defined as an allied health professional who has a bachelor's degree from an accredited college/university, has fulfilled the requirements for certification as established by the National Athletic Trainers' Association (NATA) Board of Certification, and has passed the NATA certification examination administered by the NATA Board of Certification, Inc.

The six domains of athletic training from which specified tasks are measured in the examination are:

1. Prevention of athletic injuries;
2. Recognition and evaluation of athletic injuries;
3. Management, treatment, and disposition of athletic injuries;
4. Rehabilitation of athletic injuries;
5. Organization and administration of athletic training programs; and
6. Education and counseling of athletes.

The certified athletic trainer works under the direction of a licensed physician when practicing the art and science of athletic training.

Career Opportunities

Professional preparation and certification in athletic training offer employment opportunities for practice in athletic programs at all levels of interscholastic and intercollegiate competition, sports medicine clinics, recreation departments, community and governmental agencies, professional sports, and the armed services. Career opportunities beyond the scholastic setting are available for those with a varied background of academics and practical experience. Undergraduate degree students are usually limited in employment opportunities since the degree and appropriate certification represent the minimum level of entry into the profession of athletic training.

Much of the work is physical in nature and includes manual exercise, physical examination, taping, manufacturing of protective devices, and similar duties. These activities are also technical and require a strong knowledge base and extensive decision-making skills. Undergraduate degrees, usually in athletic training, health, physical education, or exercise science are considered minimal academic credentials for eligibility to enter the profession. In addition to an undergraduate degree, professional programs require courses in human anatomy, human physiology, kinesiology/biomechanics, health, exercise physiology, and athletic training. These curricular programs also require extensive clinical affiliation with athletic teams; at least 800 hours under appropriate supervision. Successful completion of course work and clinical experience requirements allows students to sit for the athletic training certification examination. State licensure may restrict the practice of an athletic trainer within some states. Once certified, athletic trainers must continue to update their knowledge through continuing education units.

▼

The Great Athletic Supporter

Athletic trainers usually cite the daily variety, travel, personalities of the athletes and coaches, and seeing the success of their efforts as the most rewarding or enjoyable part of their profession. Surely no two days are ever alike and monotony never enters the picture. However, job stress runs high among these individuals because their job involves large time commitments and a major negative aspect of sports—that of injuries. Pressure to win and succeed in sports also falls on the shoulders of the athletic trainer, who has to be direct in his or her role as the supporter of the athlete.

Salaries

Salaries for high school athletic trainers range from $19,000 to $23,000 as a starting base. Stipends for athletic training duties, when teaching is part of the contract, range from $1,000 to $6,000 above base pay. Many communities are now being served by sports medicine clinics that hire athletic trainers. Starting salaries at the clinical setting usually range between $19,000 to $22,500. College athletic trainers are usually required to possess a master's or doctoral degree, or a license in another healthcare profession, plus experience as a certified athletic trainer. The salary range is from $18,000 to $45,000, depending on education, experience, and size of the school. Professional sports athletic trainers usually have advanced academic degrees and experience in the field. Salaries with this group vary but may start around $20,000.

Athletic trainers are needed in order to effectively meet the needs of athletes, parents, physicians, and coaches. They play an important role in the athletic arena because they are on-site, they are counselors, they are advisors, and they render a difficult-to-obtain medical service when time and the season are critical enemies. No other healthcare profession delivers its service as part of an athletic team at the site of practice or competition, nor on a daily and year-round basis. For these reasons, athletic trainers are usually known for their compassion, empathy, loyalty, and trustworthiness, and are regarded as excellent communicators and organizers.

Nature of the Profession

Athletic trainers are specialists in the prevention, recognition, management, and rehabilitation of injuries incurred by athletes. In providing these services, athletic trainers administer immediate first aid, minimize the athlete's reaction to injury, and maximize his or her physical status for return to competition. Based on knowledge of the athlete's injuries and the factors influencing them, the athletic trainer, with the attending family or team physician, develops a treatment program based on medical, exercise, and sports sciences. Athletic training includes a continual communication with the athlete, physician, coach, and family on appropriate procedures for the resumption of the injured athlete's participation in training and competition. In addition to being involved with the practical application of the athletic training service, the athletic trainer also develops knowledge of the administration of athletic training programs, in the methods appropriate for prevention and management of athletic injuries, in the purchase of related supplies and equipment, in the supervision of staff or other supportive personnel, and in the cooperative aspects of sports medicine team care.

A typical day for an athletic trainer will vary with the level of competition and other institutional requirements. Some athletic trainers are hired by the school system where they may also teach. For these athletic trainers, managing time for preparation of all the various team practices becomes a priority. Preparation includes taping, bandaging, wrapping, bracing, and similar protective measures prior to practice. During after-school practice time, injuries are evaluated and the determination is made to refer the athlete to a physician or to follow up standing orders to manage injuries of a mild nature. Usual injury management consists of a variety of hot and cold treatments and exercise. Prescriptive exercise is sometimes limited at the high school setting and athletic trainers have to be innovative in order to provide a progressive and specific exercise regimen needed to rehabilitate injured athletes. Post-practice review of injuries follows similar examination techniques and therapy. Attendance at evening competition may also be part of the daily activity of the high school athletic trainer. The healthcare services provided on-site at competition are primarily for first aid and referral. However, assistance and consultation to athletes and coaches in injury matters is also an important service provided on-site by the athletic trainer at athletic events. A typical day may not be constrained by an eight-hour clock. An athletic trainer's duties and responsibilities usually determine the amount of time s/he or she has to spend on the job.

DANNY T. FOSTER, M.A., A.T.C., is director of the Athletic Training Education Program and associate director of the Department of Athletic Training Services at the University of Iowa. Mr. Foster received his bachelor's and master's degrees from the University of Iowa and earned his athletic training certification in 1975. He is actively involved in the National Athletic Trainers' Association with the committees that review undergraduate and graduate athletic training education programs.

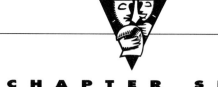

Working as a Recreational Therapist in Physical Rehabilitation Settings

Thomas K. Skalko, Ph.D., C.T.R.S.,
President, American Therapeutic Recreation Association

Understanding Recreational Therapy

The questions most frequently asked by the average person are, "What is recreational therapy?", "What do recreational therapists do?", and "Why is recreational therapy important in rehabilitation?"

Perhaps the best approach to answering such questions is to begin by trying to understand the implications physical disabilities can have on an individual's life. Imagine having a stroke, a traumatic head injury, or a spinal cord injury. How would such an injury change your life? Although the limitations imposed by such disabilities vary with the individual, the effects are far reaching. The person may or may not be able to resume work or school, to perform self-care activities, and/or be able to resume those activities that enhance his quality of life such as meaningful recreation, community events, and/or social activities.

Recreational therapy is a separate and distinct discipline that uses activities as a means of treatment for individuals with disabilities and illnesses. The **recreational therapist** uses recreational and other activities to assist the person with a disability in developing strengths and skills that help him function in the environment. For instance, a person who has received an injury to the brain may need help learning to concentrate, to interact with other people, to relearn motor skills, and/or to develop skills in order to re-enter the community and resume life. The recreational therapist plans specific activities to help the person redevelop these skills and to work toward becoming as independent as possible. The role of the recreational therapist, in regards to assisting persons with physical disabilities (and their families) to regain personal independence and control in their lives, is significant.

Becoming a Recreational Therapist

Though some people enter the field as activity aides, the entry-level requirements for a recreational therapist include a bachelor's degree in recreational therapy (also called therapeutic recreation) from an accredited college or university and national certification by the National Council for Therapeutic Recreation Certification (NCTRC).

Recreational therapy professional preparation programs require content in the human and social sciences (i.e., anatomy, physiology, human biology, psychology, etc.) and professional preparation in recreational therapy, in addition to university and college core requirements. Students are also required to complete a clinical internship under the supervision of a certified therapeutic recreation specialist. (Information on recreational therapy/therapeutic recreation professional preparation programs can be obtained from the national association listed at the end of this chapter.)

Upon completion of the bachelor preparation, a person should be eligible to sit for the National Certification Examination. This examination is given once each year at sites throughout the United States. A passing score on the examination qualifies a person for the certified therapeutic recreation specialist (C.T.R.S.) credential, which is the professional-level credential for recreational therapists.

Complementing the educational preparation, recreational therapists must be skilled at a wide variety of recreational activities, aquatic skills with certifications, crafts, expressive arts, and life skills.These skills provide the recreational therapist with the tools needed for the development of effective treatment programs.

The Employment Outlook for Recreational Therapy

According to the U.S. States Department of Labor's 1992 *Occupational Outlook Handbook*, "Employment of recreational therapists is expected to grow faster than the average for all occupations through the year 2005, because of the anticipated expansion in long-term care, physical and psychiatric rehabilitation, and services for the disabled." There are approximately 32,000 employment positions in the United States and the growth rate is projected at 39 percent through the year 2005. It is important to note that there are jobs available in a wide variety of settings working with individuals with varying types of disabilities.

Salaries for recreational therapists depend primarily upon the type of setting in which they are employed. The U.S. Department of Labor lists the average earnings for recreational therapists in the federal government to be approximately $30,559 per year for 1991. According to the 1993 *Federal Job Opportunity Listing*, entry-level recreational therapist salaries will range from $18,350 to $34,600. Salary information from the American Therapeutic Recreation Association indicates that the average salary for recreational therapists ranges from $25,557 to $42,000 annually and is based upon years of experience and educational preparation. The average annual salary for administrative positions is $36,000 to $55,000 and also depends upon the size of the department, years of experience, and educational preparation.

Most positions in recreational therapy are at the therapist level. Some therapist positions may also require supervisory duties that entail working with recreational therapy aides and volunteers. **Recreational therapy director** positions generally require graduate work in the discipline. Some individuals may choose to continue with doctoral work so that they may enter higher management positions or university instruction and research.

Working as a Recreational Therapist in Physical Rehabilitation

A career as a recreational therapist can be very rewarding. It offers opportunities for work in a range of settings, assisting people with different types of disabilities using a wide variety of activities. The recreational therapist in the physical rehabilitation setting may become engaged in activities that range from using crafts, to wheelchair sports, to basic exercise, to aquatics, to social etiquette activities and community outings. The type of activity depends on the needs of the person and the treatment goals.

The typical day of a recreational therapist will vary based upon the facility, though most days begin with a meeting of the treatment team and a review of how each patient is doing. The recreational therapist, in cooperation with other rehabilitation professionals, evaluates the status of each person on his or her case load and begins to prepare for each individual or group activity treatment session. This preparation includes being sure that the patient and professional staff are aware of the scheduled treatment program, ensuring that supplies and materials are ready, and making other arrangements as needed.

The recreational therapist involves the patient in the activity prescribed to meet the individual's treatment needs. For example, if the person has had a stroke (often times resulting in paralysis of one side of the body), the recreational therapist, in concert with a physical therapist and other treatment team members, may engage the person in a recreation activity such as swimming. This activity requires the individual, with the assistance of the recreational therapist, to use the affected limbs. The use of recreational activities offers the opportunity for individuals to regain the use of lost abilities in an enjoyable manner. Participation in successful activity experiences is more apt to help a person continue with recovery.

In another instance, the recreational therapist may assist the person with a traumatic brain injury in relearning skills needed to access various community resources. This may include relearning the use of a public transportation system or locating community resources such as the library, the recreation center, or a specific restaurant. If the person cannot return to the community and function with some level of independence, his quality of life will be adversely affected.

1991-92 Allied Health Graduates by State

Based on educational programs accredited by the Committee on Allied Health Education and Accreditation as of July 1992.
1. California, 4,572 graduates
2. Texas, 4,382
3. Pennsylvania, 2,646
4. Florida, 2,603
5. New York, 2,287
6. Ohio, 2,026
7. Illinois, 1,587
8. Michigan, 1,544
9. Georgia, 1,415
10. Alabama, 1,297
Source: *Allied Health Education Directory*

Recreational therapists play a significant role in adding to the quality of life of individuals with disabilities. They offer varied activities designed to meet the unique needs of the person with the disability.

The Future of Recreational Therapy

Although no one can predict the future, there are always indicators that offer insight into what is to come. The indicators for recreational therapy show that there will continue to be opportunities for employment in the field. The move toward community-based services and cost-effective healthcare options offers greater demand for credentialed recreational therapy professionals. The call to respond to the needs of persons with disabilities will continue in the future and there will be a demand for qualified persons to provide these services.The role of recreational therapists will continue to be crucial in the comprehensive rehabilitation of persons with physical disabilities.

For more information contact:

American Therapeutic Recreation Association
National Office
PO Box 15215
Hattiesburg, MS 39404-5125
1-800-553-0304

American Therapeutic Recreation Association
Legislative Office
1111 14th St. NW, Suite 1001
Washington, D.C. 20005-5603

▼

DR. THOMAS K. SKALKO, C.T.R.S. received his bachelor and master degrees from the University of Georgia and his doctoral degree in therapeutic recreation from the University of Maryland. Currently, Dr. Skalko is an associate professor of recreational therapy at Florida International University and president of the American Therapeutic Recreation Association.

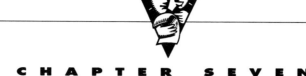

Therapeutic Recreation Specialists: The Quality of Life Professionals

Karen C. Wenzel, CTRS/CLP,
Program Director

Therapeutic recreation offers a unique career opportunity for individuals who value leisure experiences and enjoy working with people with disabilities. Employment of therapeutic recreation specialists is expected to grow much faster than the average for all occupations through the year 2000, chiefly because of anticipated expansion in the need for long-term care and physical and psychiatric rehabilitation. The U.S. Department of Labor Statistics projects that there were approximately 29,000 positions in therapeutic recreation in 1986. It is further projected that positions will grow at the rate of 20 percent through the year 2000.

What Is Therapeutic Recreation?

Therapeutic recreation is a professional service which uses recreation services to improve or maintain physical, mental, emotional, and/or social functioning to assist persons with disabilities and other limitations exercise their right to a lifestyle that focuses on functional independence, health, and well-being. Therapeutic recreation services are provided in clinical, residential, and community settings. With a degree in therapeutic recreation, you can work in a variety of agencies and organizations. The possibilities include acute care hospitals, rehabilitation centers, nursing homes, psychiatric hospitals, community recreation centers, pediatric hospitals, group homes, senior centers, community mental health centers, public and private schools, correctional facilities, and in private practice. Services are provided for individuals with a variety of disabilities, illnesses, or limitations. Individuals of all ages benefit from the services provided by the **Therapeutic Recreation Specialist (TRS).**

Comprehensive therapeutic recreation services involve a continuum of care, including:

• **Treatment**—the use of activities to remediate or rehabilitate functional abilities and to assist in diagnosis.

• **Leisure Education**—the use of activities to acquire skills, knowledge, and abilities that facilitate an independent leisure lifestyle.

• **Recreation**—providing opportunities to engage in leisure activities which enhance health, growth and development, and well-being.

The services provided by a TRS will be based upon the client's needs and interests, as well as the mandate of the agency in which services are provided. For example, in a hospital setting, where the focus is on treatment and rehabilitation, therapeutic recreation will be provided as one of the active treatments with the goal of restoring, remediating, or rehabilitating in order to improve functioning and independence and reducing or eliminating the effects of the illness or disability.

In a non-clinical setting, therapeutic recreation would more likely offer leisure education and special recreation services. Therapeutic recreation in this context would provide leisure resources and opportunities to improve or maintain health and well-being.

A Day in the Life of a Therapeutic Recreation Specialist

The day-to-day work experience of a therapeutic recreation specialist can vary dramatically, depending upon the setting and population they serve. However, all therapeutic recreation specialists conduct assessments of physical, mental, emotional, and social functioning to determine the client's needs, interests, and abilities. The TRS works with the client, family, and other specialists to design and implement an individualized treatment, education, or program plan, depending upon the setting.

A typical day of work in a hospital setting might begin with a *staffing* or treatment planning conference. Each member of the interdisciplinary treatment team, including therapeutic recreation, reviews the results of their respective assessments and a treatment plan is developed. The TRS may then go to hear a report on new admissions and updates on the current clients in his or her unit.

Typically, a TRS will be responsible for one or more group activities each day. These may include a stress management group, a high- or low-ropes course activity, a community outing, a family activity, an exercise group, or a leisure education group, just to name a few. The TRS may also meet with individual clients to conduct an assessment or to develop a leisure discharge plan. Charting client progress and communicating with other disciplines and family members are also part of a typical day. The TRS may also attend a variety of meetings on a given day: team meetings, department meetings, planning meetings, etc. In addition, the TRS is often involved in planning evening and weekend activities with clients and in planning special events and holiday activities. The services provided are designed to help clients meet the goals identified in their individual treatment plan.

A TRS working in a community recreation center also conducts assessments to determine client needs and interests. Due to the large number of individuals served, the assessments will vary in scope and intensity. Special programs and activities will be offered to meet client needs. The TRS will be responsible for adapting activities as needed or for providing adaptive equipment to enable individuals with special needs to participate. The specialist will be involved directly or indirectly in providing programs which could include: adapted aquatics, a wheelchair basketball league, a social recreational program for adults with mental retardation, a downhill skiing program for individuals with physical disabilities, special summer day camps, or adapted golf lessons.

The TRS would provide in-service training for recreation staff who will have individuals with disabilities in their programs to orient them to the needs of these individuals and promote general sensitivity. The TRS will generally seek to integrate clients into existing programs and classes when possible. This might be accomplished by coordinating a *recreation buddy* program, in which a person with a disability is matched with a non-disabled buddy who could participate alongside them and assist as needed.

An important responsibility for a TRS in a community and clinical setting is to serve as an **advocate** for individuals with disabilities. This includes addressing such issues as limited transportation resources, inaccessible facilities, and legislation which impacts people with disabilities or limitations. A TRS will frequently serve on advisory committees or consult with outside agencies to ensure that services and resources are provided for people with special needs.

Professional Preparation in Therapeutic Recreation

Therapeutic recreation is provided by professionals who are trained and certified, registered, and/or licensed to provide therapeutic recreation services. Most employers require a minimum of a bachelor's degree in therapeutic recreation or in recreation with an emphasis in therapeutic recreation. There are currently over 50 accredited schools in the United States that offer degrees in therapeutic recreation. The program itself may also be accredited by NRPA/AALR.

A therapeutic recreation degree is conferred upon successful completion of course work and an internship experience. During an internship, the student is placed in an agency they have selected and is given the opportunity to apply and practice skills learned in the classroom.

Recently, professional credentialing has become essential for employment. National certification is

A Rewarding Challenge

For most of my career, I have worked with individuals with psychiatric illnesses. However, I recently began working with people with multiple sclerosis. I have been employed in inpatient, outpatient, and now a day treatment program. I feel constantly challenged and have the opportunity for continued professional growth. The changes in healthcare delivery, which are occurring and will continue in the future, have provided the profession with challenges and opportunities. It is exciting and sometimes difficult to work as a therapeutic recreation specialist, but the opportunities are great. The opportunity to positively impact the quality of life of an individual with a disability or limitation is incredibly rewarding.

available through the National Council for Therapeutic Recreation Certification (NCTRC), an independent credentialing body. NCTRC awards the title of Certified Therapeutic Recreation Specialist (CTRS) based upon prescribed education and experience requirements and successful performance on a 200-item national examination. Some states have requirements for licensure, registration, or certification as well. Credentialing is one way to ensure that an individual has met the minimum requirements needed to safely provide therapeutic recreation services. Only certified professionals are able to refer to themselves as a CTRS.

Career Opportunities

The U.S. Bureau of Labor Statistics projects an increased need for therapeutic recreation specialists. The statistics indicate a shortage of qualified therapeutic recreation personnel and an increased demand for their services. Salary ranges for an entry-level position will vary greatly depending upon which setting you work in, which population you work with, and the part of the country in which you are working. A general salary range would be $20,000 to $25,000 per year for an entry-level position. One of the most attractive qualities of the profession is the great opportunity for variety and diversity.

The best way to find out about therapeutic recreation is to speak directly with a professional in your area. Contact your state therapeutic recreation organization or one of the national organizations serving the profession.

▼

KAREN C. WENZEL is a certified therapeutic recreation specialist. She received a bachelor of arts degree and a bachelor of science degree from the University of Colorado, Boulder, where she majored in recreation with an emphasis in therapeutic recreation and in psychology. She received her master's degree in therapeutic recreation from the University of Northern Colorado in Greeley. She worked for 10 years in psychiatric settings, initially as a therapeutic recreation specialist, then as director of therapeutic recreation, and eventually as director of rehabilitation services. She currently directs an adult day care program for MS Community Resources in Denver, CO and teaches at the University of Northern Colorado.

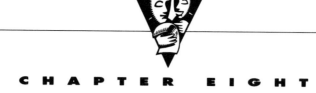

CHAPTER EIGHT

Massage Therapy: Hands-on Healing

Elliot Greene,
President, American Massage Therapy Association

One of the most frequent comments I hear massage therapists make is, "I feel fortunate to have found work I love." They feel this way because a career in **massage therapy** allows them to help people in a meaningful way with a high degree of personal contact. It provides a satisfying opportunity to express very positive values about caring and well-being in their work.

The field of massage therapy is growing rapidly in response to the public's expanding interest in forms of healthcare that promote well-being and a higher quality of life. Consequently, massage therapy has the attributes of an emerging profession undergoing a great deal of relatively rapid change. For example, professional standards for both individuals and massage training schools have markedly advanced and increased over the past five years. Standards in the field are not always uniform, though this article will point out the most *prevalent* standards.

Entering the Field of Massage Therapy

A growing majority of individuals enter the field by completing an educational training program. Some enter by taking a number of workshops from different independent instructors or studying with a practitioner in an apprenticeship. It is recommended to go through a training program at a school that offers a minimum of 500 in-class hours of instruction. A training program usually offers a more well-rounded and complete preparation for the field of massage therapy.

Programs in massage therapy generally require a high school diploma, though postsecondary education is useful. Previous studies in broad subjects such as sciences, psychology, business, and humanities is helpful. Many schools require a personal interview. Personal qualities and characteristics, such as excellent communication skills and a capacity for empathy, are important, due to the high degree of personal interaction involved in massage therapy. Schools are usually moderately to slightly selective, and some schools are beginning to have waiting lists, due to the growing number of applicants.

It is recommended to enroll at a school with a training program that is approved or accredited by a nationally recognized program. One such program is the American Massage Therapy Association's (AMTA) Commission on Massage Training Accreditation/Approval, which currently covers 58 programs. Feel free to ask a school about its accreditation or approval, along with its philosophy of teaching. Many schools offer an open house, which can be a useful way to find out more information.

The training program curriculum covers such subjects as anatomy, physiology, kinesiology, theory and practice of massage therapy, hands-on practice under faculty supervision, ethics, and business practices. Many schools offer a supervised student clinic that is open to the public. Training programs may tend to emphasize certain *styles* of massage, so it's useful to find out if a school teaches a style you feel comfortable with. Schools often offer both full- and part-time programs. Many practitioners find that their skills improve during the first few years after school because they are integrating what they have learned with hands-on practice in the field.

What You May Need Besides Your Diploma

Legal standards vary across the country. Massage therapy currently is licensed in some form by 19 states and a number of counties and cities. These licenses generally, though not in all cases, require 500 hours of training and/or passing an exam. You may want to find out what the requirements are in the area where you want to practice.

As part of the advancement of standards in the field, a national certification program was inaugurated in 1992. Similar to the "national boards" given in other healthcare fields, the exam is given at test centers across the country twice a year. Those who pass the exam become nationally certified in therapeutic massage and bodywork. Several of the states that require licensing have adopted this test for *their* licensing exam. It is expected that students will most likely take the certification exam after graduating.

Practicing Massage Therapy: Career Opportunities

Massage therapists practice in a variety of settings, such as private offices or massage therapy clinics, chiropractors or doctors offices, holistic health clinics, health club/fitness centers, spas, nursing homes/hospitals, or sports medicine/training facilities. Some massage therapists have portable equipment and work at their clients' offices or homes. Massage therapists may work as salaried or commissioned employees, independent contractors, or as self-employed practitioners in private or group settings.

Earnings vary widely, depending on the area of the country, type of practice, skills, and experience. Those who work for an hourly wage generally earn the least.

Independent contractors split their fees on a percentage basis. Usually, the percentage split is based on what services are provided for the massage therapist, such as working space, appointment-making, and providing supplies and equipment. Practitioners with their own facilities usually earn the most and have the most responsibility.

A massage therapist in a major metropolitan area may earn $30 to $60 an hour, and $25 to $50 an hour elsewhere. Those working for an hourly wage may earn less, but do not have overhead expenses. Because massage therapy is *physical* work, massage therapists commonly work less than 40 hours a week.

Massage therapy does not have the typical career *ladder*, in that advancements are not achieved through promotions. It takes much time (commonly six months to a year), effort, and persistence to build a practice. Business and entrepreneurial skills can have an impact on practice building. Income can be increased by increasing productivity, however this is limited by the relatively intensive one-on-one nature of massage therapy.

Create Your Own Career

The typical day for a massage therapist can vary due to the diversity of where massage therapy can be practiced. Besides the different practice settings mentioned above, massage can be used for a variety of purposes, such as promoting general well-being and relaxation, stress reduction, chronic muscular tension reduction, soft tissue problems recovery, and for addressing specific medical conditions. A massage therapist may devote his/her practice to only one type of massage and/or client or may work with a variety of patients.

Massage Therapy for the Future

In the future, massage therapy standards will continue to advance. Entry-level training requirements will most likely increase. As healthcare reform brings about greater acceptance for alternative forms of healthcare, massage therapists' interactions with other health professionals will increase. Massage therapy will become more integrated into wellness-oriented team approaches to healthcare. Efforts will be made, not only to advance the *science* of massage therapy, but also the *art* of massage, so that the vital caring qualities of massage continue to be part of the work. The importance of skilled, intentional touch for promoting health and well-being will finally be embraced in the healthcare system of the future.

ELLIOT GREENE, M.A., has practiced massage therapy for 20 years, maintaining a private practice in the Washington, DC area. He has lectured and taught classes and seminars across the country on various subjects related to massage therapy and body-oriented psychology. He is the president of the American Massage Therapy Association, a 16,500-member professional association for massage therapists.

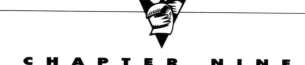

CHAPTER NINE

Careers for Minorities in Massage/Bodywork

Sherri Williamson,
President, Associated Bodywork & Massage Professionals

The **massage/bodywork** field is tremendously diverse and interesting and offers great employment potential, especially for women, minorities, and individuals who are visually or hearing impaired.

Employment Opportunities

While the majority of individuals within this vocation choose to be self-employed, there are numerous and unique opportunities for employment in a variety of settings, including airports, beauty salons, athletic clubs, spas, chiropractic offices, osteopathic physician offices, sports medicine clinics, physical therapy clinics, cruise ships, dance studios, dance touring companies, golf and country clubs, private employment by celebrities, resorts, hotels, professional athletic teams, and corporate wellness programs.

During the past 10 years, the massage/bodywork industry in the United States has seen welcomed changes. Massage/bodywork has increasingly received more recognition as a legitimate career and is less-associated with the unfortunate misuse of the term *massage* by illicit businesses. This has been a boon to individuals interested in pursuing massage/bodywork as a full-time or second career, and has opened the door to safe, helpful employment environments for women. Many individuals, tired of the corporate rat race or of working for someone else in traditional careers, are choosing massage/bodywork as a viable, alternative way to make a living. It is interesting to note that many individuals do not intentionally set out to enter into this career, but do so instead after recognizing they possess a gift of touch or as a result of an evolvement into a different lifestyle.

In addition to mastering excellent massage/bodywork techniques, the ideal candidate for massage/bodywork is physically strong and energetic, enjoys working with the public, and has an outgoing personality, non-judgmental attitude, caring, nurturing, and has a cheery disposition.

Women/Minorities/Visual and Hearing Impaired

The field of massage and bodywork is especially welcoming to women. Associated Bodywork & Massage Professionals (ABMP) estimates that 86 percent of the individuals practicing massage/bodywork today are women. This may be due, in part, to the fact that a successful massage/bodywork practitioner must have caring and nurturing qualities, an area in which women often excel. The practice of skilled touch is both an art and a science. The ability to practice both a strong and gentle touch simultaneously is both learned and innate. Many women possess this innate, artistic touch naturally. In addition, women who have raised children for several years and have found it difficult to break into other career opportunities, requiring years of training and/or experience, are finding massage/bodywork an easy and enjoyable career to develop.

Massage/bodywork skills have created unique and unlimited career opportunities for minorities as well as for the visually and hearing impaired. In many different cultures throughout history, the blind have traditionally practiced massage/bodywork. The development of an acute sense of touch has been well-documented in the visually impaired. There are several training institutions throughout the United States that assist visually impaired persons in learning massage/bodywork techniques.

Massage/bodywork is one of the few careers available to the visually impaired where they usually excel above those individuals who are not visually impaired. Similarly, hearing impaired individuals often excel in the practice of massage/bodywork.

Training

Educational requirements for entrance into the massage/bodywork field vary throughout the United States. As of 1992, only 16 states regulate the practice on a statewide basis. The remaining states either regulate the practice on a municipal basis through city/county ordinances or have no regulatory licensing.

There are over 500 massage/bodywork schools in the United States and over 40 different styles or techniques of massage/bodywork. Training periods vary from one month to two years, depending on the complexity of the practice the person wishes to pursue and the regulations within any given state or municipality. Learning a variety of massage/bodywork styles or techniques will broaden an individual's employment opportunities and provide variety to his/her work. For example, combining massage/bodywork skills with training in various spa treatments, such as hydrotherapy (underwater massage), herbal wraps, or facials, will certainly expand opportunities in spas, health clubs, and resorts. For this reason, an individual may wish to research the different earning capacities and opportunities available to those trained in various techniques.

Self-Employment

Many massage/bodywork practitioners enjoy the freedom of self-employment. The majority provide massage/bodywork in their own homes, place of business, or in the homes of their clients. Others work on an independent contractor basis in establishments such as chiropractic offices or health clubs. Still others, in what has become one of the hottest new employment opportunities in the massage/bodywork industry, provide on-site executive massage in a variety of businesses. The majority of massage/bodywork schools do not provide comprehensive education in establishing a business. Individuals interested in opening their own establishment may require additional education or information. To meet this need, ABMP provides its members with extensive information concerning the establishment and marketing of a private practice or business.

Best States for Women Entrepreneurs

Ranked by: Rate of business ownership among adult women in 1987
1. Alaska, with 84.7 businesses
2. Colorado, 72.9
3. Vermont, 65.4
4. Wyoming, 65.0
5. Montana, 60.0
6. Kansas, 56.6
7. Oregon, 56.3
8. Utah, 55.6
9. New Hampshire, 55.5
9. Hawaii, 55.5
Source: *American Demographics*

Working for Others

In situations where massage/bodywork practitioners find employment through an existing business, the practitioner is typically an employee or an independent contractor, depending on the description of the position and the structure of the business. In many situations, the massage/bodywork practitioner manages or works in a separate massage/bodywork department.

Responsibilities vary with the actual employment situation, but generally, the massage/bodywork practitioner's primary responsibility is to provide massage/bodywork services to clientele. The typical work day for a full-time massage/bodywork practitioner consists of seeing up to eight clients a day, with the average massage/bodywork session lasting 50 to 55 minutes. Depending on the support staff available, a typical day may also include preparing the room for the massage/bodywork session and performing some reception duties. In larger facilities, where support staff is available, a person may only be required to provide the service to the client, and the room preparation and other services are provided by support staff. Some establishments require their massage/bodywork practitioners to help out in other ways during slow times.

Income

The earnings for massage/bodywork vary tremendously. On the low end of the scale, $10 an hour might be the entry-level pay in a setting such as a spa or as an assistant in a physical therapy clinic. The *average* earnings would be closer to $20 an hour. Years of experience, the quality of service, and clientele loyalty can easily boost earnings to $35 to $50 per hour, particularly for those who are self-employed. In many employment situations, a base salary is set, or an individual works on a commission basis. Since much of the massage/bodywork vocation is considered to be within the hospitality industry, an individual's earnings usually depend at least partially upon tips. Earning capacity will depend somewhat upon the satisfaction of the customer.

Individuals who are self-employed or in independent contractor situations in very busy and lucrative resorts, tourist areas, or high-end spas, can earn a starting salary of $30 to $35 per hour. A few individuals in the massage/bodywork field earn upwards of $75,000 per year. Those who earn the top salaries work almost exclusively in affluent communities and are self-employed. It is unlikely that an individual would earn that amount while working for someone else.

Advancement/Career Moves

Other than being promoted to a department head or supervisor of a massage/bodywork department, promotions are not readily available in this vocation in terms of a title. However, wages generally increase to a certain level based on experience and customer satisfaction.

The opportunity for variety is unique in this vocation. Individuals can travel extensively, work on cruise ships and in resort areas, or establish private businesses within their own community. Practitioners often shift the focus of their services as their individual areas of interest change throughout the years. That focus may, for example, shift from providing basic stress-reduction massage/bodywork to providing more medically-oriented injury prevention practice. Further education would be required in order to make this transition.

Many individuals use massage/bodywork training as a stepping stone to enter chiropractic healthcare, physical therapy, or other areas of the healthcare field. Some find it a way to familiarize themselves with one-on-one client contact to determine if a medical career is of interest. Others use massage/bodywork as a way to put themselves through medical, chiropractic, or osteopathic school. Massage/bodywork is a valuable skill that can be used in a nursing, physical therapy, or chiropractic career. Some practitioners expand their massage/bodywork practice to include additional services for their clients, such as personal training, aerobics instruction, or facials.

Job Interviews

Interviews for massage/bodywork positions are usually two-fold. An interview with your potential employer allows him/her to outline the specific job description and allows you to familiarize the potential employer with your qualifications. In addition, employers at most facilities will ask you to provide a hands-on massage/bodywork demonstration, since skill levels vary greatly and the techniques desired in different settings vary. Oftentimes, the employer needs to critique the style and evaluate the strength and skill level of the applicant. Employers frequently look for an openness to learning new techniques or learning the routines necessary for a given position.

Internships are sometimes available and are a worthwhile avenue to explore.

Opportunities and requirements vary tremendously by state. In areas where no licensing is required and the requirements for practice are essentially non-existent, internships are generally easy to procure. When looking for tutelage, be sure that the credentials of the individual providing instruction are adequate.

▼

SHERRI WILLIAMSON is president of Associated Bodywork & Massage Professionals (ABMP), an international professional organization for massage/bodywork practitioners. Sherri was self-employed in Hawaii as a licensed massage therapist for nine years, where she owned and operated a successful massage business in a resort hotel. She also owned and operated a massage school approved by the State of Hawaii Department of Education.

ABMP is devoted to promoting ethical practices, fostering unification and acceptance of the profession, and protecting the right of massage and bodywork practitioners. ABMP is affiliated with over 25 organizations worldwide.

ABMP membership benefits include client and employment referral services, subscription to *Massage & Bodywork Quarterly,* comprehensive liability insurance, useful business forms for a successful practice, significant discounts on business and personal services, opportunities for savings on travel and leisure activities, affordable health insurance programs, and international networking and affiliations. ABMP members also receive valuable information on business practices, marketing and promotion, professional ethics, and contra-indications to massage and bodywork. For further information, contact Associated Bodywork & Massage Professionals, PO Box 1869, Evergreen, CO 80439-1869, (303) 674-8478.

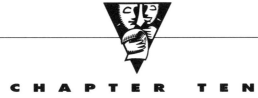

Life and Breath

Robert J. Czachowski, Ph.D.,
Director of Education, American Association for Respiratory Care

Prior to 1950, inhalation therapy was not widely accepted or practiced. It was not until 1957 that the American Medical Association proposed that schools of inhalation therapy should be established. Since then, the profession has evolved dramatically and educational opportunities have expanded significantly.

Today, respiratory care practitioners (RCP) who specialize in the diagnosis, care, and treatment of patients with breathing disorders will intervene whenever it is a matter of life and breath.

Work and Work Settings

Respiratory care practitioners work under physician direction in various healthcare settings. They are found on the staffs of critical care hospitals, skilled nursing facilities, rehabilitation centers, and home healthcare companies.

In the area of diagnosis, RCP's measure the capacity of a patient's lungs to determine if there is impaired function. By comparing these measurements with normal readings for a person of the same age, height, weight, and sex, the RCP can determine whether lung deficiencies exist. In order to determine the amounts of oxygen and carbon dioxide in a patient's blood, RCP's draw arterial blood samples. The sample is placed in a blood gas analyzer, and the result relayed to the physician.

Patients treated range from premature infants whose lungs are not fully developed to the very old whose lungs are diseased. Treatment can vary from giving temporary relief to an asthmatic or a patient with emphysema to emergency care of victims of strokes, heart failure, drowning, or shock. The three most common treatments are the administration of oxygen or oxygen mixtures, chest physiotherapy, or the administration of aerosol medications.

Oxygen and oxygen mixtures are administered in various ways. An increased quantity of oxygen can be administered by placing a delivery device, either a mask or a cannula (a small tube), on the patient and setting the oxygen flow prescribed by the physician. In more extreme cases, when a patient can't breathe on his own, the RCP would connect the patient to a ventilator, a machine which delivers pressurized air into the lungs. A tube is inserted into the patient's trachea, or windpipe, which is connected to the ventilator. The RCP sets the rate, volume, and concentration of the air entering the patient's lungs.

Chest physiotherapy is used on patients suffering from lung diseases like cystic fibrosis and on patients following surgery when anesthesia may have depressed respiration. In chest physiotherapy, the patient's rib cage is thumped and vibrated and the patient is instructed to cough. This procedure stimulates the lungs to expand and helps clear them of congestion. This procedure helps prevent respiratory illnesses which could complicate recovery.

Aerosols, which are liquid medications suspended in a gas that forms a mist, are also administered by RCP's. In some cases, patients are instructed on how to administer and inhale the aerosol themselves. In either case, to be effective, the medicine must be properly administered.

Monitoring patients who are using oxygen or ventilators is a routine part of the work day. If readings are abnormal, or if a patient is having difficulty breathing, adjustments must be made. The practitioner alerts the physician and adjusts the equipment according to the physician's order. Equipment is continually checked to ensure that there are no complications and all systems are functionally operational.

More and more sophisticated breathing equipment is being utilized by patients in their homes. Teaching patients and their families care and maintenance of this equipment is an integral part of the practitioner's job. Many of these people will receive home respiratory care for the remainder of their lives. Routine home visits by the therapist ensure proper use, care, and cleaning of the equipment.

Specialization among RCP's is growing with the acquisition of additional skills. Working with newborn and premature infants and treatment and rehabilitation of cardiopulmonary patients are only two areas of specialty training. Management of respiratory care departments and teaching are other areas in which RCP's are involved.

Entry into Practice

Licensure, certification, and registration are methods used to establish skill levels and competence of practitioners. Currently, 34 states and Puerto Rico have licensure laws. Licensure is a prerequisite for employment.

Certification and registration are voluntary processes whereby the National Board for Respiratory Care (NBRC) administers standardized examinations attesting to an individual's clinical skills and knowledge. Everyone entering the profession takes the certifying examination which leads to the designation, Certified Respiratory Therapy Technician (CRTT). A subsequent examination, open only to CRTT's who meet education and experience requirements, results in the designation, Registered Respiratory Therapist (RRT).

Normally, practitioners advance from the treatment of general patients to critical care patients. Additional skills and experience are required to provide respiratory care for patients with significant problems in the organ systems, such as heart or kidneys.

Hospital respiratory care departments operate around the clock, providing patient care, requiring evening, night, and weekend work. A great deal of time is spent walking to, and standing at, patients' beds. Since RCP's work with needles and patients' blood, the risk of AIDS or hepatitis B infection exists, but normal precautions reduce this threat significantly.

Earnings

The starting salaries for certified respiratory therapy technicians average $20,500 per year. Registered respiratory therapists average $24,200 per year. Individuals who reach the position of program director in a hospital average $40,000. Salaries vary dramatically by geographic region and work setting.

1992 Estimated Entry Level Salaries

1. Anesthesiologist's assistant, $60,000
2. Medical assistant, $15,059
3. Occupational therapist, $30,737
4. Physician assistant, $38,826
5. Respiratory therapist, $24,934
6. Surgeon assistant, $41,300

Source: *Allied Health Education Directory*

Employment Outlook

There are currently about 81,000 respiratory care practitioners working in hospitals. Another 20,000 work in skilled nursing facilities, rehabilitation facilities, home healthcare, education, and sales.

The Bureau of Labor Statistics has projected a 52 percent increase in demand for practitioners by the year 2000. This need is attributed to a substantial increase in the older population, which will increase the incidence of cardiopulmonary disease. Additionally, advances in treating victims of heart attacks, accident victims, and premature infants will increase the requirement for RCP's. The projected rapid growth in the number of AIDS patients will also require more respiratory care practitioners since lung disease most often accompanies AIDS.

Training and Other Qualifications

Formal training is necessary for entry into the field. Accredited programs are found at more than 425 colleges, universities, and vocational-technical schools.

Program length varies at different schools, and outcome degrees range from associate to bachelor's degrees.

Respiratory care practitioners should be sensitive to patients' physical and psychological needs. They must be most attentive to detail, follow instructions, and work as a member of a team. Operating complex respiratory therapy equipment requires mechanical ability and manual dexterity.

High school students considering a career in respiratory care should be encouraged to take courses in biology, mathematics, chemistry, and physics. A working knowledge of science and mathematics is essential. The use of percentages, fractions, exponents, and algebra, as well as the metric and English systems of measuring, is important. Computing medication dosages and calculating gas concentrations are two examples of the need for knowledge of science and mathematics.

Curriculum

Actual training as a respiratory care practitioner is available only in an accredited formal program of didactic, laboratory, and clinical preparation. Biological and physical sciences basic to understanding the functioning of the human breathing system, such as anatomy, physiology, medical terminology, chemistry, mathematics, microbiology, physics, therapeutic procedures, clinical medicine, and clinical expressions are a part of every program. The program of study also includes social sciences basic to understanding how to relate with patients—such as psychology, communication skills, and medical ethics. Clinical training in routine and special procedures applicable to pediatric, adult, and geriatric patients is also provided.

The educational preparation and job experience of respiratory care practitioners are an excellent foundation for advancement in the healthcare professions. With additional education, there is potential for employment as a perfusionist, anesthetist, physical therapist, or nurse.

Respiratory care practitioners are involved in a wide variety of life-saving and life-supporting situations working side-by-side with other members of the healthcare team. Their expertise is in demand and the opportunities to expand their knowledge and skills is limitless. This is, *indeed*, a career with a future.

▼

ROBERT J. CZACHOWSKI received his bachelor of science degree from Marquette University, Milwaukee, WI. He obtained an MBA from Boston University, Boston, MA, and a Ph.D. in adult and continuing education from Texas A & M University, College Station, TX. He serves as director of education for the American Association for Respiratory Care, a membership organization of more than 36,000 respiratory care practitioners, headquartered in Dallas, TX. He has been involved in the education and training of allied health personnel for almost 29 years.

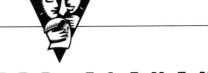

An Expanding Need for Physician Assistants

Lisa Mustone Alexander, MPH, PA-C,
Director, Physician Assistant Program, George Washington
University Medical Center

Like so many people, I was drawn to the medical profession at an early age. It wasn't, however, until I was in high school that a television program introduced me to the specific healthcare career that I would ultimately pursue. The program was about a physician assistant (commonly known as a PA) who was serving the needs of a medically underserved Hispanic neighborhood in a large metropolitan area. I was fascinated. I searched the profession and, as they say, *found my niche*.

A Short History

The physician assistant profession has broadened in scope since its inception at Duke University in 1965. In the mid-1960s, physicians and educators recognized that there was a shortage and an uneven distribution of primary care physicians. Dr. Eugene Stead, the physician credited with originating the PA concept, saw the military medic as an ideal person to be trained as a *physician extender*. The first PAs were former Navy corpsmen who completed an intensive two-year medical training program. Dr. Stead envisioned these new healthcare providers as serving the needs of rural populations in much the same way as the *country doctor* used to do.

PAs Practice Medicine

Today, physician assistants serve in a far broader set of circumstances. They still meet the healthcare needs of rural population—approximately a third of all PAs work in towns with fewer than 50,000 residents. Physician assistants are also found in urban areas in settings such as HMOs, hospitals, community health care clinics, and public health departments. They even serve on the White House medical staff. Over 70 percent of all physician assistants work in clinics and physician's offices and just under 30 percent work in hospitals.

In all of these settings, PAs provide patients with a wide range of primary healthcare services that would otherwise be provided by physicians. A physician assistant performs physical examinations, provides patient education, diagnoses illnesses, and establishes and carries out treatment for a multitude of primary care medical problems. PAs might also be involved in suturing wounds, setting broken bones, applying casts, and assisting in surgery or other technical procedures that augment the services provided by physicians. In most states, physician assistants can also write prescriptions.

By law, all physician assistants are *dependent* practitioners. They must work with a supervising physician. It is not necessary, however, for the physician and PA to always be located in the same building or even the same town. Most state laws, in fact, provide for supervision to occur via the telephone or other means of telecommunications. This way, a PA can work in a site remote from the supervising physician. It is not uncommon in many rural or frontier areas for the supervising physician to be located over 100 miles away.

This is one reason why PA education prepares a student to deal with many medical emergencies. Some physician assistants specialize in particular areas of medicine, such as surgery or orthopedics. In addition to the traditional clinical role, experienced PAs have found professional challenges in other related areas, such as education, clinical research, and administration. A wealth of advancement opportunities available to experienced PAs also help make this career exciting and personally satisfying.

Education

The physician assistant profession is a challenging and dynamic vocation, and the competition to get into a PA program is fierce. In 1992, there were four applicants for every PA program opening. There are over 50 accredited physician assistant programs throughout the United States graduating approximately 1,600 men and women each year. They are located at medical schools, teaching hospitals, colleges and universities, and through the armed services. To meet the growing demand for PAs, more programs are being created each year, enabling more applicants to begin their training.

Applicants with diverse backgrounds, not just those who are already in the healthcare field, are encouraged to enter this profession. However, most programs require that applicants have a minimum of two years of college credit and some healthcare experience prior to admission. Many applicants are former emergency medical technicians, nurses, or other allied health professionals.

At the George Washington University PA Program in Washington, DC, where I serve as director, there is no such thing as the *typical* applicant. Students range from the individual who has completed the traditional pre-med route in college, to the woman who has decided she would like to enter the field of medicine at what many term the *mid-career* point of her life, to the previously trained healthcare professional who wishes to expand his/her role in medicine. Nationally, 19 percent of all PA students are from an ethic minority group, and 60 percent of all PA students are women.

Due to the close working relationship physician assistants have with physicians, a PA's education is designed to complement that of a medical student's education. In fact, physician assistants are often in the same classes as medical students. One of the main differences between the two types of programs is not the core content of the curriculum, but the *amount of time* spent in school. A PAs education is approximately two-thirds that of a medical student's program—102 weeks versus 153.

> Earning potential is another attraction of this profession. Starting salaries for physician assistants nationally range from $35,000 to $40,000 and increase with years of experience, type of clinical practice, and geographic location. A number of PAs report salaries over $100,000.

In the first year, PA students spend most of their time in the classroom obtaining an in-depth understanding of the medical sciences—anatomy, microbiology, physiology, psychology. The second year is spent in clinical rotations where students have direct patient contact. Students spend time learning family medicine, internal medicine, emergency medicine, pediatrics, surgery, and orthopedics, to name a few of thespecialties.

Depending upon the program, physician assistants graduate with a certificate of completion or a baccalaureate degree. Nine of the accredited PA programs also offer a master's degree or master's option.

Graduation

A physician assistant's education doesn't end with graduation. Nearly all states require PAs to pass a national certifying examination before they can begin practicing. The exam, open only to graduates of accredited PA programs, is given each year by an independent organization established to assure the competency of physician assistants.

To maintain national certification, physician assistants must complete 100 hours of continuing medical education (CMEs) every two years. A PA must also take the recertification exam every six years. Only those with current certification can use the credentials Physician Assistant-Certified (PA-C) after their name.

Financing

Like most education programs, the cost of attending a PA program is a concern for prospective students. Although PA education costs are high, it is an excellent investment for one's future. Scholarships, loan sources, and other creative ways to finance an education exist for this field. Tuition assistance is also available through many hospitals and other healthcare facilities in exchange for a commitment to join the staff of those institutions after graduating. The U.S. Public Health Service also sponsors a scholarship program for physician assistants in exchange for time served as a PA in the Health Service at the completion of the program. Some states also offer financial assistance programs.

The American Academy of Physician Assistants (AAPA) publishes a financial aid information booklet that identifies some of the national and state financial aid sources. It is an excellent starting point to identifying ways to finance a PA education.

Demand

There is a bright future for the men and women who select a career as a physician assistant. Currently, the demand for PAs is greater than ever. There are six job openings for every new graduate, and the U.S. Department of Labor predicts there will be a 44 percent increase in the number of PA positions between 1990 and the year 2005. Part of the reason for the increase in demand is because of the quality of care provided by physician assistants. Federal studies have concluded that PAs provide care that is *equivalent* in quality to the care provided by physicians, and PAs have demonstrated their clinical effectiveness in terms of patient acceptance.

There are currently over 25,000 physician assistants, more than double the number just 10 years ago. In some rural areas, where physicians are in short supply, PAs serve as the only providers of healthcare, conferring with their supervising physicians and other medical professionals as needed or required by law. Many hospitals, faced with a shortage of physician residents (new medical school graduates), employ physician assistants in medical and surgical departments.

Physician assistants have been practicing medicine for over 25 years. They are widely recognized as filling an important role in the healthcare field. Coupled with an abundance of jobs offering competitive salaries, there couldn't be a better time to become a physician assistant!

LISA MUSTONE ALEXANDER, PA-C, is director of the Physician Assistant Program at the George Washington University Medical Center. For more information about physician assistants, write to the American Academy of Physician Assistants, 950 North Washington Street, Alexandria, VA 22314, or call (703) 836-2272.

Surgical Physician Assistant: The Rising Star of the Surgical Team

The American Association of Surgeon Assistants

The **surgical physician assistant** is an intermediate-level healthcare provider who supplements the care provided to patients by the surgeon.

What Does a Surgeon Assistant Do?

As a dependent practitioner, the surgical physician assistant (SA) can fulfill important needs of the patient and a surgical practice. Surgical physician assistants perform physical examinations and order and interpret diagnostic tests. Other tasks and functions of a surgeon assistant may include eliciting a detailed and accurate health history from the patient, performing an appropriate physical examination, recording and presenting data to the supervising surgeon, performing or assisting in routine laboratory work and related diagnostic studies, performing therapeutic procedures, helping the supervising surgeon in making hospital rounds, recording patient progress notes, executing orders, preparing comprehensive case summaries, and assisting in operative procedures.

The quality and quantity of patient services is directly enhanced by the surgical physician assistant through the improved availability and continuity of care and the liaison between healthcare providers. The utilization of the surgical physician assistant allows for the enhanced focus of the surgeon's time and expertise on more rigorous patient care demands.

History of the Surgeon Assistant Profession

In the mid `60s, the concept of an assistant to the surgeon took form within the establishment of the nation's first surgeon assistant program by Dr. John Kirklin at the University of Alabama at the Birmingham Medical Center.

Until 1989, separate educational essentials were in place for surgeon assistant programs. In that year, however, through a consensus with the Committee on Allied Health Education and Accreditation (CAHEA), the American College of Surgeons and the Association of Physician Assistant Programs unified to comprise one single document—*Essentials and Guidelines for an Accredited Educational Program for the Physician Assistant*—containing the guidelines for both surgeon assistant programs and primary care physician assistant programs. Currently, primary care programs are adopting curricula representing more surgical training, and the surgeon assistant programs are modifying their curricula to include more education in primary care.

Is a Surgeon Assistant a Physician Assistant?

A surgeon assistant is *indeed* a **physician assistant** (PA). The generic physician assistant works dependently with the supervision of a physician, usually a primary care physician. The surgeon assistant works dependently with the supervision of a surgeon. The premise of assisting the physician by performing patient care, or surgical procedures, to free the physician for more complex problems, is the same for PAs and SAs. Both PAs and SAs are skilled in the basic medical sciences and in functions such as compiling medical histories and performing physical examinations. The SA must be able to take patient histories, perform physical examinations, assist at operations, and participate in the postoperative care of the patient. To act in this capacity, the SA must be more than an *operative* assistant.

Education and Training

Surgical physician assistants are prepared with specialized education and training in surgery. There are three CAHEA-approved undergraduate surgeon assistant training programs in the nation, each two years in length.

Clinical didactic instruction includes the study of medical nomenclature, anatomy, physiology, pathophysiology, pharmacology, the fundamentals of general surgery and surgical patient care, asepsis, radiographic interpretation, electrocardiogram recording technique and interpretation, pulmonary function testing, inhalation therapy, and communications. The supervised clinical practice components of the curriculum are designed to develop the students' increasing competencies in eliciting a health history and in performing a physical examination, in providing assistance to the surgeon during surgery, and in performing preoperative and postoperative care procedures under the tutelage and supervision of the surgeon. Also included is a period of instruction that focuses on the care of acutely injured patients within an emergency care service.

The curriculum of a surgeon assistant program is structured much like a primary care physician assistant program with a didactic phase followed by a clinical practicum. In a surgeon assistant program, the emphasis is on clinical and technical sciences. The clinical experience of a surgeon assistant is gained in general and specialty surgical services and in the emergency department. Both surgeon assistants and physician assistants are skilled in the basic medical sciences and in functions such as compiling medical histories and performing physical examinations.

The American Medical Association's *Directory of Allied Health Careers* provides a summary of each of the undergraduate surgeon assistant programs. Additional information on the specific undergraduate programs is available from each training program and from the Association of Physician Assistant Programs (APAP). The three undergraduate surgeon assistant programs currently in existence are at:

- University of Alabama School of Medicine
- Cornell University Medical College (NY)
- Cuyahoga Community College (OH)

In addition, there are eight postgraduate surgical residency training programs, approximately one year in length, for physician assistant graduates of primary care programs:

- Montefiore Medical Center (NY)
- Norwalk/Yale PA Surgical Residency Program (CT)
- Sinai Hospital of Baltimore (MD)
- St. Vincent's Medical Center (NY)
- Geisinger Medical Center (PA)
- Martin Luther King Jr./Drew Medical Center (CA)
- Butterworth Hospital/Western Michigan University (MI)
- Mayo Foundation (MN)

The American College of Surgeons has actively participated in shaping and supporting the physician assistant/surgeon assistant profession. The College cooperates with other physician and physician assistant organizations to maintain the educational standards by which PA and SA programs are accredited. The College is also represented on the national certifying commission and has a long-standing liaison with the American Association of Surgeon Assistants (AASA).

Certification of Surgeon Assistants

Currently, 49 states, the District of Columbia, and Guam recognize and permit surgeon assistants and physician assistants to practice. Certified surgeon assistants and physician assistants may work for federal institutions in the state of New Jersey. In Missouri and Mississippi, the scope of a PA's practice is determined by the physician's delegatory authority. In addition, 41 states require graduation from an approved surgeon assistant or physician assistant program to practice.

Passage of the National Commission for the Certification of Physician Assistants (NCCPA) National Certification Examination is required by 39 states before practicing. Recertification is required by nine states to continue practice. Further information on the certification and recertification of physician assistants is available from the National Commission on Certification of Physician Assistants, Inc.

Eligibility to sit for the NCCPA National Certifying Examination is contingent upon first successfully completing a CAHEA-approved surgeon assistant/physician assistant program.

Individual states are responsible for the regulation of physician assistant practice within their states. For specific information regarding the regulation of physician assistants in a particular state, contact that state's medical licensing board, or the American Academy of Physician Assistants.

How Many PA's and SA's Are There?

In the *1985 Physician Assistant Role Delineation Study*, by Willis, Cyr, Schafft, and Steinbrueck, approximately 17 percent of a sample survey of over 1,400 respondents worked in general surgery or a surgical subspecialty. In 1987, there were nearly 20,000 generic physician assistants, including surgeon assistants and surgical physician assistants in the nation. This would calculate to over 3,000 generic physician assistants working in a surgical specialty or subspecialty. The actual total number of graduates of surgeon assistant programs in the country is less than 1,000.

Surgeon assistants and physician assistants with surgical skills are in high demand. A national survey showed a 33 percent increase in the number of physician assistants working in surgical specialties. This growth is due to several factors, including:

- New Medicare coverage for PA's assisting in surgery.

- The proven ability of PA's to provide high quality pre- and post-operative patient care, reducing the morbidity and mortality rates.

- The contributions of PA's toward increased practice productivity.

Many physician assistants working in surgery are graduates of *primary care* PA programs. They have a broad, solid base of medical and patient care knowledge. They may have obtained additional surgical training through postgraduate residency programs or by working with surgeons. A 1990 survey by the AAPA estimated that 21 percent of practicing physician assistants work in surgical settings.

Personal Qualifications

Essential qualities for the assistant to the surgeon include good interpersonal relations, a capacity for calm and reasoned judgement in meeting emergencies, an awareness and understanding of one's professional role, an orientation towards service, and a level of intelligence commensurate with the performance of one's professional skills. In addition, the surgeon assistant *must* maintain respect for the person and privacy of the patient.

The Surgeon Assistant as First Assistant

According to the 1993 Regents of the American College of Surgeons' *Statement on Qualifications for Surgical Privileges in Approved Hospitals*, the first assistant to the surgeon, during a surgical operation, should be trained and capable of participating and actively assisting the surgeon to establish a good working team. The first assistant provides aid in exposure, hemostasis, and other technical functions, which will help the surgeon carry out a safe operation with optimal results for the patient. This role varies considerably with the surgical operation, specialty area, and type of hospital.

In some hospitals in this country, there may not be specifically trained and readily available surgical assistants in the operating room. The first assistant's role in such institutions has traditionally been filled by a variety of individuals from diverse backgrounds. Designation of an individual most appropriate for this purpose within the bylaws of the hospital medical staff is the responsibility of the surgeon.

The American College of Surgeons supports the concept, that ideally, the first assistant to the surgeon at the operating table should be a qualified surgeon or resident in a surgical education program approved by the appropriate residency review committee and accredited under the Accreditation Council for Graduate Medical Education. It is a principle of surgical education and care that residents at appropriate levels of training should be provided with opportunities to assist and participate in operations. Other physicians experienced in assisting the responsible surgeon may participate when a trained surgeon or a resident in an accredited program is not available.

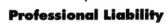

Professional Liability

A 1986 review of medical malpractice claims involving the country's 20,000 physician assistants revealed fewer than a dozen reported cases over the past 20 years. Historically, PAs have been regarded as extremely valuable in decreasing physician liability. Therefore, unlike some other non-physician healthcare providers, SA's have not experienced difficulty in obtaining malpractice insurance, either on their own or through their employers. The cost of professional liability insurance for SA's and PA's is relatively low. A one-million dollar policy offered to members of the American Academy of Physician Assistants, for example, would cost a surgeon assistant from $2,500 to $4,200 per year, depending upon geographic location.

Attainment of this ideal in all hospitals is recognized as impractical. In some circumstances, it is necessary to utilize appropriately trained non-physicians to serve as first assistants to qualified surgeons. Surgeon assistants or physician assistants with additional surgical training may be employed if they meet national standards.

THE AMERICAN ASSOCIATION OF SURGEON ASSISTANTS (AASA) was founded in 1973 as the official organization representing student and graduate surgeon assistants and physician assistants who work in surgery. Its objectives are to encourage communication and discussion, to achieve academic and clinical excellence among its members, and to promote surgeon assistants in the medical community. In the years since the association's establishment, the original mission of the AASA has remained unchanged in encouraging, through its programs, excellence in service to the medical profession and the patients it serves.

As the profession has grown, the association has responded to the changing needs of surgeon assistants and physician assistants in surgery. AASA goals include the continued encouragement of professional excellence and integrity, and the education of the medical and lay communities of the role of the surgeon assistant in providing quality healthcare as members of the surgical team.

The association publishes a newsletter and grants various awards to SA's and surgical PA's. These honors include the AASA President's Award, the John W. Kirklin M.D. Award for Professional Excellence, and the Editor's Award of Merit (presented to the author(s) of the best scientific article of the year in the association's quarterly newsletter). Corporate support makes possible three annual student scholarships, one for each of the three CAHEA-accredited SA programs.

For the future, AASA anticipates continued growth. Its membership can expect continuing professional representation, strengthening in its medical education programs, and a broadening in services offered.

C H A P T E R   T H I R T E E N

Medical Assistantship: One of America's Fastest-Growing Careers

Annette H. Heyman, R.M.A., R.T. (R),
Director, American Registry of Medical Assistants

The common definition of **medical assistant** is one who assists the physician in the care and treatment of the patient. Actually, a medical assistant is one who performs his/her duties within the overall classification of allied health, that is: those trained in medical assisting, R.N., L.P.N., the technologies—radiology, medical laboratory, respiratory, surgery; the aides—nurses, occupational therapy, physical therapy; emergency medical technicians, etc.

Duties of the Medical Assistant

Medical assistants perform clinical, laboratory, and administrative duties generally in the physician's office. Most physicians hire at least one medical assistant whose tasks may vary with the size and kind of practice.

Preparing the patients for examinations, they take vital signs, height, weight, temperature, pulse, and respirations. They may get the medical history and record answers in the patient's file. They arrange medical instruments and hand them to the physician as the examination proceeds.

Medical assistants help with first aid, collect and process specimens, and perform ordered tests. They may draw blood for examination and perform electrocardiograms; they may help with minor surgery, remove sutures, or change dressings on wounds. The medical assistant may also instruct the patient on diet, medicines, or special procedures before laboratory tests, surgery, or x-rays.

The medical assistant keeps the examining rooms in order before and after each patient enters and leaves—cleans/sterilizes or discards any instruments used, and changes and disposes of any used linens and examination gowns.

As the physician's *right hand*, these professionals act as receptionists, greet patients, schedule appointments, process the mail, prepare and maintain patient medical records, record data on physicals and surgery referrals, and arrange hospital admissions. They type medical reports, keep files up-to-date in order to meet legal requirements, process health insurance forms, keep financial records, send invoices, and take payments. Assistants may manage personnel, do payroll for the office staff, negotiate leases, and obtain equipment and supplies. A medical assistant serves as a liaison between the physician and others, such as representatives of drug companies and medical supply companies.

Working Conditions, Hours, Earnings

Medical assistants may be employed in medical offices and clinics, hospitals, nursing homes, or laboratories. Working hours depend on the physician's specialty and schedule of the facility. Most work 35 to 40 hours a week but the hours may vary to include very early or very late hours or weekends. In an emergency, they may have to stay on the job past regular hours and will either be compensated for the additional hours worked or be given compensatory time off. Salary may be between $8,000 - $25,000 per year, averaging $18,000, but varies with education, credentials, experience, and geographic location.

Since much of their work is with people and often those who are very ill, the prospective medical assistants must determine if they can deal with these problems and stresses.

Personal Characteristics

The medical assistant must be pleasant and courteous to patients and co-workers, must be able to follow instructions, and, since most of the patients they encounter are ill or uneasy, the medical assistant must be patient and compassionate. S/he must be able to communicate both orally and in writing, be accurate in all phases of his/her work, and maintain confidentiality.

Disabled workers may be able to be accommodated and should contact their school or employment counselors, state office of vocational rehabilitation, or state department of labor.

Education and Training

A high school diploma or equivalent is required to enter the field. Training may be obtained on the job, but specific specialties within the allied health field have definite requirements of education, training, and/or licensure in order to be allowed to practice.

The general medical assistant program may be chosen from a nine-month to two-year course given by vocational schools, community colleges, and some business schools. Two-year programs result in associate degrees while nine-month and one-year programs grant certificates or diplomas. The certificate program, in general, consists of approximately 700 to 750 hours of classroom study plus 200 to 250 hours of externship during which time practical experience and training in the actual office setting is achieved—generally without pay, although if the student performs very satisfactory work, the physician may offer some compensation. This is also determined by the arrangements made between the school and the physician.

Medical assisting programs are accredited by the Committee on Allied Health Education and Accreditation (CAHEA) and the Accrediting Bureau of Health Education Schools (ABHES), both agencies being recognized by the U.S. Department of Education.

Suggested Curriculum and Credentials

Some of the suggested course material include: biology, physiology, anatomy; office procedures: typing and transcription, computer skills, case history writing, bookkeeping, and insurance forms; medical records: record keeping, procedural and diagnosis coding, transcription, filing, medical terminology, business English, medical office correspondence, and mail handling; administrative procedures: communication and telephone skills, appointment scheduling, office management, office supplies, inventory control, and medical ethics; laboratory procedures: basal metabolism, specimen collection, urinalysis, microscope, blood drawing and analysis, quality control, and other testing done in offices; first aid; CPR; clinical assisting: patient preparation, vital signs, sterilization and instruments, bacteriology, nutrition, safety in the office, emergencies, bandaging, drugs and drug laws, injection techniques, and the metric system.

> **1991-92 Allied Health Graduates by Occupation**
>
> 1. Anesthesiologist's assistant, 28 graduates
> 2. Medical assistant, 6,902
> 3. Occupational therapist, 2,900
> 4. Physician assistant, 1,433
> 5. Surgeon assistant, 49
>
> Source: *Allied Health Education Directory*

Graduates of accredited medical assisting programs and medical assistants with a minimum of 12 months of experience may be registered, with recommendation from their employer, through the American Registry of Medical Assistants or American Medical Technologists. Certification is available through the American Association of Medical Assistants. They may use the initials R.M.A. and C.M.A., respectively. A state license is generally not required of the medical assistant except for those performing x-rays. Nurses, and in some states, assistants must pass a test for giving injections or drawing blood.

Before committing to a course of study in medical assisting, the student may wish to *try it on for size*, that is, volunteer as an aide or *candy striper* in a hospital or clinic, nursing home, or doctor's office to see what it is like to assist with the ill, disabled, or frightened person, and to confront the hands-on care required; help out as a typist, filing clerk, office *go-pher* in the medical office or medical record room. These situations and experiences may help to determine if the work is for them—if they want to spend the rest of their working life in this field.

Certification vs. Registration

Over the years, there has been much confusion over the difference between certification and registration. The medical assistant may choose to be certified (C.M.A.) or registered (R.M.A.) depending upon the organization to which one belongs. They are both voluntary and national credentials indicating that the person is qualified to perform the duties of a medical assistant.

The C.M.A. is given by the Certifying Board of the American Association of Medical Assistants Organization, while the R.M.A. is a generic term used by ARMA since 1950 and by the American Medical Technologists since 1984.

Neither federal nor state governments require a medical assistant to be either certified or registered in order to practice. Some states do require a license, however, to practice within certain specialties.

An examination is given by the other two organizations in order to belong. Members of the American Registry of Medical Assistants must be recommended either by their employer after having a minimum of one year's training on the job or by the director or instructor of the school from which they graduated in a course of medical assisting. Neither the federal nor state government requires a medical assistant to have been formally trained to be employed at this time. Graduation from an accredited program benefits the student by providing proof of completion of a program that meets nationally accepted standards, recognition of their education by their professional peers, and eligibility for registration or certification.

Receiving a recommendation from an employer indicates that not only does s/he pass upon the training that has been received in the facility, but upon the ability of that person to do the job for which s/he has trained. In fact, some of those recommendations that ARMA has received have been glowing tributes.

Hopefully, through accrediting efforts, medical assisting will be elevated into a true profession and our employer-physicians will recognize their value. At ARMA, we have seen the fruits of our labors in many sections of the country where physicians think so highly of their assistants—of our members—that they will only hire someone who is registered.

It is our hope that this feeling will grow and develop throughout the country. Our members can help by *talking us up*, by recommending more new people into our group, by educating the physicians to their status, and by constantly exhibiting the highest standards and ethics on the job and in their everyday life.

Employment Outlook

Medical assisting is the second fastest growing occupation according to the U.S. Department of Labor, 1992 report. Health insurance, Medicare, and Medicaid make medical care available to more people and with the number of physicians increasing, more staff members will be needed to run their offices. The growing volume of paperwork related to government requirements will also contribute to the demand for medical assistants. The growth of outpatient clinics and Health Maintenance Organizations (HMOs), the increase in population, and greater numbers of older people requiring more medical care will also increase the job opportunities for the medical assistant.

Those medical assistants who have graduated from an accredited program, are registered or certified, have had experience, and are skilled in the use of word processors and computers, will be preferred by physicians and have an advantage over others without this background. Opportunities within the field include clinical medical assistant, administrative medical assistant, medical receptionist, medical insurance biller, medical bookkeeper, medical transcriber, and laboratory assistant.

Advancement for those who wish to continue their education and training is great. The medical assistant may advance to become office manager or instructor, or may transfer to a larger office, clinic, or hospital, where they can expand their skills and earn higher salaries.

Some medical assistants continue training or acquire skills in another field and may then transfer to these fields or practice their combined skills in a hospital or clinic. This is known as cross-training, that is, training for more than one occupation. Many medical assistants continue their studies to become nurses or excel in the laboratory to become laboratory or medical technologists, phlebotomists, or other specialties, while others enter the teaching field as biology teachers or instructors of medical assistants.

With their wide range of studies as a background and if they wish to leave the direct medical profession, the medical assistant may even accept a variety of other employment opportunities in areas such as secretarial, transcription, insurance, dental and veterinary assisting, general office work, computers, and word processing.

A Typical Working Day

The day of a medical assistant is anything but routine and rarely dull. Although the salary is not as great as that of other professions, the satisfaction of helping in the care and management of the patients is well worth the effort expended. You must decide if it is better to be happy in the job and receive less pay or receive a higher salary and be unhappy in your day-to-day work life. Generally, those who remain in the field consider it to be very fulfilling and are satisfied with a job well done.

The physician assistant (PA), in contrast to the medical assistant (MA), provides routine patient services traditionally performed by a physician, such as interviewing and writing up medical histories, performing physical exams, ordering laboratory tests and x-rays, examining the lab tests, prescribing certain drugs, and referring patients while working under the supervision of doctors. They present their findings to the doctor who determines the proper course of treatment.

The PA assists the doctor in conducting hospital rounds, develops and implements patient management plans, and performs routine diagnostic procedures. They usually do not choose a specialty until they work with a doctor who is a specialist, although there are special programs such as surgeon's assistant and child health associate.

The PA may be found in doctor's offices, hospitals, clinics, HMOs, student health services, community health centers, nursing homes, correctional facilities, and in the military.

General college preparation is recommended with a two-year undergraduate major in sciences required. The certificate program is 24 to 28 months; a bachelor of science program is four years. Admission to many programs requires some patient care experience. Healthcare experience as a military corpsman, nurse, or other allied health worker may substitute for some college.

Certification through the National Committee on Certification of Physician Assistants is required in order to practice and PA's must be licensed by their state board of medical examiners.

▼

ANNETTE H. HEYMAN, R.M.A., R.T.(R) lives in Springfield, MA, and received a B.S. in physiology from the University of Massachusetts, Amherst; certification as laboratory and x-ray technician from Eastern School for Physicians' Aides, Inc., NY; registered as a radiologic technologist in diagnostic radiology; registered as medical assistant with the American Registry of Medical Assistants; received ME.d. from Springfield College, Springfield, MA, and certified with the Commonwealth of Massachusetts as teacher of secondary education in biology; was department head of the Radiology Department, Western Massachusetts Hospital, Westfield, MA. After 40 years, Ms. Heyman has retired but maintains her license to practice from the state of Massachusetts. She has been a board member of ARMA since 1950, progressing from secretary general to director (1988-present).

CHAPTER FOURTEEN

Chiropractic: A "High Touch" Healthcare Career

John Healy,
Director of Communications, Northwestern
College of Chiropractic

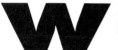 hat is the top-rated healthcare career of the 1990s? The answer isn't a dentist, or an optometrist, or a physical therapist.

It's a **doctor of chiropractic**. Chiro-*what*? Chiropractic. The career is currently the second-highest paying in healthcare, as well as the second-largest healing profession in the world, with more than 40,000 doctors of chiropractic currently practicing in the United States.

What Is Chiropractic Healthcare?

Chiropractic is *high touch*, rather than *high tech*, primary healthcare that treats millions of Americans every year. It is a conservative form of treatment that emphasizes the *whole* patient, *all* the body systems, and the discovery and healing of the *cause* of the disease, not just its symptoms.

Its holistic approach to human health is based on the premise that the relationship between structure and function in the human body is a significant health factor and that relationships between the spinal column and the nervous system contribute to the disease process. In contrast with traditional medicine of today, chiropractic successfully treats many health problems without the use of prescription drugs and major surgery.

A recent poll in *Time* magazine found that only about one out of three Americans has visited a doctor of chiropractic in his/her lifetime. This is beginning to change, however, partially because of groundbreaking scientific studies conducted at research centers in many of the chiropractic colleges in the country. That is part of the reason why chiropractic is the top-rated healthcare career of the 1990s—because of its nearly *unlimited* growth potential.

In fact, many famous athletes swear that their chiropractor is the only way they can continue playing sports. Joe Montana, the San Francisco 49ers star quarterback, visits a chiropractor weekly. In 1991, golf professional Payne Stewart was troubled by a strained lower back in the weeks prior to the competition. It began to seriously affect his golf game, and he considered pulling out of the U.S. Open. Instead, he sought help for his back from a chiropractor, and he went on to win the U.S. Open tournament, winning hundreds of thousands of dollars.

That growth will be shared by each doctor in the profession, because almost all chiropractors own their own clinics. Being one's own boss has been an attractive part of a chiropractic career for many people. *You* are the one who decides how successful you will become. It is one of the few professions where your future is pretty much in *your* hands.

In addition, you'll find a chiropractor in just about every community, especially in the Midwest. Thus, whether you want to pursue a career in a large city or a small town, you'll have a chance to make a go of your career as a chiropractor in a location you pick. It's not like a lot of jobs, where you have to move someplace you hate to find a job in the profession you're trained in.

Career Preparation

If you're interested in helping people with their health problems—and wouldn't mind enjoying a comfortable living while doing so—then you might consider a career as a chiropractor. There are currently 14 colleges in North America that offer degrees as a doctor of chiropractic. The colleges are accredited by the same organization that accredits places like the University of Minnesota and Notre Dame.

Getting into a chiropractic college requires a minimum of two academic years of college credit toward a baccalaureate degree with a core group of 60 credit hours. You should take plenty of science classes in subjects like biology, chemistry, and physics. That goes for those who are still in high school. Take science classes—they'll be extremely useful once you begin working on your doctor of chiropractic degree.

Specialties

There is a wide range of areas that you can specialize in if you become a doctor of chiropractic. Some focus on working with sports injuries, with expectant mothers and young children, or with the elderly. Others specialize in treating headaches (without using medication) or helping companies reduce employee injuries. In fact, this is a rapidly growing area for chiropractors. Many companies are asking chiropractors to come into their workplace to evaluate their job sites and look for ways to reduce injuries to workers with repetitive motion jobs.

However, be sure to also take psychology, English, communications, and other humanities or social science classes. Interpersonal communication has always been a strength for chiropractors, with many patients pointing to this communication as one of the major reasons they visit chiropractors.

Students who are pursuing a doctor of chiropractic degree at one of the 14 chiropractic colleges in North America generally take 10 15-week trimesters that total more than 4,400 hours of classroom, laboratory, and clinical experience. Those 10 trimesters usually take three-and-a-half to four years. Tuition ranges from $3,500 to $4,000 per trimester and books and supplies are extra. A variety of financial aid options are available to students, including grants, loans, and hundreds of scholarship opportunities.

An education at a chiropractic college doesn't consist of just all classroom lectures and laboratory work. Chiropractic colleges pride themselves on integrating hands-on clinical experience into the educational curriculum. Through internships in college clinics, which serve the public, plus internships with private doctors of chiropractic, students at chiropractic colleges receive extensive training in caring for patients who suffer from a great variety of health problems.

It is in the college's clinics that students hone their *adjusting* skills. This involves realigning the spinal column, which chiropractors believe has a great deal of impact on the health of the human body. When it is *out of alignment*, the body's natural defenses to ward off disease and illness are lowered, and a person is more likely to become sick. Therefore, chiropractors ensure that the spine is in proper alignment so that the body stays in a state of *homeostasis* or balance.

Salaries

After about five years in practice, doctors who own their own clinic generally earn close to $70,000. It's not uncommon for doctors of chiropractic to average six figures after 10 years in practice.

History of Chiropractic Care

Where exactly did chiropractic originate? It's a surprise to many people when they learn that chiropractic's roots trace from the physicians of ancient Greece, and has close links with the healthcare traditions of China, Japan, and the Indians of North and Central America. Hippocrates, the ancient Greek physician who lent his name to the oath taken by traditional doctors, practiced healthcare that included many chiropractic methods. Even in his time, Hippocrates' holistic approach was in conflict with rival doctrines that centered on the *disease* rather than the *patient*.

Chiropractic took its first step, as a formal method of healthcare, near the turn of the century. In 1895, Daniel David Palmer was a frontier doctor in Davenport, IA, using a form of hypnotherapy, as well as *laying on the hands*. He was highly critical of the confusion that existed in the healing practices of the day and was concerned that the drugs and potions in common use actually caused toxic stress in patients.

In September of that year, the first beneficiary of chiropractic treatment walked into Dr. Palmer's office. Harvey Lillard, the building's maintenance man, suffered from severe hearing impairment. Through examination, Dr. Palmer determined that the vertebra in Lillard's upper spine was out of place. The vertebra was painful, and Lillard confirmed that his hearing loss and the pain in his back had both begun at the same time. Dr. Palmer reasoned that if the vertebra were put back into place, the patient's hearing would be restored. He, therefore, repositioned the bone and Lillard's hearing returned to normal.

The experience led Mr. Palmer to begin to search for the mechanical laws governing the spine, and his experience with more patients and other types of disorders led to the development of chiropractic treatment. Most of the basic concepts and clinical practices that would make up chiropractic had already been established informally by the late 19th Century, but through his study, Dr. Palmer rediscovered a set of principles that was to serve as the foundation for the development of the science.

For more information on working toward a degree as a doctor of chiropractic, contact the Northwestern College of Chiropractic. If you're simply interested in learning more about chiropractic, contact the American Chiropractic Association.

▼

JOHN HEALY, director of communications at Northwestern College of Chiropractic in Bloomington, MN, received his B.S. in journalism at the University of Oregon. He drew *extensively* on interviews with doctors of chiropractic in private practice, as well as faculty members of the college, while writing this article.

CHAPTER FIFTEEN

Dietitian...A Hot Career in the '90s

Pam Michael, MBA, RD,
Membership Coordinator, The American Dietetic Association

I f you are looking for a career that is exciting, dynamic, and challenging and also offers many opportunities for employment, then you may want to consider a career as a dietitian. Dietitians are experts in food and nutrition who apply their knowledge of nutrition to improve the public's health and well being. Dietitians work in healthcare, education, and research. They also work in sports and fitness facilities, government agencies, restaurant management, food companies, and in private practice. Job responsibilities vary depending on the area of dietetics practice.

Job Outlook

According to the U.S. Bureau of Labor Statistics, employment of dietitians is expected to grow faster than the average profession through the year 2000. This growth will be more noticeable in areas of public health, consulting, and business.

Areas of Dietetics Practice

Dietitians can be found in a variety of settings. **Management dietitians** work in healthcare institutions, schools, cafeterias, and restaurants. They are responsible for personnel management, menu planning, budgeting, and purchasing. They direct food service systems where large quantities of meals are prepared and served. With more and more Americans recognizing the importance of good nutrition, management dietitians increasingly play a key role wherever food is served.

Clinical dietitians are a vital part of the medical team in hospitals, nursing homes, health maintenance organizations, and other healthcare facilities. They work with doctors, nurses, and therapists to help speed patients' recovery and lay the groundwork for long-term health. A typical day may involve reviewing medical charts, assessing a patient/client's nutritional status, making recommendations to the healthcare team regarding nutritional care, and instructing patients/clients and their families on special diets necessary to promote health. Opportunities for advancement are available by choosing a particular area of nutrition, such as diabetes, heart, or pediatrics.

Community dietitians work in public and home health agencies, daycare centers, health and recreation clubs, and in government-funded programs that feed and counsel families, the elderly, pregnant women, children, and disabled or underprivileged individuals. Community dietitians educate and counsel these individuals, as well as use their training in clinical nutrition to ensure that government nutrition programs meet the nutrition standards for which the programs were designed. Wherever proper nutrition can help improve quality of life, they reach out to the public to teach, monitor, and advise.

Educator dietitians work in colleges, universities, and community or technical schools, teaching future doctors, nurses, dietitians, and dietetic technicians the sophisticated science of foods and nutrition. Besides giving lectures, educators write lesson plans, supervise, and counsel students in their on-site practical experiences. Many say they enjoy their role as mentors who bring qualified students into the exciting field of dietetics.

Research dietitians work in government agencies, food and pharmaceutical companies, and in major universities and medical centers. They conduct or direct experiments to answer critical nutrition questions, and find alternative foods or dietary recommendations for the public. Research dietitians' activities also include writing grants to request funds for research opportunities, interviewing potential subjects for studies, and collecting, analyzing, and interpreting research data.

Consultant dietitians work full- or part-time, usually under contract with a healthcare facility or in their own private practice. Consultant dietitians in private practice perform nutrition screening and assessment of their own clients and those referred to them by a physician. They offer advice on weight loss, cholesterol reduction, and a variety of other diet-related concerns. Those under contract with healthcare facilities often consult with food service managers, providing expertise on food sanitation and safety procedures, budgeting, and portion control. Other clients include athletes, company employees, and nursing home residents.

Business dietitians work in food and nutrition related industries. They work in product development, sales, marketing, advertising, public relations, purchasing, and in many other capacities that enable companies to satisfy consumers' growing interest in nutrition.

Credentials and Education

Most dietitians obtain the professional credential, registered dietitian (RD), for career advancement and a wider variety of employment opportunities. Many employers require the RD credential as a prerequisite for employment as a dietitian.

In order to become a registered dietitian, individuals must complete either of the following pathways:

Pathway 1: An American Dietetic Association (ADA) Coordinated Program. This includes a bachelor's or master's degree program in dietetics *and* supervised practice program (a minimum of 900 hours of supervised practice).

Pathway 2: An ADA approved bachelor's degree dietetics program *followed* by an ADA approved/accredited supervised practice program (which is completed at another institution). The supervised practice program, dietetic internship, or AP4 (approved preprofessional practice program) generally is completed in 9 to 24 months. Although most supervised practice programs are full-time programs, several allow students to complete the experience on a part-time basis. Many internships or AP4's also combine the supervised practice experience with the completion of a master's degree. *Author's note: Because of the competitive nature of the supervised practice programs, some students may not be selected for a position at these programs.*

After completing either pathway, students are eligible to take the Registration Examination for Dietitians. Upon passing the exam, individuals may use the title Registered Dietitian, and the credentials RD after their name. Once registered, dietitians must also complete continuing education (75 hours accumulated over 5 years) throughout their professional career.

Dietitians may also need to qualify for and adhere to state licensure laws. These requirements, which are generally determined by the state government's regulatory agency, may vary from the ADA's requirements for registration. If a dietitian meets the state's guidelines to practice, s/he may use the title, LD, for Licensed Dietitian.

Experienced dietitians can advance into assistant, associate, and/or director positions within a dietetics department in a healthcare facility. These positions may or may not require additional education. Clinical dietitians may choose to advance their career by specializing in nutrition support, kidney disease, diabetes, heart disease, pediatrics, or gerontology. Research or educator dietitian positions generally require completion of an advanced degree (master's or doctoral).

Preparation

Individuals interested in becoming a dietitian can prepare for the college curriculum by taking math, chemistry, and biology classes. Science courses and nutrition are heavily emphasized in the ADA approved/accredited bachelor's degree dietetics program. Additional required college courses include restaurant and institutional management, psychology, English, and business classes.

Salary Information

Salaries for registered dietitians vary depending on geographical location, scope of responsibility, and supply of practitioners. According to The American Dietetic Association 1991 Membership Database, of those registered dietitians who have been employed full-time in dietetics for one year after registration, (entry-level practitioners), 74 percent reported annual gross incomes between $20,000-30,000; 21 percent reported annual gross incomes between $30,000-40,000.

Working as a Dietitian

Dietitians work both independently and also with groups, such as a healthcare team. Individuals who want to become a dietitian should have an interest in food, nutrition, and health, and also enjoy working with people. Because of the varied job responsibilities, dietitians need to be efficient, creative, and flexible. Other characteristics include patience, tact, and strong organizational skills to identify and solve problems expediently.

Most full-time dietitians work 40 hours a week, which may include working on the weekends. Part-time employment is also available, and both part or full-time clinical or food service administrative dietitians may work varied shifts. Although rigorous activity is not usually included in a dietitian's job description, administrative dietitians generally work with large, heavy food preparation equipment.

Where to Get More Information

The American Dietetic Association is the world's largest organization of food and nutrition professionals, including dietitians, nutritionists, and dietetic technicians. Individuals enrolled in the ADA approved/accredited dietetics programs are eligible to join ADA as affiliate members. In addition, brochures on ADA offers careers in dietetics and a list of ADA approved/accredited education programs (free of charge). Call or write The American Dietetic Association, 216 W. Jackson Blvd., Chicago, IL 60606-6995, 1-800-877-1600 for more information.

▼

PAM MICHAEL, MBA, RD works as a membership coordinator at The American Dietetic Association. She manages ADA's membership recruitment and retention activities, and is also the contact person at ADA for information about careers in dietetics. Prior to ADA, she was the nutrition program director at a physician's private practice clinic. She has also worked in private practice, providing nutrition consultation to a long-term care facility. As an out-patient dietitian in a major medical center, she worked both in the community and in several clinics conducting prenatal and weight loss classes.

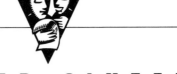

Dental Hygiene: A "Polished" Profession

Sheranita L. Hemphill, RDH,
Assistant Professor, Dental Hygiene Department,
Sinclair Community College

A registered dental hygienist (RDH) is a licensed member of the healthcare delivery system and assumes responsibility for providing oral health care as determined by the state dental practice acts. Hygienists perform a variety of functions in several different roles. In the traditional role of clinician the hygienist is typically employed in a dental office setting. Duties in this environment include:

- health history recording
- oral examinations
- head and neck examinations
- radiographic examinations
- topical fluoride applications
- periodontal and dental charting
- sealant applications
- impression taking
- client education
- clinical and historical data assessments
- presentation of findings to the attending dentists

A Typical Day in the Office

In the dental office setting, the hygienist is a member of the dental *team*. The team is characteristically composed of the hygienist, dentist, dental assistant, dental lab technician, and office manager. A typical day may begin with the hygienist reviewing the schedule of appointments. The treatment area is then prepared for the first client. Universal infection control procedures are followed to prevent cross-contamination of disease, both before and after each client. Next, the client is escorted to the treatment area and the appointment procedures begin.

Clients are asked screening questions to determine the need for potential interventions prior to dental hygiene services, and the initial vital signs are recorded. Data is revised and recorded as necessary in the patient's permanent record.

Next, the hygienist examines the oral cavity, noting and recording significant clinical findings. All findings are reported to the attending dentist for follow-up care. Dental hygienists may *interpret* findings, but the attending dentist *diagnoses* conditions. Treatment planning follows, which consists of determining the client's individual oral hygiene needs.

▼
On the Go

Patient needs vary, as will oral healthcare services. In a typical day, the hygienist may perform scaling and root planing to remove deposits from the teeth; apply dental sealants for children; discuss nutrition with a new mother; take radiographs (x-rays) of several patients; take impressions for study casts; work with "special needs" clients; and provide individualized dental education to everyone!

How Much Education Is Required?

Two years of secondary education within an accredited dental hygiene program is the *minimum* academic preparation. The program curriculum provides for a well-rounded educational experience and general studies courses usually transfer to other universities. The ultimate objective of a dental hygiene program is the education of a dental hygienist who, as a member of the dental team and healthcare delivery system, can assume responsibilities for providing client care as determined by the state practice acts.

How Do I Apply to a Dental Hygiene Program?

Contact the office of admissions at the institution of interest and request an application for admission into the dental hygiene program. There are approximately 200 dental hygiene programs throughout the country. The application procedures may vary, depending upon the institution, however, the process is easily initiated with a phone call to the college or university of choice.

What Courses Are Required?

The curriculum consists of courses in concentrated dental hygiene topics and in the physical and social sciences, including the humanities. Specific dental hygiene courses may vary in title due to institutional preferences, however, the content of each dental hygiene program is standardized through the accreditation process. The following is an example of the course titles in a typical dental hygiene program. The following is not intended to be a complete list of the dental hygiene program courses:

• Introduction to Dental Hygiene

- Head and Neck Anatomy
- Dental Hygiene Techniques
- Oral Pathology
- Dental Radiology
- Dental Office Emergencies
- Clinical Dental Hygiene
- Dental Materials
- Periodontics
- Community Dental Health
- Dental Health Education
- Dental Practice Administration

Courses in the general sciences include:

- Anatomy and Physiology
- Sociology
- Biochemistry
- English Composition
- Nutrition
- Pathophysiology
- Allied Health Math
- General Psychology
- Interpersonal Communication

Careers in the business industry typically require additional education and sales experience. Hygienists may position themselves for independent consulting, contracting, management, and product sales employment opportunities with manufacturers of dental-related products. Such positions may require training periods, flexible hours, travel, weekend conventions, paperwork, and good organizational skills.

What About Compensation and Benefits?

Compensation varies with the position and geographic location. Hygienists may receive remuneration for services by salary, percentage compensation, or a combination of both. According to a survey on staff salaries and benefits in *Dental Management* magazine recently, *hygienist salaries are at an all-time high.* More than 600 dentists nationwide responded to questions on what they pay in wages and benefits to RDHs. Daily wages for RDHs vary from a low of $111 in the East South Central states (Mississippi, Alabama, Tennessee, and Kentucky) to a high of $184 in the Pacific states. New England averages were at a daily rate of $152. Bonus payments are also available in some practices as a remuneration benefit.

Characteristics of an Ideal Dental Hygienist

There are several key characteristics of a successful dental hygiene candidate. These characteristics are all related to and affect treatment outcomes, success with patient compliance, and the performance of the student and future dental hygienist. A key characteristic for the candidate is **versatility.** This is essential because the dental hygiene profession is service-oriented. It exists to provide services to and for a very diverse population.

Skills essential to success in the profession include **dexterity** and **good communications.** Dexterity is necessary because the provision of hands-on technical skills is basic to successful clinical performance. Verbal and non-verbal communication skills are fundamental to the presentation of information that routinely occurs with clients, other healthcare workers, and in group settings.

Recognition and **appreciation of cultural differences** demonstrates a mature personality (one that fares well in *any* service-oriented profession). Good **time management skills, interpersonal skills,** and **initiative** are also conducive to success in this profession.

If you are interested in pursuing a career in dental hygiene, recall that the curriculum of the dental hygiene profession is designed to assist students in developing and refining skills indispensable to success in the profession.

What Are the Entry-Level Jobs?

Career opportunities at the associate degree level and/or certificate level include clinical practice in: dental offices; special needs facilities; governmental institutions, such as the armed services; correctional institutions; specialty dental practices; and in the insurance industry.

What Other Opportunities Exist?

With additional education, dental hygienists are employed in public health settings, such as state and local departments of health. Job variety exists and leadership potential is a must. Administrative positions are available for hygienists who possess and enjoy managerial skills. Entry-level positions within the public health setting might include involvement in the administration of projects, involving the assessment, planning, implementation, and evaluation of community health programs.

Many hygienists pursue additional training in the field of education and/or dental hygiene. As a dental hygiene educator, hygienists may teach classes on public health, nutrition, special needs dental patients, and/or other dental hygiene classes. They may also assist in teaching second-year clinical dental hygiene classes. A position as a dental hygiene instructor typically requires a master's degree and teaching experience.

How Does a Dental Hygienist Become Licensed?

In addition to the successful completion of the program requirements, the following must be fulfilled to satisfy state, regional, and national requirements: successful passage of the national board examination; successful passage of the regional boards (if applicable); and successful passage of the state examination.

The **national** board is an examination that covers the following subject areas: anatomic sciences, biochemistry/physiology and nutrition, microbial and immunology, pathology, pharmacology, patient assessment, radiology, management of dental hygiene care, periodontology, preventive agents, supportive treatment, and community health. This exam occurs relatively close to the end of the student hygienists' tenure in the program. It consists of one full day of testing that resembles the SAT or ACT testing format. Each candidate is charged a fee to sit for this exam.

The **regional** board examination is intended to determine the qualifications of licensure candidates in dental hygiene. The examination is conducted regionally and consists of two parts. First, a written exam consisting of a combination of slides and multiple choice questions is administered. Second, a practical exam that assesses the students' ability to provide scaling and root planing procedures (hard and soft deposit removal) is conducted. The candidate is charged a fee for this exam as well.

The Future of Dental Hygiene

The population's growth, need, and demand for dental hygiene services will pave the way for the continued expansion of the dental hygiene profession. *Healthy People 2000,* a government report detailing future health goals for the nation, revealed a staggering need for dental and dental hygiene services. The current administration, in its attempt to find solutions to cost and non-cost barriers to healthcare, is becoming increasingly cognizant of the under-utilization of healthcare workers. Better use of dental hygiene services has the potential to positively impact the barriers to access of these services. Consumers serve as an additional vehicle for increasing the utilization of dental hygiene services. They are more prevention-oriented and are demanding access to quality care. The reduction and/or elimination of barriers to dental hygiene services will increase the utilization of services which will expand the profession of dental hygiene.

SHERANITA HEMPHILL, RDH received an associate's degree in applied science in dental hygiene at Sinclair Community College and a B.S. in health education at the University of Dayton, both of which are located in Dayton, OH. She is currently completing her graduate degree. Nine months out of the year, she works as an assistant professor in the Dental Hygiene Department at Sinclair Community College, and in the summer months, she works as a substitute dental hygienist—and loves it!

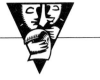

CHAPTER SEVENTEEN

The Pharmacist: Not Just Behind the Counter

Anna C. Kowblansky, R.Ph.,
Officer, American Pharmaceutical Association,
Academy of Pharmacy Practice and Management

The profession of pharmacy is exciting and rewarding and offers a broad variety of opportunities for students who want to serve the healthcare needs of a community. There are so many different areas of pharmacy practice to choose from that a **pharmacist** can always find a challenge in the profession. If one area of practice, such as community pharmacy, becomes routine and non-challenging, changing practice sites to a hospital pharmacy or in the pharmaceutical industry is not unreasonable. In fact, throughout a pharmacist's career, he or she can change the type and location of practice several times.

Pharmacy Education

To obtain a license to practice pharmacy in the United States, a student must fulfill the prepharmacy school requirements. This involves one or two years at a university or junior college. The courses for prepharmacy could include: biology, chemistry, algebra, psychology, sociology, physics, and some liberal arts classes. Each pharmacy school has its own prepharmacy requirements, so it is a good idea to check this out with a specific college of pharmacy.

Following prepharmacy, a student applies to a school of pharmacy. Presently, there are 75 schools or colleges of pharmacy in the United States. To obtain a list of the different schools, see your school counselor or librarian or contact the American Association of Colleges of Pharmacy. There are some basic differences between the schools of pharmacy. The length of education may vary from three to five years and the degrees awarded vary according to length of education. A bachelor's degree takes fewer years to obtain than a doctor of pharmacy degree.

Additional education and graduate degrees are also available after a student completes basic pharmacy education. A student can pursue a master's or doctorate degree in pharmacy administration or pharmaceutical sciences, or study business and obtain an M.B.A. A pharmacist can also obtain more clinical pharmacy education by entering a one-year postpharmacy residency program. This is often in a hospital setting, and the young practitioner develops a broad range of specialized skills in such areas as clinical services, drug information, quality control, drug distribution services, and product formulation.

In order to receive a license to practice pharmacy, a graduate of a pharmacy school must take a state board examination. Each state offers such an exam, and once you are licensed in one state, you can reciprocate to almost any other state to practice pharmacy. This means that most states will recognize and accept the state board examination that you passed in your own state.

Pharmacy Career Opportunities

Community Pharmacy

There are various locations where a community pharmacist can work. These include the independent community pharmacy (remembered as the corner drug store to some), the small chain pharmacy, or the large chain pharmacy. The practice of pharmacy in each of these locations is similar, because the pharmacist deals directly with the patient. However, each location has its own different opportunities and challenges.

Independent community pharmacists are often on the cutting edge of many major innovations within the profession. From computers and patient counseling to home healthcare and intravenous nutritional and pharmaceutical services, independent pharmacists are continually exploring new ways to serve their patients' needs and build thriving businesses in the communities. Independent pharmacists can set up their business in medical buildings, shopping centers, office buildings, and free-standing pharmacies. They serve patients in the community who come to their pharmacy to have a prescription filled or to simply obtain healthcare information. The independent pharmacist also serves patients in nursing homes, hospices, and in private homes.

In the Beginning

The history of pharmacy practice has its roots in community practice—the local neighborhood pharmacist. Although many pharmacists have gone on to practice in other settings, the neighborhood or community pharmacist is still recognized all across the country.

The independent pharmacist must have business knowledge. Owning a business means making numerous decisions about how to run the business and how to serve the patients. The pharmacist/owner must decide if the pharmacy will focus only on prescription and healthcare services or have a broader assortment of products. There are many opportunities to create a unique pharmacy practice—the only limitation is one's imagination.

Chain pharmacies are the fastest growing setting for pharmacy practice. It offers abundant opportunities in both professional and managerial positions. Computers are an integral part of chain pharmacy practice. An increasing number of chain pharmacies are linked together via computer. This is a real benefit for the patient because any pharmacist in the chain can link that patient's drug information to another pharmacy in the chain via computer.

Opportunities in a chain pharmacy include managerial positions. The career path usually begins at the store level. Working as a pharmacist, you can take on pharmacy management responsibilities followed by store management activities. Subsequent positions in a pharmacy chain would be at the district, regional, and corporate levels. Many chain companies have management development programs to assist a pharmacist who aspires to a managerial position.

Hospital Pharmacy

Pharmacy practice in a hospital setting can be quite diverse and challenging. Hospital pharmacists monitor a patient's drug therapy, prepare intravenous medications, oversee drug administration, and make purchasing decisions. One unique aspect of hospital pharmacy practice is that the pharmacist has access to each patient's complete medical record, which provides a clear understanding of the diagnosis and why a patient is taking a certain medication. With access to laboratory test results and diagnostic information, the hospital pharmacist often consults with the doctor about the patient's drug therapy.

Another way hospital pharmacy practice is unique is through the *team* approach to healthcare. Within a pharmacy department, pharmacists team up with technicians to provide efficient pharmacy services. Technicians often perform the drug distribution tasks, such as placing the medications into each patient's medication drawer and preparing intravenous admixtures. This frees up the pharmacist for broader clinical responsibilities. This teamwork continues outside the pharmacy department as the pharmacist works with nurses and doctors to provide quality patient care.

Hospital pharmacy practice is becoming increasingly more specialized. Pharmacists receive specialized training in such areas as pediatrics, geriatrics, nutritional support, oncology, nuclear medicine, and drug information. There are many areas for career advancement in hospital pharmacy. Pharmacists can advance to management positions within the pharmacy department or may choose to broaden their experience through transfers to other hospitals.

Consultant Pharmacy

The **consultant pharmacist** provides a specialized service to nursing homes or long-term care facilities. This pharmacist is a community pharmacist who has broadened his or her activities to include drug therapy monitoring and drug information services for those patients in long-term care facilities. Consultant pharmacists have a wide array of skills as clinicians, managers, educators, communicators, and overseers of drug therapy, depending on individual practice areas.

The information services consultant pharmacists offer include advice about ordering, storing, administering, and maintaining drug records. These pharmacists have an expertise in identifying drug therapy problems and resolving those problems using their clinical skills. The consultant pharmacist has an expertise in information services.

Academia

Some pharmacists choose to work in academic settings. These pharmacists are teachers, who have specialized in a certain area of pharmacy. However, teaching is only *one* part of the **academic pharmacist**. Most are involved in service and research activities as well. A typical day for a faculty member may include teaching a class, serving on a college or university committee, working with several graduate students on research projects, and working on a specific research project.

Academia is very attractive and satisfying to those who favor autonomy. *You* have control of your day-to-day activities. For the most part, you have the freedom to choose what and how you want to teach. Also, it is up to you to initiate and conduct research projects and to decide what types of service you will provide to the academic and professional committees. One of the requisites for a successful career in academia is a graduate or professional practice degree.

Pharmaceutical Industry

A career in the pharmaceutical industry generally requires communication skills, general business skills, or specific research skills. Numerous career areas are available for pharmacists within a pharmaceutical company. Pharmaceutical sales is generally regarded as the simplest way for pharmacists to enter the industry. This is often a very good place to begin to learn more about career paths first hand and to gain practical business experience. Many companies will subsidize higher education programs for sales representatives who are interested in pursuing graduate degrees that will help further their careers.

Other Areas

There are a variety of other interesting career opportunities in the pharmaceutical industry. Many companies have departments which maintain communication with professional groups, such as medical or pharmacy associations, or with government agencies such as state Medicare boards. Another career area is pharmaceutical corporation law. Some pharmacists go to law school after they complete their pharmacy education. Many with pharmacy backgrounds are employed by the industry, both in legal practice and in areas that require a legal background. Those pharmacists interested in research activities can find a career in pharmaceutical manufacturing. These positions often require higher education in pharmaceutical sciences.

Summary

The opportunities for pharmacists are numerous and limitless. Many pharmacists start out their career in one area of practice and then make a career change after several years. That's what makes pharmacy so much fun. You will never get bored with the profession. If the work you are doing begins to get routine and you want more of a challenge on your career, you can change your focus down another career path. If you want a first-hand perspective, visit your neighborhood community pharmacist and ask some questions.

ANNA C. KOWBLANSKY, R.Ph., M.S. received her bachelor of science degree in pharmacy from the University of Illinois at Chicago College of Pharmacy and a master's of science degree in management from DePaul University in Chicago, IL. She presently owns her own pharmaceutical consultant firm working with pharmacy associations and the pharmaceutical industry. She is an elected officer of the American Pharmaceutical Association, Academy of Pharmacy Practice and Management, Administrative Practice Section.

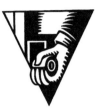

THE JOB
SEARCH
PROCESS

Getting Started:
Self-Evaluation and Career Objectives

etting a job may be a relatively simple one-step or couple of weeks process or a complex, months-long operation.

Starting, nurturing and developing a career (or even a series of careers) is a lifelong process.

What we'll be talking about in the five chapters that together form our Job Search Process are those basic steps to take, assumptions to make, things to think about if you want a job—especially a first job in some area of allied health. But when these steps—this process—are applied and expanded over a lifetime, most if not all of them are the same procedures, carried out over and over again, that are necessary to develop a successful, lifelong, professional career.

What does all this have to do with putting together a resume, writing a cover letter, heading off for interviews and the other "traditional" steps necessary to get a job? Whether your college graduation is just around the corner or a far distant memory, you will continuously need to focus, evaluate and re-evaluate your response to the ever-changing challenge of your future: Just what do you want to do with the rest of your life? Whether you like it or not, you're all looking for that "entry-level opportunity."

You're already one or two steps ahead of the competition—you're sure you want to pursue a career in allied health. By heeding the advice of the many professionals who have written chapters for this *Career Directory*—and utilizing the extensive entry-level job, organization, and career resource listings we've included—you're well on your way to fulfilling that dream. But there are some key decisions and time-consuming preparations to make if you want to transform that hopeful dream into a real, live job.

The actual process of finding the right company, right career path and, most importantly, the right first job, begins long before you start mailing out resumes to potential employers. The choices and decisions you make now are not irrevocable, but this first job will have a definite impact on the career options you leave yourself. To help you make some of the right decisions and choices along the way (and avoid some of the most notable traps and pitfalls), the following chapters will lead you through a series of organized steps. If the entire job search process we are recommending here is properly executed, it will undoubtedly help you land exactly the job you want.

If you're currently in high school and hope, after college, to land a job in the healthcare industry, then attending the right college, choosing the right major, and getting the summer work experience many companies look for are all important steps. Read the section of this *Career Directory* that covers the particular field and/or job specialty in which you're interested—many of the contributors have recommended colleges or graduate programs they favor.

If you're hoping to jump right into any of these fields without a college degree or other professional training, our best and only advice is—don't do it. As you'll soon see in the detailed information included in the **Job Opportunities Databank,** there are not that many job openings for students without a college degree or training. Those that do exist are generally clerical and will only rarely lead to promising careers.

The Concept of a Job Search Process

As we've explained, a job search is not a series of random events. Rather, it is a series of connected events that together form the job search process. It is important to know the eight steps that go into that process:

1. Evaluating yourself

Know thyself. What skills and abilities can you offer a prospective employer? What do you enjoy doing? What are your strengths and weaknesses? What do you want to do?

2. Establishing your career objectives

Where do you want to be next year, three years, five years from now? What do you ultimately want to accomplish in your career and your life?

3. Creating a company target list

How to prepare a "Hit List" of potential employers—researching them, matching their needs with your skills and starting your job search assault. Preparing company information sheets and evaluating your chances.

4. Networking for success

Learning how to utilize every contact, every friend, every relative, and anyone else you can think of to break down the barriers facing any would-be healthcare professional. How to organize your home office to keep track of your communications and stay on top of your job campaign.

5. Preparing your resume

How to encapsulate years of school and little actual work experience into a professional, selling resume. Learning when and how to use it.

6. Preparing cover letters

The many ordinary and the all-too-few extraordinary cover letters, the kind that land interviews and jobs.

7. Interviewing

How to make the interview process work for you—from the first "hello" to the first day on the job.

8. Following up

Often overlooked, it's perhaps the most important part of the job search process.

We won't try to kid you—it is a lot of work. To do it right, you have to get started early, probably quite a bit earlier than you'd planned. Frankly, we recommend beginning this process one full year prior to the day you plan to start work.

So if you're in college, the end of your junior year is the right time to begin your research and preparations. That should give you enough time during summer vacation to set up your files and begin your library research.

Whether you're in college or graduate school, one item may need to be planned even earlier—allowing enough free time in your schedule of classes for interview preparations and appointments. Waiting until your senior year to "make some time" is already too late. Searching for a full-time job is itself a full- time job! Though you're naturally restricted by your schedule, it's not difficult to plan ahead and prepare for your upcoming job search. Try to leave at least a couple of free mornings or afternoons a week. A day or even two without classes is even better.

Otherwise, you'll find yourself, crazed and distracted, trying to prepare for an interview in the ten-minute period between classes. Not the best way to make a first impression and certainly not the way you want to approach an important meeting.

The Self-Evaluation Process

Learning about who you are, what you want to be, what you can be, are critical first steps in the job search process and, unfortunately, the ones most often ignored by job seekers everywhere, especially students eager to leave the ivy behind and plunge into the "real world." But avoiding this crucial self-evaluation can hinder your progress and even damage some decent prospects.

Why? Because in order to land a job with a company at which you'll actually be happy, you need to be able to identify those firms and/or job descriptions that best match your own skills, likes, and strengths. The more you know about yourself, the more you'll bring to this process and the more accurate the "match-ups." You'll be able to structure your presentation (resume, cover letter, interviews, follow up) to stress your most marketable skills and talents (and, dare we say it, conveniently avoid your weaknesses?). Later, you'll be able to evaluate potential employers and job offers on the basis of your own needs and desires. This spells the difference between waking up in the morning ready to enthusiastically tackle a new day of challenges and shutting off the alarm in the hopes the day (and your job) will just disappear.

Creating Your Self-Evaluation Form

If your self-evaluation is to have any meaning, you must first be honest with yourself. This self-evaluation form should help you achieve that goal by providing a structured environment to answer these tough questions.

Take a sheet of lined notebook paper. Set up eight columns across the top—Strengths, Weaknesses, Skills, Hobbies, Courses, Experience, Likes, Dislikes.

Now, fill in each of these columns according to these guidelines:

Strengths: Describe personality traits you consider your strengths (and try to look at them as an employer would)—e.g., persistence, organization, ambition, intelligence, logic, assertiveness, aggression, leadership, etc.

Weaknesses: The traits you consider glaring weaknesses—e.g., impatience, conceit, etc. Remember: Look at these as a potential employer would. Don't assume that the personal traits you consider weaknesses will necessarily be considered negatives in the business world. You may be "easily bored," a trait that led to lousy grades early on because teachers couldn't keep you interested in the subjects they were teaching. Well, many entrepreneurs need ever-changing challenges. Strength or weakness?

Skills: Any skill you have, whether you think it's marketable or not. Everything from basic business skills—like typing and word processing—to computer or teaching experience and foreign language literacy. Don't forget possibly obscure but marketable skills like "good telephone voice."

Hobbies: The things you enjoy doing that, more than likely, have no overt connection to career objectives. These should be distinct from the skills listed above, and may include activities such as reading, games, travel, sports, and the like. While these may not be marketable in any general sense, they may well be useful in specific circumstances.

Courses: All the general subject areas (history, literature, etc.) and/or specific courses you've taken which may be marketable, you really enjoyed, or both.

Experience: Just the specific functions you performed at any part-time (school year) or full-time (summer) jobs. Entries may include "General Office" (typing, filing, answering phones, etc.), "Doctor's Office Assistant," "Retail Clerk" etc.

Likes: List all your "likes," those important considerations that you haven't listed anywhere else yet. These might include the types of people you like to be with, the kind of environment you prefer (city, country, large places, small places, quiet, loud, fast-paced, slow-paced) and anything else which hasn't shown up somewhere on this form. Try to think of "likes" that you have that are related to the job you are applying for. For example, if you're applying for a job at a major corporation, mention that you enjoy reading the Wall St. Journal. However, try not to include entries which refer to specific jobs or companies. We'll list those on another form.

Dislikes: All the people, places and things you can easily live without.

Now assess the "marketability" of each item you've listed. (In other words, are some of your likes, skills or courses easier to match to a allied health job description, or do they have little to do with a specific job or company?) Mark highly marketable skills with an "H." Use "M" to characterize those skills which may be marketable in a particular set of circumstances, "L" for those with minimal potential application to any job.

Referring back to the same list, decide if you'd enjoy using your marketable skills or talents as part of your everyday job—"Y" for yes, "N" for no. You may type 80 words a minute but truly despise typing or worry that stressing it too much will land you on the permanent clerical staff. If so, mark typing with an "N." (Keep one thing in mind— just because you dislike typing shouldn't mean you absolutely won't accept a job that requires it. Almost every professional job today requires computer-based work that make typing a plus.)

Now, go over the entire form carefully and look for inconsistencies.

To help you with your own form, there's a sample one on the following page that a job-hunter might have completed.

The Value of a Second Opinion

There is a familiar misconception about the self-evaluation process that gets in the way of many new job applicants—the belief that it is a process which must be accomplished in isolation. Nothing could be further from the truth. Just because the family doctor tells you you need an operation doesn't mean you run right off to the hospital. Prudence dictates that you check out the opinion with another physician. Getting such a "second opinion"—someone else's, not just your own—is a valuable practice throughout the job search process, as well.

So after you've completed the various exercises in this chapter, review them with a friend, relative, or parent—just be sure it's someone who knows you well and cares about you. These second opinions may reveal some aspects of your self-description on which you and the rest of the world differ. If so, discuss them, learn from them and, if necessary, change some conclusions. Should everyone concur with your self-evaluation, you will be reassured that your choices are on target.

Establishing Your Career Objective(s)

For better or worse, you now know something more of who and what you are. But we've yet to establish and evaluate another important area—your overall needs, desires and goals. Where are you going? What do you want to accomplish?

If you're getting ready to graduate from college or graduate school, the next five years are the most critical period of your whole career. You need to make the initial transition from college to the workplace, establish yourself in a new and completely

Strength	Weakness	Skill	Hobby	Course	Experience	Like	Dislike
Marketable?							
Enjoy?							
Marketable?							
Enjoy?							
Marketable?							
Enjoy?							

unfamiliar company environment, and begin to build the professional credentials necessary to achieve your career goals.

If that strikes you as a pretty tall order, well, it is. Unless you've narrowly prepared yourself for a specific profession, you're probably most ill-prepared for any real job. Instead, you've (hopefully) learned some basic principles—research and analytical skills that are necessary for success at almost any level—and, more or less, how to think.

It's tough to face, but face it you must: No matter what your college, major, or degree, all you represent right now is potential. How you package that potential and what you eventually make of it is completely up to you. It's an unfortunate fact that many companies will take a professional with barely a year or two experience over any newcomer, no matter how promising. Smaller firms, especially, can rarely afford to hire someone who can't begin contributing immediately.

So you have to be prepared to take your comparatively modest skills and experience and package them in a way that will get you interviewed and hired. Quite a challenge.

There are a number of different ways to approach such a task. If you find yourself confused or unable to list such goals, you might want to check a few books in your local library that have more time to spend on the topic of "goal-oriented planning."

But Is the Healthcare Industry Right for You?

Presuming you now have a much better idea of yourself and where you'd like to be, let's make sure some of your basic assumptions are right. We presume you purchased this *Career Directory* because you're considering a career in some area of allied health. Are you sure? Do you know enough about the industry as a whole and the particular part you're heading for to decide whether it's right for you? Probably not. So start your research now—learn as much about your potential career field as you now know about yourself.

Start with the essays in the Advice for the Pro's section—these will give you an excellent overview of the allied health and therapy industry, some very specialized (and growing) areas, and some things to keep in mind as you start on your career search. They will also give you a relatively simplified, though very necessary, understanding of just what people who work in all these areas of healthcare actually do.

Other sources you should consider consulting to learn more about this business are listed in the Career Resources section of this book.

In that section, we've listed trade associations and publications associated with allied health and therapy professions (together with many other resources that will help your job search. (Consult the front of this directory for a complete description of the Career Resource section.) Where possible in the association entries, we've included details on educational information they make available, but you should certainly consider writing each of the pertinent associations, letting them know you're interested in a career in their area of specialization and would appreciate whatever help and advice they're willing to impart. You'll find many sponsor seminars and conferences throughout the country, some of which you may be able to attend.

The trade publications are dedicated to the highly specific interests of allied health professionals. These magazines are generally not available at newsstands, but you may be able to obtain back issues at your local library (most major libraries have extensive collections of such journals) or by writing to the magazines' circulation/subscription departments. We've also included regional and local magazines.

You may also try writing to the publishers and/or editors of these publications. State in your cover letter what area of healthcare you're considering and ask them for whatever help and advice they can offer. But be specific. These are busy professionals and they do not have the time or the inclination to simply "tell me everything you can about working at a clinic."

If you can afford it now, we strongly suggest subscribing to whichever trade magazines are applicable to the specialty you're considering. If you can't subscribe to all of them, make it a point to regularly read the copies that arrive at your local public or college library.

These publications may well provide the most imaginative and far-reaching information for your job search. Even a quick perusal of an issue or two will give you an excellent feel for the industry. After reading only a few articles, you'll already get a handle on what's happening in the field and some of the industry's peculiar and particular jargon. Later, more detailed study will aid you in your search for a specific job.

Authors of the articles themselves may well turn out to be important resources. If an article is directly related to your chosen specialty, why not call the author and ask some questions? You'd be amazed how willing many of these professionals will be to talk to you and answer your questions, and the worst they can do is say no. (But *do* use common sense—authors will not *always* respond graciously to your invitation to "chat about the business." And don't be *too* aggressive here.)

You'll find such research to be a double-edged sword. In addition to helping you get a handle on whether the area you've chosen is really right for you, you'll slowly learn enough about particular specialties, companies, the industry, etc., to actually sound like you know what you're talking about when you hit the pavement looking for your first job. And nothing is better than sounding like a pro—except being one.

Allied Health Is It. Now What?

After all this research, we're going to assume you've reached that final decision—you really do want a career in some aspect of allied health. It is with this vague certainty that all too many of you will race off, hunting for any firm willing to give you a job. You'll manage to get interviews at a couple and, smiling brightly, tell everyone you meet, "I want a career in healthcare." The interviewers, unfortunately, will all ask the same awkward question—"What *exactly* do you want to do at our company?"—and that will be the end of that.

It is simply not enough to narrow your job search to a specific industry. And so far, that's all you've done. You must now establish a specific career objective—the job you want to start, the career you want to pursue. Just knowing that you "want to get into allied health" doesn't mean anything to anybody. If that's all you can tell an interviewer, it demonstrates a lack of research into the industry itself and your failure to think ahead.

Interviewers will *not* welcome you with open arms if you're still vague about your career goals. If you've managed to get an "informational interview" with an executive whose company currently has no job openings, what is he or she supposed to do with your resume after you leave? Who should he or she send it to for future consideration? Since *you* don't seem to know exactly what you want to do, how's he or she going to figure it out? Worse, that person will probably resent your asking him or her to function as your personal career counselor.

Remember, the more specific your career objective, the better your chances of finding a job. It's that simple and that important. Naturally, before you declare your objective to the world, check once again to make sure your specific job target matches the skills and interests you defined in your self-evaluation. Eventually, you may want to state such an objective on your resume, and "To obtain an entry-level position as an occupational therapist at a mid-sized therapy clinic," is quite a bit better than "I want a career in healthcare." Do not consider this step final until you can summarize your job/career objective in a single, short, accurate sentence.

Targeting Prospective Employers and Networking For Success

As you move along the job search path, one fact will quickly become crystal clear—it is primarily a process of **elimination**: your task is to consider and research as many options as possible, then—for good reasons—**eliminate** as many as possible, attempting to continually narrow your focus.

Your Ideal Company Profile

Let's establish some criteria to evaluate potential employers. This will enable you to identify your target companies, the places you'd really like to work. (This process, as we've pointed out, is not specific to any industry or field; the same steps, with perhaps some research resource variations, are applicable to any job, any company, any industry.)

Take a sheet of blank paper and divide it into three vertical columns. Title it "Target Company—Ideal Profile." Call the lefthand column "Musts," the middle column "Preferences," and the righthand column "Nevers."

We've listed a series of questions below. After considering each question, decide whether a particular criteria *must* be met, whether you would simply *prefer* it or *never* would consider it at all. If there are other criteria you consider important, feel free to add them to the list below and mark them accordingly on your Profile.

1. What are your geographical preferences? (Possible answers: U.S., Canada, International, Anywhere). If you only want to work in the U.S., then "Work in United States" would be the entry in the "Must" column. "Work in Canada or Foreign Country" might be the first entry in your "Never" column. There would be no applicable entry for this question in the "Preference" column. If, however, you will consider working in two of the three, then your "Must" column entry

might read "Work in U.S. or Canada," your "Preference" entry—if you preferred one over the other—could read "Work in U.S.," and the "Never" column, "Work Overseas."

2. If you prefer to work in the U.S. or Canada, what area, state(s) or province(s)? If overseas, what area or countries?

3. Do you prefer a large city, small city, town, or somewhere as far away from civilization as possible?

4. In regard to question three, any specific preferences?

5. Do you prefer a warm or cold climate?

6. Do you prefer a large or small company? Define your terms (by sales, income, employees, offices, etc.).

7. Do you mind relocating right now? Do you want to work for a firm with a reputation for *frequently* relocating top people?

8. Do you mind travelling frequently? What percent do you consider reasonable? (Make sure this matches the normal requirements of the job specialization you're considering.)

9. What salary would you *like* to receive (put in the "Preference" column)? What's the *lowest* salary you'll accept (in the "Must" column)?

10. Are there any benefits (such as an expense account, medical and/or dental insurance, company car, etc.) you must or would like to have?

11. Are you planning to attend graduate school at some point in the future and, if so, is a tuition reimbursement plan important to you?

12. Do you feel that a formal training program is necessary?

13. If applicable, what kinds of specific accounts would you prefer to work with? What specific products?

It's important to keep revising this new form, just as you should continue to update your Self-Evaluation Form. After all, it contains the criteria by which you will judge every potential employer. Armed with a complete list of such criteria, you're now ready to find all the companies that match them.

Targeting Individual Companies

To begin creating your initial list of targeted companies, start with the **Job Opportunities Databank** in this directory. We've listed many major therapy facilities and hospitals, most of which were contacted by telephone for this edition. These listings provide a plethora of data concerning the companies' overall operations, hiring practices, and other important information on entry-level job opportunities. This latter information includes key contacts (names), the average number of entry-level people they hire each year, along with complete job descriptions and requirements.

One word of advice. You'll notice that some of the companies list "0" under average entry-level hiring. This is more a reflection of the current economic times than a long-range projection. These companies have hired in the past, and they will again in the future. We have listed these companies for three reasons: 1) to present you with the overall view of prospective employers; 2) because even companies that don't plan to do any hiring will experience unexpected job openings; and 3) things change, so as soon as the economy begins to pick up, expect entry-level hiring to increase again.

We have attempted to include information on those major firms that represent many of the entry-level jobs out there. But there are, of course, many other companies of all sizes and shapes that you may also wish to research. In the Career Resources section, we have listed other reference tools you can use to obtain more information on the companies we've listed, as well as those we haven't.

▼

Ask the Person Who Owns One

Some years ago, this advice was used as the theme for a highly successful automobile advertising campaign. The prospective car buyer was encouraged to find out about the product by asking the (supposedly) most trustworthy judge of all—someone who was already an owner.

The Other Side of the Iceberg

You are now better prepared to choose those companies that meet your own list of criteria. But a word of caution about these now-"obvious" requirements—they are not the only ones you need to take into consideration. And you probably won't be able to find all or many of the answers to this second set of questions in any reference book—they are known, however, by those persons already at work in the industry. Here is the list you will want to follow:

Promotion

If you are aggressive about your career plans, you'll want to know if you have a shot at the top. Look for companies that traditionally promote from within.

Training

Look for companies in which your early tenure will actually be a period of on-the-job training, hopefully ones in which training remains part of the long-term process. As new techniques and technologies enter the workplace, you must make sure you are updated on these skills. Most importantly, look for training that is craft- or function-oriented—these are the so-called **transferable skills**, ones you can easily bring along with you from job-to-job, company-to-company, sometimes industry-to-industry.

Salary

Some industries are generally high paying, some not. But even an industry with a tradition of paying abnormally low salaries may have particular companies or job functions (like sales) within companies that command high remuneration. But it's important you know what the industry standard is.

Benefits

Look for companies in which health insurance, vacation pay, retirement plans, 401K accounts, stock purchase opportunities, and other important employee benefits are extensive—and company paid. If you have to pay for basic benefits like medical coverage yourself, you'll be surprised at how expensive they are. An exceptional benefit package may even lead you to accept a lower- than-usual salary.

Unions

Make sure you know about the union situation in each industry you research. Periodic, union-mandated salary increases are one benefit nonunion workers may find hard to match.

Making Friends and Influencing People

Networking is a term you have probably heard; it is definitely a key aspect of any successful job search and a process you must master.

Informational interviews and **job interviews** are the two primary outgrowths of successful networking.

Referrals, an aspect of the networking process, entail using someone else's name, credentials and recommendation to set up a receptive environment when seeking a job interview.

All of these terms have one thing in common: Each depends on the actions of other people to put them in motion. Don't let this idea of "dependency" slow you down, however. A job search *must* be a very pro-active process—*you* have to initiate the action. When networking, this means contacting as many people as you can. The more you contact, the better the chances of getting one of those people you are "depending" on to take action and help you out.

So what *is* networking? How do you build your own network? And why do you need one in the first place? The balance of this chapter answers all of those questions and more.

Get your telephone ready. It's time to make some friends.

Not the World's Oldest Profession, But...

Networking is the process of creating your own group of relatives, friends, and acquaintances who can feed you the information you need to find a job—identifying where the jobs are and giving you the personal introductions and background data necessary to pursue them.

If the job market were so well-organized that details on all employment opportunities were immediately available to all applicants, there would be no need for such a process. Rest assured the job market is *not* such a smooth-running machine—most applicants are left very much to their own devices. Build and use your own network wisely and you'll be amazed at the amount of useful job intelligence you will turn up.

While the term networking didn't gain prominence until the 1970s, it is by no means a new phenomenon. A selection process that connects people of similar skills, backgrounds, and/or attitudes—in other words, networking—has been in existence in a variety of forms for centuries. Attend any Ivy League school and you're automatically part of its very special centuries-old network.

And it works. Remember your own reaction when you were asked to recommend someone for a job, club or school office? You certainly didn't want to look foolish, so you gave it some thought and tried to recommend the best-qualified person that you thought would "fit in" with the rest of the group. It's a built-in screening process.

Creating the Ideal Network

As in most endeavors, there's a wrong way and a right way to network. The following tips will help you construct your own wide-ranging, information-gathering, interview-generating group—*your* network.

Diversify

Unlike the Harvard or Princeton network—confined to former graduates of each school—your network should be as diversified and wide-ranging as possible. You never know who might be in a position to help, so don't limit your group of friends. The more diverse they are, the greater the variety of information they may supply you with.

Don't Forget...

...to include everyone you know in your initial networking list: friends, relatives, social acquaintances, classmates, college alumni, professors, teachers, your dentist, doctor, family lawyer, insurance agent, banker, travel agent, elected officials in your community, ministers, fellow church members, local tradesmen, and local business or social club officers. And everybody they know!

Be Specific

Make a list of the kinds of assistance you will require from those in your network, then make specific requests of each. Do they know of jobs at their company? Can they introduce you to the proper executives? Have they heard something about or know someone at the company you're planning to interview with next week?

The more organized you are, the easier it will be to target the information you need and figure out who might have it. Begin to keep a business card file or case so you can keep track of all your contacts. A small plastic case for file cards that is available at any discount store will do nicely. One system you can use is to staple the card to a 3 x 5 index card. On the card, write down any information about that contact that you might need later—when you talked to them, job leads they provided, specific job search advice, etc. You will then have all the information you need about each company or contact in one easily accessible location.

Learn the Difference...

...between an **informational** interview and a **job** interview. The former requires you to cast yourself in the role of information gatherer; *you* are the interviewer and knowledge is your goal—about an industry, company, job function, key executive, etc. Such a meeting with someone already doing what you soon hope to be doing is by far the best way to find out everything you need to know—before you walk through the door and sit down for a formal job interview, at which time your purpose is more sharply defined: to get the job you're interviewing for.

If you learn of a specific job opening during an informational interview, you are in a position to find out details about the job, identify the interviewer and, possibly, even learn some things about him or her. In addition, presuming you get your contact's permission, you may be able to use his or her name as a referral. Calling up the interviewer and saying, "Joan Smith in your human resources department suggested I contact you regarding openings for assistant editors," is far superior to "Hello. Do you have any job openings at your magazine?"

(In such a case, be careful about referring to a specific job opening, even if your contact told you about it. It may not be something you're supposed to know about. By presenting your query as an open-ended question, you give your prospective employer the option of exploring your background without further commitment. If there is a job there and you're qualified for it, you'll find out soon enough.)

Don't Waste a Contact

Not everyone you call on your highly-diversified networking list will know about a job opening. It would be surprising if each one did. But what about *their* friends and colleagues? It's amazing how everyone knows someone who knows someone. Ask—you'll find that someone.

Value Your Contacts

If someone has provided you with helpful information or an introduction to a friend or colleague, keep him or her informed about how it all turns out. A referral that's panned out should be reported to the person who opened the door for you in the first place. Such courtesy will be appreciated—and may lead to more contacts. If someone has nothing to offer today, a call back in the future is still appropriate and may pay off.

The lesson is clear: Keep your options open, your contact list alive. Detailed records of your network—whom you spoke with, when, what transpired, etc.—will help you keep track of your overall progress and organize what can be a complicated and involved process.

Informational Interviews

So now you've done your homework, built your network, and begun using your contacts. It's time to go on your first informational interview.

A Typical Interview

You were, of course, smart enough to include John Fredericks, the bank officer who handled your dad's mortgage, on your original contact list. He knew you as a bright and conscientious college senior; in fact, your perfect three-year repayment record on the loan you took out to buy that '67 Plymouth impressed him. When you called him, he was happy to refer you to his friend, Carol Jones, a human resources manager at a large local therapy clinic. Armed with permission to use Fredericks' name and recommendation, you wrote a letter to Carol Jones, the gist of which went something like this:

> *I am writing at the suggestion of Mr. John Fredericks at Fidelity National Bank. He knows of my interest in a therapy career and, given your position at RehabWorks, Inc., thought you might be able to help me gain a better understanding of this specialized field and the career opportunities it presents.*
>
> *While I am majoring in occupational therapy, I know I need to speak with professionals such as yourself to learn how to apply my studies to a work environment. If you could spare a half hour to meet with me, I'm certain I would be able to get enough information about this specialty to give me the direction I need.*
>
> *I'll call your office next week in the hope that we can schedule a meeting.*

Send a copy of this letter to Mr. Fredericks at the bank—it will refresh his memory should Ms. Jones call to inquire about you. Next step: the follow-up phone call. After you get Ms. Jones' secretary on the line, it will, with luck, go something like this:

> *"Hello, I'm Paul Smith. I'm calling in reference to a letter I wrote to Ms. Jones requesting an appointment."*
>
> *"Oh, yes. You're the young man interested in occupational therapy. Ms. Jones can see you on June 23rd. Will 10 A.M. be satisfactory?"*
>
> *"That's fine. I'll be there."*

Well, the appointed day arrives. Well-scrubbed and dressed in your best (and most conservative) suit, you are ushered into Ms. Jones' office. She offers you coffee (you decline) and says that it is okay to light up if you wish to smoke (you decline). The conversation might go something like this:

> *Ms. Jones relaxes. She realizes this is a knowledge hunt you are on, not a thinly-veiled job interview. Your approach has kept her off the spot—she doesn't have to be concerned with making a hiring decision. You've already gotten high marks for not putting her on the defensive.*

You: "Thank you for seeing me, Ms. Jones. I know you are busy and appreciate your taking the time to talk with me."

Jones: "Well it's my pleasure since you come so highly recommended. I'm always pleased to meet someone interested in my field."

You: "As I stated in my letter, my interest in occupational therapy is very real, but I'm having trouble seeing how all of my studies will adapt to the work environment. I think I'll be much better prepared to evaluate future job offers if I can learn more about your experiences. May I ask you a few questions about RehabWorks?"

Jones: "Fire away, Paul".

You: "I have a few specific questions I'd like to ask. First, at a company such as yours, where does an entry-level person start?"

Jones: "In this company, you would be assigned to an experienced therapist to work as that person's assistant for the first month of your employment. This gives you a chance to see the way we work and to become comfortable with our facilities. After that, if you had progressed well, you would begin seeing patients on your own."

You: "Where and how fast does someone progress after that?"

Jones: "Obviously, that depends on the person, but given the proper aptitude and ability, that person would simply get more responsibilities to handle. How well you do all along the way will determine how far and how fast you progress."

You: "What is the work environment like—is it pretty hectic?"

Jones: "We try to keep the work load at an even keel. The comfort of our workers is of prime importance to us. Excessive turnover is costly, you know. But this is an exciting business, and things change sometimes minute-to-minute. It's not a profession for the faint-hearted!"

You: "If I may shift to another area, I'd be interested in your opinion about therapy careers in general and what you see as the most likely areas of opportunity in the foreseeable future. Do you think this is a growth career area, despite the many changes that have occurred in the last 18 months?"

Jones: "Well, judging by the hiring record of our company, I think you'll find it's an area worth making a commitment to. At the entry level, we've hired a number of new people in the past three or four years. There always seems to be opportunities, though it's gotten far more competitive."

You: "Do you think someone with my qualifications and background could get started in occupational therapy? Perhaps a look at my resume. would be helpful to you." *(Give it to Ms. Jones.)*

Jones: "Your course work looks appropriate. I especially like the internships you've held every summer. I think you have a real chance to break into this field. I don't think we're hiring right now, but I know a couple of firms that are looking for bright young people with qualifications like yours. Let me give you a couple of phone numbers." *(Write down names and phone numbers.)*

You: "You have been very generous with your time, but I can see from those flashing buttons on your phone that you have other things to do. Thank you again for taking the time to talk with me."

Jones: "You're welcome."

After the Interview

The next step should be obvious: **Two** thank-you letters are required, one to Ms. Jones, the second to Mr. Fredericks. Get them both out immediately. (And see the chapter on writing letters if you need help writing them.)

Keeping Track of the Interview Trail

Let's talk about record keeping again. If your networking works the way it's supposed to, this was only the first of many such interviews. Experts have estimated that the average person could develop a contact list of 250 people. Even if we limit your initial list to only 100, if each of them gave you one referral, your list would suddenly have 200 names. Presuming that it will not be necessary or helpful to see all of them, it's certainly possible that such a list could lead to 100 informational and/or job interviews! Unless you keep accurate records, by the time you're on No. 50, you won't even remember the first dozen!

So get the results of each interview down on paper. Use whatever format with which you're comfortable. You should create some kind of file, folder, or note card that is an "Interview Recap Record." If you have access to a personal computer, take advantage of it. It will be much easier to keep you information stored in one place and well-organized. Your record should be set up and contain something like the following:

Name: RehabWorks, Inc.
Address: 333 E. 54th St., Rochester, NY 10000
Phone: (212) 555-4000
Contact: Carol Jones
Type of Business: Occupational therapy
Referral Contact: Mr. Fredericks, Fidelity National Bank
Date: July 30, 1993

At this point, you should add a one-or two-paragraph summary of what you found out at the meeting. Since these comments are for your eyes only, you should be both objective and subjective. State the facts—what you found out in response to your specific questions—but include your impressions—your estimate of the opportunities for further discussions, your chances for future consideration for employment.

"I Was Just Calling To..."

Find any logical opportunity to stay in touch with Ms. Jones. You may, for example, let her know when you graduate and tell her your grade point average, carbon her in on any letters you write to Mr. Fredericks, even send a congratulatory note if her company's year-end financial results are positive or if you read something in the local paper about her department. This type of follow up has the all-important effect of keeping you and your name in the forefront of others' minds. Out of sight *is* out of mind. No matter how talented you may be or how good an impression you made, you'll have to work hard to "stay visible."

There Are Rules, Just Like Any Game

It should already be obvious that the networking process is not only effective, but also quite deliberate in its objectives. There are two specific groups of people you must attempt to target: those who can give you information about an industry or career area and those who are potential employers. The line between these groups may often blur. Don't be concerned—you'll soon learn when (and how) to shift the focus from interviewer to interviewee.

To simplify this process, follow a single rule: Show interest in the field or job area under discussion, but wait to be asked about actually working for that company. During your informational interviews, you will be surprised at the number of times the person you're interviewing turns to you and asks, "Would you be interested in...?" Consider carefully what's being asked and, if you *would* be interested in the position under discussion, make your feelings known.

If the Process Scares You

Some of you will undoubtedly be hesitant about, even fear, the networking process. It is not an unusual response—it is very human to want to accomplish things "on your own," without anyone's help. Understandable and commendable as such independence might seem, it is, in reality, an impediment if it limits your involvement in this important process. Networking has such universal application because **there is no other effective way to bridge the gap between job applicant and job.** Employers are grateful for its existence. You should be, too.

Whether you are a first-time applicant or reentering the work force now that the children are grown, the networking process will more than likely be your point of entry. Sending out mass mailings of your resume and answering the help-wanted ads may well be less personal (and, therefore, "easier") approaches, but they will also be far less effective. The natural selection process of the networking phenomenon is your assurance that water does indeed seek its own level—you will be matched up with companies and job opportunities in which there is a mutual fit.

Six Good Reasons to Network

Many people fear the networking process because they think they are "bothering" others with their own selfish demands. Nonsense! There are good reasons—six of them, at least—why the people on your networking list will be happy to help you:

Why Should You Network?

- To unearth current information about the industry, company and pertinent job functions. Remember: Your knowledge and understanding of broad industry trends, financial health, hiring opportunities, and the competitive picture are key.
- To investigate each company's hiring policies—who makes the decisions, who the key players are (personnel, staff managers), whether there's a hiring season, whether they prefer applicants going direct or through recruiters, etc.
- To sell yourself—discuss your interests and research activities—and leave your calling card, your resume.
- To seek out advice on refining your job search process.
- To obtain the names of other persons (referrals) who can give you additional information on where the jobs are and what the market conditions are like.
- To develop a list of follow-up activities that will keep you visible to key contacts.

1. **Some day you will get to return the favor.** An ace insurance salesman built a successful business by offering low-cost coverage to first-year medical students. Ten years later, these now-successful practitioners remembered the company (and person) that helped them when they were just getting started. He gets new referrals every day.

2. **They, too, are seeking information.** An employer who has been out of school for several years might be interested in what the latest developments in the classroom are. He or she may be hoping to learn as much from you as you are from them, so be forthcoming in offering information. This desire for new information may be the reason he or she agreed to see you in the first place.

3. **Internal politics.** Some people will see you simply to make themselves appear powerful, implying to others in their organization that they have the authority to hire (they may or may not), an envied prerogative.

4. **They're "saving for a rainy day".** Executives know that it never hurts to look and that maintaining a backlog of qualified candidates is a big asset when the floodgates open and supervisors are forced to hire quickly.

5. **They're just plain nice.** Some people will see you simply because they feel it's the decent thing to do or because they just can't say "no."

6. **They are looking themselves.** Some people will see you because they are anxious to do a friend (whoever referred you) a favor. Or because they have another friend seeking new talent, in which case you represent a referral they can make (part of their own continuing network process). You see, networking never does stop—it helps them and it helps you.

Before you proceed to the next chapter, begin making your contact list. You may wish to keep a separate sheet of paper or note card on each person (especially the dozen or so you think are most important), even a separate telephone list to make your communications easier and more efficient. However you set up your list, be sure to keep it up to date—it won't be long before you'll be calling each and every name on the list.

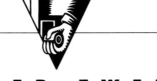

Preparing Your Resume

Your resume is a one-page summary of you—your education, skills, employment experience and career objective(s). It is not a biography, but a "quick and dirty" way to identify and describe you to potential employers. Most importantly, its real purpose is to sell you to the company you want to work for. It must set you apart from all the other applicants (those competitors) out there.

So, as you sit down to formulate your resume, remember you're trying to present the pertinent information in a format and manner that will convince an executive to grant you an interview, the prelude to any job offer. All resumes must follow two basic rules—excellent visual presentation and honesty—but it's important to realize that different career markets require different resumes. The resume you are compiling for your career in allied health is different than one you would prepare for a finance career. As more and more resume "training" services become available, employers are becoming increasingly choosy about the resumes they receive. They expect to view a professional presentation, one that sets a candidate apart from the crowd. Your resume has to be perfect and it has to be specialized—clearly demonstrating the relationship between your qualifications and the job you are applying for.

An Overview of Resume Preparation

- **Know what you're doing**—your resume is a personal billboard of accomplishments. It must communicate your worth to a prospective employer in specific terms.
- **Your language should be action-oriented,** full of "doing"-type words. And less is better than more—be concise and direct. Don't worry about using complete sentences.

- **Be persuasive.** In those sections that allow you the freedom to do so, don't hesitate to communicate your worth in the strongest language. This does not mean a numbing list of self-congratulatory superlatives; it does mean truthful claims about your abilities and the evidence (educational, experiential) that supports them.

- **Don't be cheap or gaudy.** Don't hesitate to spend the few extra dollars necessary to present a professional-looking resume. Do avoid outlandish (and generally ineffective) gimmicks like oversized or brightly-colored paper.

- **Find an editor.** Every good writer needs one, and you are writing your resume. At the very least, it will offer you a second set of eyes proofreading for embarrassing typos. But if you are fortunate enough to have a professional in the field—a recruiter or personnel executive—critique a draft, grab the opportunity and be immensely grateful.

- **If you're the next Michelangelo,** so multitalented that you can easily qualify for jobs in different career areas, don't hesitate to prepare two or more completely different resumes. This will enable you to change the emphasis on your education and skills according to the specific career objective on each resume, a necessary alteration that will correctly target each one.

- **Choose the proper format.** There are only three we recommend—chronological, functional, and targeted format—and it's important you use the one that's right for you.

Considerations in the Electronic Age

Like most other areas of everyday life, computers have left their mark in the resume business. There are the obvious changes—the increased number of personal computers has made it easier to produce a professional-looking resume at home—and the not so obvious changes, such as the development of resume databases.

There are two kinds of resume databases: 1) An internal file maintained by a large corporation to keep track of the flood of resumes it gets each day (*U.S. News and World Report* stated that Fortune 50 companies receive more than 1,000 unsolicited resumes a day and that four out of every five are thrown away after a quick review). 2) Commercial databases that solicit resumes from job-seekers around the United States and make them available to corporations, who pay a fee to search the database.

Internal Databases Mean Some of the Old Rules Don't Apply

The internal databases maintained by large companies are changing some of the time-honored traditions of resume preparation. In the past, it was acceptable, even desirable, to use italic type and other eye-catching formats to make a resume more visually appealing. Not so today. Most of the companies that have a database enter resumes into it by using an optical scanner that reads the resume character by character and automatically enters it into the database. While these scanners are becoming more and more sophisticated, there are still significant limits as to what they can recognize and interpret.

What does this mean to you? It means that in addition to the normal screening process that all resumes go through, there is now one more screening step that determines if the scanner will be able to read your resume. If it can't, chances are your resume is going to be one of the four that is thrown away, instead of the one that is kept. To enhance the chances of your resume making it past this scanner test, here are some simple guidelines you can follow:

- Use larger typefaces (nothing smaller than 12 point), and avoid all but the most basic typefaces. Among the most common are Times Roman and Helvetica.

- No italics or underlining, and definitely no graphic images or boxes.

- Do not send copies. Either print a fresh copy out on your own printer, or take the resume to a print shop and have it professionally copied onto high-quality paper. Avoid dot matrix printers.

- Use 8 1/2 x 11 paper, unfolded. Any words that end up in a crease will not be scannable.

- Use only white or beige paper. Any other color will lessen the contrast between the paper and the letters and make it harder for the scanner to read.

- Use only a single column format. Scanners read from right to left on a page, so two- or three-columns formats lead to nonsensical information when the document is scanned.

- While it is still appropriate to use action words to detail your accomplishments (initiated, planned, implemented, etc.), it is also important to include precise technical terms whenever possible as well. That's because databases are searched by key words, and only resumes that match those key words will be looked at. For example, if a publishing company was seeking someone who was experienced in a desktop publishing, they might search the database for all occurrences of "PageMaker" or "Ventura," two common desktop publishing software packages. If your resume only said "Successfully implemented and oversaw in-house desktop publishing program," it would be overlooked, and you wouldn't get the job!

National Databases: Spreading Your Good Name Around

Commercial resume databases are also having an impact on the job search process in the 1990s, so much so that anyone about to enter the job market should seriously consider utilizing one of these services.

Most of these new services work this way: Job-seekers send the database company a copy of their resume, or they fill out a lengthy application provided by the company. The information is then loaded into the company's computer, along with hundreds of other resumes from other job-seekers. The cost of this listing is usually nominal—$20 to $50 for a six- to 12-month listing. Some colleges operate systems for their graduates that are free of charge, so check with your placement office before utilizing a commercial service.

Once in the system, the resumes are available for viewing by corporate clients who have openings to fill. This is where the database companies really make their money—depending on the skill-level of the listees and the professions covered, companies can pay thousands of dollars for annual subscriptions to the service or for custom searches of the database.

Worried that your current employer might just pull up *your* resume when it goes searching for new employees? No need to be—most services allow listees to designate companies that their resume should not be released to, thus allowing you to conduct a job search with the peace of mind that your boss won't find out!

One warning about these services—most of them are new, so do as much research as you can before paying to have your resume listed. If you hear about a database you think you might want to be listed in, call the company and ask some questions:

- How long have they been in business?
- What has their placement rate been?
- What fields do they specialize in? (In other words, will the right people even *see* your resume?)
- Can you block certain companies from seeing your resume?
- How many other resumes are listed in the database? How many in your specialty?
- Is your experience level similar to that of other listees in the database?

The right answers to these questions should let you know if you have found the right database for you.

To help you locate these resume databases, we have listed many of them in the **Career Resources** chapter of this book.

The Records You Need

Well, now that you've heard all the dos and don'ts and rules about preparing a resume, it's time to put those rules to work. The resume-writing process begins with the assembly and organization of all the personal, educational, and employment data from which you will choose the pieces that actually end up on paper. If this information is properly organized, writing your resume will be a relatively easy task, essentially a simple process of just shifting data from a set of the worksheets to another, to your actual resume. At the end of this chapter, you'll find all the forms you need to prepare your resume, including worksheets, fill-in-the-blanks resume forms, and sample resumes.

As you will soon see, there is a great deal of information you'll need to keep track of. In order to avoid a fevered search for important information, take the time right now to designate a single location in which to store all your records. My recommendation is either a filing cabinet or an expandable pocket portfolio. The latter is less expensive, yet it will still enable you to sort your records into an unlimited number of more- manageable categories.

Losing important report cards, citations, letters, etc., is easy to do if your life's history is scattered throughout your room or, even worse, your house! While copies of many of these items may be obtainable, why put yourself through all that extra work? Making good organization a habit will ensure that all the records you need to prepare your resume will be right where you need them when you need them.

For each of the categories summarized below, designate a separate file folder in which pertinent records can be kept. Your own notes are important, but keeping actual report cards, award citations, letters, etc. is even more so. Here's what your record-keeping system should include:

Transcripts (Including GPA and Class Rank Information)

Transcripts are your school's official record of your academic history, usually available, on request, from your high school's guidance office or college registrar's office. Your college may charge you for copies and "on request" doesn't mean "whenever you want"—you may have to wait some time for your request to be processed (so **don't** wait until the last minute!).

Your school-calculated GPA (Grade Point Average) is on the transcript. Most schools calculate this by multiplying the credit hours assigned to each course times a numerical grade equivalent (e.g., "A" = 4.0, "B" = 3.0, etc.), then dividing by total credits/courses taken. Class rank is simply a listing of GPAs, from highest to lowest.

Employment Records

Details on every part-time or full-time job you've held, including:

- Each employer's name, address and telephone number
- Name of supervisor
- Exact dates worked
- Approximate numbers of hours per week
- Specific duties and responsibilities
- Specific skills utilized and developed
- Accomplishments, honors
- Copies of awards, letters of recommendation

Volunteer Activities

Just because you weren't paid for a specific job—stuffing envelopes for the local Democratic candidate, running a car wash to raise money for the homeless, manning a drug hotline—doesn't mean that it wasn't significant or that you shouldn't include it on your resume.

So keep the same detailed notes on these volunteer activities as you have on the jobs you've held:

- Each organization's name, address and telephone number
- Name of supervisor
- Exact dates worked

- Approximate numbers of hours per week
- Specific duties and responsibilities
- Specific skills utilized
- Accomplishments, honors
- Copies of awards, letters of recommendation

Extracurricular Activities

List all sports, clubs, or other activities in which you've participated, either inside or outside school. For each, you should include:

- Name of activity/club/group
- Office(s) held
- Purpose of club/activity
- Specific duties/responsibilities
- Achievements, accomplishments, awards

If you were a long-standing member of a group or club, also include the dates that you were a member. This could demonstrate a high-level of commitment that could be used as a selling point.

Honors and Awards

Even if some of these honors are previously listed, specific data on every honor or award you receive should be kept, including, of course, the award itself! Keep the following information in your awards folder:

- Award name
- Date and from whom received
- What it was for
- Any pertinent details

Military Records

Complete military history, if pertinent, including:

- Dates of service
- Final rank awarded
- Duties and responsibilities
- All citations and awards
- Details on specific training and/or special schooling
- Skills developed
- Specific accomplishments

At the end of this chapter are seven **Data Input Sheets**. The first five cover employment, volunteer work, education, activities, and awards and are essential to any resume. The last two—covering military service and language skills—are important if, of course, they apply to you. I've only included one copy of each but, if you need to, you can copy the forms you need or simply write up your own using these as models.

Here are some pointers on how to fill out these all- important Data Sheets:

Employment Data Input Sheet: You will need to record the basic information—employer's name, address, and phone number; dates of employment; and supervisor's name—for your own files anyway. It may be an important addition to your networking list and will be necessary should you be asked to supply a reference list.

Duties should be a series of brief action statements describing what you did on this job. For example, if you worked as a hostess in a restaurant, this section might read: "Responsible for the delivery of 250 meals at dinner time and the supervision of 20 waiters and busboys. Coordinated reservations. Responsible for check and payment verification."

Skills should enumerate specific capabilities either necessary for the job or developed through it.

If you achieved *specific results*—e.g., "developed new filing system," "collected over $5,000 in previously-assumed bad debt," "instituted award-winning art program," etc.—or *received any award, citation or other honor*—"named Employee of the Month three times," "received Mayor's Citation for Innovation," etc.—make sure you list these.

Prepare one employment data sheet for each of the last three positions you have held; this is a basic guideline, but you can include more if relevant. Do not include sheets for short-term jobs (i.e., those that lasted one month or less).

Volunteer Work Data Input Sheet: Treat any volunteer work, no matter how basic or short (one day counts!), as if it were a job and record the same information. In both cases, it is especially important to note specific duties and responsibilities, skills required or developed and any accomplishments or achievements you can point to as evidence of your success.

Educational Data Input Sheet: If you're in college, omit details on high school. If you're a graduate student, list details on both graduate and undergraduate coursework. If you have not yet graduated, list your anticipated date of graduation. If more than a year away, indicate the numbers of credits earned through the most recent semester to be completed.

Activities Data Input Sheet: List your participation in the Student Government, Winter Carnival Committee, Math Club, Ski Patrol, etc., plus sports teams and/or any participation in community or church groups. Make sure you indicate if you were elected to any positions in clubs, groups, or on teams.

Awards And Honors Data Input Sheet: List awards and honors from your school (prestigious high school awards can still be included here, even if you're in graduate school), community groups, church groups, clubs, etc.

Military Service Data Input Sheet: Many useful skills are learned in the armed forces. A military stint often hastens the maturation process, making you a more attractive candidate. So if you have served in the military, make sure you include details in your resume. Again, include any computer skills you gained while in the service.

Language Data Input Sheet: An extremely important section for those of you with a real proficiency in a second language. And do make sure you have at least conversational fluency in the language(s) you list. One year of college French doesn't count, but if you've studied abroad, you probably are fluent or proficient. Such a talent could be invaluable, especially in today's increasingly international business climate.

While you should use the Data Input Sheets to summarize all of the data you have collected, do not throw away any of the specific information—report cards, transcripts, citations, etc.—just because it is recorded on these sheets. Keep all records in your files; you'll never know when you'll need them again!

Creating Your First Resume

There are many options that you can include or leave out. In general, we suggest you always include the following data:

1. Your name, address and telephone number
2. Pertinent educational history (grades, class rank, activities, etc.) Follow the grade point "rule of thumb"—mention it only if it is above 3.0.
3. Pertinent work history
4. Academic honors
5. Memberships in organizations
6. Military service history (if applicable)

You have the option of including the following:

1. Your career objective
2. Personal data
3. Hobbies
4. Summary of qualifications
5. Feelings about travel and relocation (Include this if you know in advance that the job you are applying for requires it. Often times, for future promotion, job seekers **must** be willing to relocate

And you should never include the following:

1. Photographs or illustrations (of yourself or anything else) unless they are required by your profession—e.g., actors' composites
2. Why you left past jobs

3. References
4. Salary history or present salary objectives/requirements (if salary history is specifically requested in an ad, it may be included in your cover letter)

Special note: There is definitely a school of thought that discourages any mention of personal data—marital status, health, etc.—on a resume. While I am not vehemently opposed to including such information, I am not convinced it is particularly necessary, either.

As far as hobbies go, I would only include such information if it were in some way pertinent to the job/career you're targeting, or if it shows how well-rounded you are. Your love of reading is pertinent if, for example, you are applying for a part-time job at a library. But including details on the joys of "hiking, long walks with my dog and Isaac Asimov short stories" is nothing but filler and should be left out.

Maximizing Form and Substance

Your resume should be limited to a single page if possible. A two-page resume should be used **only** if you have an extensive work background related to a future goal. When you're laying out the resume, try to leave a reasonable amount of "white space"—generous margins all around and spacing between entries. It should be typed or printed (not Xeroxed) on 8 1/2" x 11" white, cream, or ivory stock. The ink should be black. Don't scrimp on the paper quality—use the best bond you can afford. And since printing 100 or even 200 copies will cost only a little more than 50, if you do decide to print your resume, *over*estimate your needs and opt for the highest quantity you think you may need. Prices at various "quick print" shops are not exorbitant and the quality look printing affords will leave the impression you want.

Use Power Words for Impact

Be brief. Use phrases rather than complete sentences. Your resume is a summary of your talents, not a term paper. Choose your words carefully and use "power words" whenever possible. "Organized" is more powerful than "put together;" "supervised" better than "oversaw;" "formulated" better than "thought up." Strong words like these can make the most mundane clerical work sound like a series of responsible, professional positions. And, of course, they will tend to make your resume stand out. Here's a starter list of words that you may want to use in your resume:

accomplished	applied	built	composed
achieved	approved	calculated	computed
acted	arranged	chaired	conceptualized
adapted	assembled	changed	conducted
addressed	assessed	classified	consolidated
administered	assigned	collected	contributed
advised	assisted	communicated	coordinated
allocated	attained	compiled	critiqued
analyzed	budgeted	completed	defined

delegated	implemented	overhauled	rewrote
delivered	improved	oversaw	saved
demonstrated	initiated	participated	scheduled
designed	installed	planned	selected
determined	instituted	prepared	served
developed	instructed	presented	sold
devised	introduced	presided	solved
directed	invented	produced	started
discovered	issued	programmed	streamlined
drafted	launched	promoted	studied
edited	learned	proposed	suggested
established	lectured	publicized	supervised
estimated	led	ran	systematized
evaluated	litigated	recommended	taught
executed	lobbied	recruited	tested
expanded	made	regulated	trained
fixed	managed	remodeled	updated
forecast	marketed	renovated	upgraded
formulated	mediated	reorganized	utilized
gathered	negotiated	researched	won
gave	obtained	restored	wrote
generated	operated	reviewed	
guided	organized	revised	

Choose the Right Format

There is not much mystery here—your background will generally lead you to the right format. For an entry-level job applicant with limited work experience, the chronological format, which organizes your educational and employment history by date (most recent first) is the obvious choice. For older or more experienced applicants, the functional—which emphasizes the duties and responsibilities of all your jobs over the course of your career, may be more suitable. If you are applying for a specific position in one field, the targeted format is for you. While I have tended to emphasize the chronological format in this chapter, one of the other two may well be the right one for you.

A List of Do's and Don't's

In case we didn't stress them enough, here are some rules to follow:

- **Do** be brief and to the point—Two pages if absolutely necessary, one page if at all possible. Never longer!

- **Don't** be fancy. Multicolored paper and all-italic type won't impress employers, just make your resume harder to read (and easier to discard). Use plain white or ivory paper, black ink and an easy-to-read standard typeface.

- **Do** forget rules about sentences. Say what you need to say in the fewest words possible; use phrases, not drawn-out sentences.

- **Do** stick to the facts. Don't talk about your dog, vacation, etc.

- **Don't** ever send a resume blind. A cover letter should always accompany a resume and that letter should always be directed to a specific person.

- **Don't** have any typos. Your resume must be perfect—proofread everything as many times as necessary to catch any misspellings, grammatical errors, strange hyphenations, or typos.

- **Do** use the spell check feature on your personal computer to find errors, and also try reading the resume backwards—you'll be surprised at how errors jump out at you when you do this. Finally, have a friend proof your resume.

- **Do** use your resume as your sales tool. It is, in many cases, as close to you as an employer will ever get. Make sure it includes the information necessary to sell yourself the way you want to be sold!

- **Do** spend the money for good printing. Soiled, tattered or poorly reproduced copies speak poorly of your own self-image. Spend the money and take the time to make sure your resume is the best presentation you've ever made.

- **Do** help the reader, by organizing your resume in a clear-cut manner so key points are easily gleaned.

- **Don't** have a cluttered resume. Leave plenty of white space, especially around headings and all four margins.

- **Do** use bullets, asterisks, or other symbols as "stop signs" that the reader's eye will be naturally drawn to.

On the following pages, I've included a "fill-in-the-blanks" resume form so you can construct your own resume right away, plus one example each of a chronological, functional, and targeted resume.

EMPLOYMENT DATA INPUT SHEET

Employer name: _____

Address: _____

Phone: _____ Dates of employment: _____

Hours per week: _____ Salary/Pay: _____

Supervisor's name and title: _____

Duties: _____

_____

_____

Skills utilized: _____

_____

_____

_____

Accomplishments/Honors/Awards: _____

_____

_____

_____

Other important information: _____

_____

_____

_____

_____

VOLUNTEER WORK DATA INPUT SHEET

Organization name:_____

Address: _____

Phone: _____ Dates of activity: _____

Hours per week: _____

Supervisor's name and title: _____

Duties: _____

_____

_____

Skills utilized: _____

_____

_____

_____

Accomplishments/Honors/Awards: _____

_____

_____

_____

Other important information: _____

_____

_____

_____

HIGH SCHOOL DATA INPUT SHEET

School name: _____

Address: _____

Phone: _____ Years attended: _____

Major studies: _____

GPA/Class rank: _____

Honors: _____

Important courses: _____

_____

_____

_____

OTHER SCHOOL DATA INPUT SHEET

School name: _____

Address: _____

Phone: _____ Years attended: _____

Major studies: _____

GPA/Class rank: _____

Honors: _____

Important courses _____

_____

_____

_____

_____

COLLEGE DATA INPUT SHEET

College: _____

Address: _____

Phone: _____ Years attended:_____

Degrees earned: _____ Major: _____Minor: _____

Honors: _____

Important courses: _____

_____

_____

_____

_____

GRADUATE SCHOOL DATA INPUT SHEET

College: _____

Address: _____

Phone: _____ Years attended:_____

Degrees earned: _____ Major: _____Minor: _____

Honors: _____

Important courses: _____

_____

_____

_____

_____

MILITARY SERVICE DATA INPUT SHEET

Branch: _____

Rank (at discharge): _____

Dates of service: _____

Duties and responsibilities: _____

_____

_____

_____

Special training and/or school attended: _____

_____

_____

_____

Citations or awards: _____

_____

_____

_____

Specific accomplishments: _____

_____

_____

_____

_____

ACTIVITIES DATA INPUT SHEET

Club/activity: _____Office(s) held: _____

Description of participation: _____

_____

_____

Duties/responsibilities: _____

_____

Club/activity: _____Office(s) held: _____

Description of participation: _____

_____

_____

Duties/responsibilities: _____

_____

Club/activity: _____Office(s) held: _____

Description of participation: _____

_____

_____

Duties/responsibilities: _____

_____

_____

_____

AWARDS AND HONORS DATA INPUT SHEET

Name of Award or Citation: _____

From Whom Received: _____ Date: _____

Significance: _____

_____

Other pertinent information: _____

_____

Name of Award or Citation: _____

From Whom Received: _____ Date: _____

Significance: _____

_____

Other pertinent information: _____

_____

Name of Award or Citation: _____

From Whom Received: _____ Date: _____

Significance: _____

_____

Other pertinent information: _____

_____

LANGUAGE DATA INPUT SHEET

Language: _____

___Read   ___Write   ___Converse

Background (number of years studied, travel, etc.) _____

_____

_____

_____

Language: _____

___Read   ___Write   ___Converse

Background (number of years studied, travel, etc.) _____

_____

_____

_____

Language: _____

___Read   ___Write   ___Converse

Background (number of years studied, travel, etc.) _____

_____

_____

_____

FILL-IN-THE-BLANKS RESUME OUTLINE

Name: _____

Address: _____

City, state, ZIP Code: _____

Telephone number: _____

OBJECTIVE: _____

_____

_____

_____

_____

SUMMARY OF QUALIFICATIONS: _____

_____

_____

_____

EDUCATION

GRADUATE SCHOOL: _____

Address: _____

City, state, ZIP Code: _____

Expected graduation date:_____Grade Point Average: _____

Degree earned (expected):_____Class Rank: _____

Important classes, especially those related to your career: _____

_____

_____

_____

_____

_____

_____

_____

COLLEGE: _____

Address: _____

City, state, ZIP Code: _____

Expected graduation date:_____Grade Point Average: _____

Class rank:_____Major:_____Minor:_____

Important classes, especially those related to your career: _____

_____

_____

_____

_____

_____

_____

_____

_____

HIGH SCHOOL: _____

Address: _____

City, state, ZIP Code: _____

Expected graduation date: _____Grade Point Average: _____

Class rank: _____

Important classes, especially those related to your career: _____

_____

_____

_____

_____

_____

_____

_____

HOBBIES AND OTHER INTERESTS (OPTIONAL) _____

_____

_____

_____

_____

_____

_____

_____

_____

EXTRACURRICULAR ACTIVITIES (Activity name, dates participated, duties and responsibilities, offices held, accomplishments): _____

_____

_____

_____

_____

_____

_____

_____

AWARDS AND HONORS (Award name, from whom and date received, significance of the award and any other pertinent details): _____

_____

_____

_____

_____

_____

_____

_____

_____

_____

WORK EXPERIENCE. Include job title, name of business, address and telephone number, dates of employment, supervisor's name and title, your major responsibilities, accomplishments, and any awards won. Include volunteer experience in this category. List your experiences with the most recent dates first, even if you later decide not to use a chronological format.

_____

_____

_____

_____

_____

_____

_____

_____

_____

_____

_____

_____

_____

_____

_____

REFERENCES. Though you should *not* include references in your resume, you do need to prepare a separate list of at least three people who know you fairly well and will recommend you highly to prospective employers. For each, include job title, company name, address, and telephone number. Before you include anyone on this list, make sure you have their permission to use their name as a reference and confirm what they intend to say about you to a potential employer.

1. _____

_____

_____

2. _____

_____

_____

3. _____

_____

_____

4. _____

_____

_____

5. _____

_____

_____

SAMPLE RESUME - CHRONOLOGICAL

JESSICA C. CAROL

457 Oak Drive
Kansas City, MO 64111
(816) 453-8794

EDUCATION

Bachelor of Science in **Occupational Therapy**
Rockhurst College   Kansas City, MO
May, 1994   GPA: 3.9   **Summa Cum Laude**

Associate Degree in **Occupational Therapy**
Pallotine Community College   Kansas City, MO
June, 1992   GPA: 3.6   **Cum Laude**

FIELD PLACEMENTS
9/93 - 11/93

City Institute for Children   Kansas City, MO
Three month rotation: Evaluated skills and abilities of patients, consulted with other members of medical team, and developed individual programs to help patients develop skill level goals.

6/93 - 8/93

Kingswood Psychiatric Hospital   Rockhurst, MO
Three month rotation: Assisted teenaged patients to accommodate to their disabilities. Kept notes and patient records.

EMPLOYMENT
9/92 - 5/93

Rockhurst Day Care Center   Kansas City, MO
Play Leader: Developed/implemented lesson plans and activity schedules for children of various ages.

9/91 - 8/92

Assistant: Learned to deal with challenging age appropriate behaviors and difficult situations.

HONORS

Dean's List
Insignis Scholarship
National Honor Society

CERTIFICATION

Scheduled to take OTR exam in November, 1994

ACTIVITIES

Water Aerobics, YWCA Instructor
Intramural Soccer Team
On-going interest in health and physical fitness

SAMPLE RESUME - FUNCTIONAL

NIKKI KENHOLD
17354 Herman Drive
Albuquerque, NM 87105
(415) 002-3496

OBJECTIVE   Entry level position in the **Field of Dietetics**.

EDUCATION   University of New Mexico   Albuquerque, NM
      Bachelor of Science in Human Nutrition
      May, 1994
      GPA: 3.5
      Honors: Cum Laude Dean's List
      ADA approved Internship in Dietetics

      Associate Degree in Nursing
      June, 1987

ACADEMIC EXPERIENCE

Familiar with renal and intravenous nutrition support. Senior research project covering the *Problems of Cholesterol*.

HEALTH CARE BACKGROUND

Five years in major health care system.
Participant in yearly community Health-O-Rama.

COMMUNICATIONS ABILITY

Professional working relationship with diverse populations.
Spanish language proficient.

**EMPLOYMENT
HISTORY**
9/92 - 9/93   Western County Health Department   Albuquerque, NM
      ADA approved Internship

7/87 - 8/92   General Hospital   Las Cruces, NM
      LPN

LICENSES   ADA Registry Eligible, July, 1994
      LPN, 1988, State of New Mexico, #01234

**PROFESSIONAL
AFFILIATES**   State Dietetic Student Association

ACTIVITIES   Rackham Choir, 1990-Present
      Classical Guitarist
      Avid Reader of Historical Novels

REFERENCES   Furnished Upon Request

SAMPLE RESUME - TARGETED

RITA W. EDWARDS

Local
W. Quad #728
Detroit, MI 48221
(313) 682-3340

Permanent
562 Luke Rd.
Ferndale, MI 48220
(313) 539-0021

CAREER GOAL

Private Periodontal Practice

**ACADEMIC
BACKGROUND**

Bachelor of Science in Dental Hygiene
University of Detroit Mercy
Detroit, MI
December, 1993   Summa Cum Laude

**EDUCATIONAL
EXPERIENCE**

- Assisted/observed in periodontal surgical procedures.
- Completed 75 light, 25 medium, & 10 heavy calculus scaling and polishing.
- Performed medical/dental histories, intra/extra oral examinations and vital signs to include blood pressures on 110 patients.
- Completely scaled and root planed 25 patients with active periodontal disease.
- Exposed, developed, and mounted dental radiographs.
- Provided in-service training in dental health to staff personnel of three nursing homes.
- Performed dental hygiene treatment on residents of nursing homes.
- Dried, etched, and placed 10 pit and fissure sealants.
- Assigned to assist and observe in the following rotation:
  Oral Surgery, Endodontics, Periodontics, Pediatrics, Operative, Prosthetics.

EXPERIENCE
Summer, 1992

E. F. Horan, DDS   Detroit, MI
Chair-Side Assistant: Responsible for being second pair of hands for the dentist, including handing instruments to the dentist.

5/89- 8/91

B. Purifoy-Seldon, DDS   Ferndale, MI
Receptionist: Received patients, performed insurance billing, managed administrative needs of small dental office.

CERTIFICATION

RDH, May, 1994
RDA, May, 1994
CDA, May, 1990

**EXTRA-
CURRICULAR**

American Dental Hygienist Association, Student Chapter
Red Cross Volunteer
Science Tutor, University Volunteer
Enjoy yoga, aerobics, and jogging.

CHAPTER TWENTY-ONE

Writing Better Letters

Stop for a moment and review your resume draft. It is undoubtedly (by now) a near-perfect document that instantly tells the reader the kind of job you want and why you are qualified. But does it say anything personal about you? Any amplification of your talents? Any words that are ideally "you?" Any hint of the kind of person who stands behind that resume?

If you've prepared it properly, the answers should be a series of ringing "no's"—your resume should be a mere sketch of your life, a bare-bones summary of your skills, education, and experience.

To the general we must add the specific. That's what your letters must accomplish—adding the lines, colors, and shading that will help fill out your self-portrait. This chapter will cover the kinds of letters you will most often be called upon to prepare in your job search. There are essentially nine different types you will utilize again and again, based primarily on what each is trying to accomplish. One well-written example of each is included at the end of this chapter.

Answer these Questions

Before you put pencil to paper to compose any letter, there are five key questions you must ask yourself:

- **Why** are you writing it?
- To **Whom**?
- **What** are you trying to accomplish?
- **Which** lead will get the reader's attention?
- **How** do you organize the letter to best accomplish your objectives?

Why?

There should be a single, easily definable reason you are writing any letter. This reason will often dictate what and how you write—the tone and flavor of the letter—as well as what you include or leave out.

Have you been asked in an ad to amplify your qualifications for a job and provide a salary history and college transcripts? Then that (minimally) is your objective in writing. Limit yourself to following instructions and do a little personal selling—but very little. Including everything asked for and a simple, adequate cover letter is better than writing a "knock 'em, sock 'em" letter and omitting the one piece of information the ad specifically asked for.

If, however, you are on a networking search, the objective of your letter is to seek out contacts who will refer you for possible informational or job interviews. In this case, getting a name and address—a referral—is your stated purpose for writing. You have to be specific and ask for this action.

You will no doubt follow up with a phone call, but be certain the letter conveys what you are after. Being vague or oblique won't help you. You are after a definite yes or no when it comes to contact assistance. The recipient of your letter should know this. As they say in the world of selling, at some point you have to ask for the order.

Who?

Using the proper "tone" in a letter is as important as the content—you wouldn't write to the owner of the local meat market using the same words and style as you would employ in a letter to the director of personnel of a major company. Properly addressing the person or persons you are writing to is as important as what you say to them.

Always utilize the recipient's job title and level (correct title and spelling are a **must**). If you know what kind of person they are (based on your knowledge of their area of involvement) use that knowledge to your advantage as well. It also helps if you know his or her hiring clout, but even if you know the letter is going through a screening stage instead of to the actual person you need to contact, don't take the easy way out. You have to sell the person doing the screening just as convincingly as you would the actual contact, or else you might get passed over instead of passed along! Don't underestimate the power of the person doing the screening.

For example, it pays to sound technical with technical people—in other words, use the kinds of words and language which they use on the job. If you have had the opportunity to speak with them, it will be easy for you. If not, and you have formed some opinions as to their types then use these as the basis of the language you employ. The cardinal rule is to say it in words you think the recipient will be comfortable hearing, not in the words you might otherwise personally choose.

What?

What do you have to offer that company? What do you have to contribute to the job, process or work situation that is unique and/or of particular benefit to the recipient of your letter.

For example, if you were applying for a sales position and recently ranked number one in a summer sales job, then conveying this benefit is logical and desirable. It is a factor you may have left off your resume. Even if it was listed in the skills/accomplishment section of the resume, you can underscore and call attention to it in your letter. Repetition, when it is properly focused, can be a good thing.

Which?

Of all the opening sentences you can compose, which will immediately get the reader's attention? If your opening sentence is dynamic, you are already 50 percent of the way to your end objective—having your entire letter read. Don't slide into it. Know the point you are trying to make and come right to it. One word of caution: your first sentence **must** make mention of what led you to write—was it an ad, someone at the company, a story you saw on television? Be sure to give this point of reference.

How?

While a good opening is essential, how do you organize your letter so that it is easy for the recipient to read in its entirety? This is a question of *flow*—the way the words and sentences naturally lead one to another, holding the reader's interest until he or she reaches your signature.

If you have your objective clearly in mind, this task is easier than it sounds: Simply convey your message(s) in a logical sequence. End your letter by stating what the next steps are—yours and/or the reader's.

One More Time

Pay attention to the small things. Neatness still counts. Have your letters typed. Spend a few extra dollars and have some personal stationery printed.

And most important, make certain that your correspondence goes out quickly. The general rule is to get a letter in the mail during the week in which the project comes to your attention or in which you have had some contact with the organization. I personally attempt to mail follow-up letters the same day as the contact; at worst, within 24 hours.

When to Write

- To answer an ad
- To prospect (many companies)
- To inquire about specific openings (single company)
- To obtain a referral
- To obtain an informational interview
- To obtain a job interview
- To say "thank you"
- To accept or reject a job offer
- To withdraw from consideration for a job

In some cases, the letter will accompany your resume; in others, it will need to stand alone. Each of the above circumstance is described in the pages that follow. I have included at least one sample of each type of letter at the end of this chapter.

Answering an Ad

Your eye catches an ad in the Positions Available section of the Sunday paper for an occupational therapist. It tells you that the position is in a large therapy clinic and that, though some experience would be desirable, it is not required. Well, you possess *those* skills. The ad asks that you send a letter and resume to a Post Office Box. No salary is indicated, no phone number given. You decide to reply.

Your purpose in writing—the objective (why?)—is to secure a job interview. Since no person is singled out for receipt of the ad, and since it is a large company, you assume it will be screened by Human Resources.

Adopt a professional, formal tone. You are answering a "blind" ad, so you have to play it safe. In your first sentence, refer to the ad, including the place and date of publication and the position outlined. (There is a chance that the company is running more than one ad on the same date and in the same paper, so you need to identify the one to which you are replying.) Tell the reader what (specifically) you have to offer that company. Include your resume, phone number, and the times it is easiest to reach you. Ask for the order—tell them you'd like to have an appointment.

Blanket Prospecting Letter

In June of this year you will graduate from a four-year college with a degree in occupational therapy. You seek a position (internship or full-time employment) at a major therapy center. You have decided to write to 50 top centers and hospitals, sending each a copy of your resume. You don't know which, if any, have job openings.

Such blanket mailings are effective given two circumstances: 1) You must have an exemplary record and a resume which reflects it; and 2) You must send out a goodly number of packages, since the response rate to such mailings is very low.

A blanket mailing doesn't mean an impersonal one—you should always be writing to a specific executive. If you have a referral, send a personalized letter to that person. If not, do not simply mail a package to the Human Resources department; identify the department head and *then* send a personalized letter. And make sure you get on the phone and follow up each letter within about ten days. Don't just sit back and wait for everyone to call you. They won't.

Just Inquiring

The inquiry letter is a step above the blanket prospecting letter; it's a "cold-calling" device with a twist. You have earmarked a company (and a person) as a possibility in your job search based on something you have read about them. Your general research tells you that it is a good place to work. Although you are not aware of any specific openings, you know that they employ entry-level personnel with your credentials.

While ostensibly inquiring about any openings, you are really just "referring yourself" to them in order to place your resume in front of the right person. This is what I would call a "why not?" attempt at securing a job interview. Its effectiveness depends on their actually having been in the news. This, after all, is your "excuse" for writing.

Networking

It's time to get out that folder marked "Contacts" and prepare a draft networking letter. The lead sentence should be very specific, referring immediately to the friend, colleague, etc. "who suggested I write you about..." Remember: Your objective is to secure an informational interview, pave the way for a job interview, and/or get referred to still other contacts.

This type of letter should not place the recipient in a position where a decision is necessary; rather, the request should be couched in terms of "career advice." The second paragraph can then inform the reader of your level of experience. Finally, be specific about seeking an appointment.

Unless you have been specifically asked by the referring person to do so, you will probably not be including a resume with such letters. So the letter itself must highlight your credentials, enabling the reader to gauge your relative level of experience. For entry-level personnel, education, of course, will be most important.

For an Informational Interview

Though the objectives of this letter are similar to those of the networking letter, they are not as personal. These are "knowledge quests" on your part and the recipient will most likely not be someone you have been referred to. The idea is to convince the reader of the sincerity of your research effort. Whatever selling you do, if you do any at all, will arise as a consequence of the meeting, not beforehand. A positive response to this type of request is in itself a good step forward. It is, after all, exposure, and amazing things can develop when people in authority agree to see you.

Thank-You Letters

Although it may not always seem so, manners do count in the job world. But what counts even more are the simple gestures that show you actually care—like writing a thank-you letter. A well-executed, timely thank-you note tells more about your personality than anything else you may have sent, and it also demonstrates excellent follow-through skills. It says something about the way you were brought up—whatever else your resume tells them, you are, at least, polite, courteous and thoughtful.

Thank-you letters may well become the beginning of an all-important dialogue that leads directly to a job. So be extra careful in composing them, and make certain that they are custom made for each occasion and person.

The following are the primary situations in which you will be called upon to write some variation of thank-you letter:

1. After a job interview
2. After an informational interview

3. Accepting a job offer

4. Responding to rejection: While optional, such a letter is appropriate if you have been among the finalists in a job search or were rejected due to limited experience. Remember: Some day you'll *have* enough experience; make the interviewer want to stay in touch.

5. Withdrawing from consideration: Used when you decide you are no longer interested in a particular position. (A variation is usable for declining an actual job offer.) Whatever the reason for writing such a letter, it's wise to do so and thus keep future lines of communication open.

IN RESPONSE TO AN AD

10 E. 89th Street
New York, NY 10028
October 22, 1993

The *New York Times*
PO Box 7520
New York, NY 10128

Dear Sir or Madam:

This letter is in response to your advertisement for a physician assistant which appeared in the October 18th issue of the *New York Times.*

I have the qualifications you are seeking. I graduated from American University with a B.S. in biology and from the Thomas Jefferson University Physician Assistant Program. I am also NCCPA certified.

I held an internship at Maryville Hospital for two summers, and have been working for over a year at the St. Luke Community Health Care Clinic. I am a member of the National Society of Physician Assistants and frequently contribute to my local NSPA chapter newsletter.

My resume is enclosed. I would like to have the opportunity to meet with you personally to discuss your requirements for the position. I can be reached at (212) 785-1225 between 8:00 a.m. and 5:00 p.m. and at (212) 785-4221 after 5:00 p.m. I look forward to hearing from you.

Sincerely,

Karen Weber

Enclosure: Resume

PROSPECTING LETTER

Kim Kerr
8 Robutuck Hwy.
Hammond, IN 54054
555-875-2392

October 22, 1993

Mr. Fred Jones
Personnel Director
Alcott Community Hospital
Sports Medicine Clinic
Chicago, Illinois 91221

Dear Mr. Jones:

The name of Alcott Hospital's Sports Medicine Clinic continually pops up in our classroom discussions of outstanding sports medicine facilities. Given my interest in physical therapy as a career and sports medicine as a specialty, I've taken the liberty of enclosing my resume.

As you can see, I have just completed a very comprehensive master's program at Warren University majoring in physical therapy with a minor in exercise physiology. Though my resume does not indicate it, I will be graduating in the top 10% of my class, with honors.

I will be in the Chicago area on November 29 and will call your office to see when it is convenient to arrange an appointment.

Sincerely yours,

Kim Kerr

INQUIRY LETTER

42 7th Street
Ski City, Vermont 85722
October 22, 1993

Dr. Michael Maniaci
Executive Director
Pinnacle Sports Training Center
521 West Elm Street
Indianapolis, IN 83230

Dear Dr. Maniaci:

I just completed reading the article in the January issue of *Fitness* on your facility's expansion to the East Coast. Congratulations!

Your innovative approach to recruiting minorities is of particular interest to me because of my background in athletic training and minority recruitment.

I am interested in learning more about your work as well as the possibilities of joining your firm. My qualifications include:

- M.S. in Physical Therapy
- Research on minority recruitment
- Physical Therapy Seminar participation (Univ. of Virginia)
- Reports preparation on exercise physiology, kinesiology, and minorities

I will be in Indiana during the week of November 22 and hope your schedule will permit us to meet briefly to discuss our mutual interests. I will call your office next week to see if such a meeting can be arranged.

I appreciate your consideration.

Sincerely yours,

Ronald W. Sommerville

NETWORKING LETTER

Rochelle A. Starky
42 Bach St., Musical City, IN 20202   317-555-1515

October 22, 1993

Dr. Michelle Fleming
Executive Director
Heights Pediatric Hospital
42 Jenkins Avenue
Fulton, Mississippi 23232

Dear Dr. Fleming:

Sam Kinney suggested I write to you. I am interested in an entry-level medical assistant position in a healthcare facility, and Sam felt it would be mutually beneficial for us to meet and talk.

I have an associate's degree from Musical City Community College's medical assisting program and have just over one year of part-time experience in a children's hospital. I also worked for two years in a clerical capacity at the Norfolk Health Clinic in my town.

I know from Sam how similar our backgrounds are—the same training, the same interests. And, of course, I am aware of how successfully you have managed your career—three promotions in four years!

As I begin my job search during the next few months, I am certain your advice would help me. Would it be possible for us to meet briefly? My resume is enclosed.

I will call your office next week to see when your schedule would permit such a meeting.

Sincerely,

Rochelle A. Starky

16 NW 128th Street
Raleigh, NC 757755
October 22, 1992

Ms. Jackie B. McClure
General Manager
Goldmine Dental Center
484 Smithers Road
Awkmont, North Carolina 76857

Dear Ms. McClure:

I'm sure a good deal of the credit for your center's 23% growth of patients last year is attributable to the highly-motivated and knowledgeable staff you have recruited during the last three years. I hope to obtain a dental hygiene position with a facility just as committed to growth.

I have four years of dental assisting experience, which I acquired while working my way through college. I believe this experience, as well as my associate's degree in applied science in dental hygiene from Raleigh University have properly prepared me for a career in dental hygiene.

As I begin my job search, I am trying to gather as much information and advice as possible before applying for positions. Could I take a few minutes of your time next week to discuss my career plans? I will call your office on Monday, October 29, to see if such a meeting can be arranged.

I appreciate your consideration and look forward to meeting you.

Sincerely,

Karen R. Burns

Lazelle Wright
921 West Fourth Street
Steamboat, Colorado 72105
303-310-3303

November 22, 1993

Dr. James R. Payne
Managing Director
Bradley Finch Chiropractic Clinic
241 Snowridge
Ogden, Utah 72108

Dear Dr. Payne:

Jinny Bastienelli was right when she said you would be most helpful in advising me on a career in chiropractic care.

I appreciated your taking the time from your busy schedule to meet with me. Your advice was most helpful and I have incorporated your suggestions into my resume. I will send you a copy next week.

Again, thanks so much for your assistance. As you suggested, I will contact Joe Simmons at the Jensen Chiropractic Clinic next week in regard to a possible opening with his facility.

Sincerely,

Lazelle Wright

AFTER A JOB INTERVIEW

1497 Lilac Street
Old Adams, MA 01281
November 22, 1993

Mr. Rudy Delacort
Director of Personnel
Ann Grace Hospital
175 Boylston Avenue
Ribbit, Massachusetts 02857

Dear Mr. Delacort:

Thank you for the opportunity to interview yesterday for the nursing assistant position. I enjoyed meeting with you and Dr. Cliff Stoudt and learning more about Ann Grace.

Your facility appears to be growing in a direction which parallels my interests and goals. The interview with you and your staff confirmed my initial positive impressions of Ann Grace, and I want to reiterate my strong interest in working for you.

I am convinced my prior experience as a nurses aide at the Fellowes Nursing Home in Old Adams, participation in several healthcare seminars conducted by the National Nurses Organization, and my college training in nursing would enable me to progress steadily through your training program and become a productive member of your staff.

Again, thank you for your consideration. If you need any additional information from me, please feel free to call.

Yours truly,

Harold Beaumont

cc: Dr. Cliff Stoudt
    Pediatrics

ACCEPTING A JOB OFFER

1497 Lilac Street
Old Adams, MA 01281
November 22, 1993

Mr. Rudy Delacort
Director of Personnel
Ann Grace Hospital
175 Boylston Avenue
Ribbit, Massachusetts 01281

Dear Mr. Delacort:

I want to thank you and Dr. Stoudt for giving me the opportunity to work for Ann Grace. I am very pleased to accept the position as a nursing assistant with your geriatrics ward. The position entails exactly the kind of work I want to do, and I know that I will do a good job for you.

As we discussed, I shall begin work on January 5, 1994. In the interim, I shall complete all the necessary employment forms, obtain the required physical examination and locate housing.

I plan to be in Ribbit within the next two weeks and would like to deliver the paperwork to you personally. At that time, we could handle any remaining items pertaining to my employment. I'll call next week to schedule an appointment with you.

Sincerely yours,

Harold Beaumont

cc: Dr. Cliff Stoudt
    Geriatrics

WITHDRAWING FROM CONSIDERATION

1497 Lilac Street
Old Adams, MA 01281
October 22, 1993

Mr. Rudy Delacort
Director of Personnel
Ann Grace Hospital
175 Boylston Avenue
Ribbit, Massachusetts 01281

Dear Mr. Delacort:

It was indeed a pleasure meeting with you and Dr. Stoudt last week to discuss your needs for a nursing assistant. Our time together was most enjoyable and informative.

As I discussed with you during our meetings, I believe one purpose of preliminary interviews is to explore areas of mutual interest and to assess the fit between the individual and the position. After careful consideration, I have decided to withdraw from consideration for the position.

I want to thank you for interviewing me and giving me the opportunity to learn about your needs. You have a fine staff and I would have enjoyed working with them.

Yours truly,

Harold Beaumont

cc: Dr. Cliff Stoudt
    Geriatrics

IN RESPONSE TO REJECTION

1497 Lilac Street
Old Adams, MA 01281
November 22, 1993

Mr. Rudy Delacort
Director of Personnel
Ann Grace Hospital
175 Boylston Avenue
Ribbit, Massachusetts 01281

Dear Mr. Delacort:

Thank you for giving me the opportunity to interview for the nursing assistant position. I appreciate your consideration and interest in me.

Although I am disappointed in not being selected for your current vacancy, I want you to know that I appreciated the courtesy and professionalism shown to me during the entire selection process. I enjoyed meeting you, Dr. Cliff Stoudt, and the other members of your staff. My meetings confirmed that Ann Grace would be an exciting place to work and build a career.

I want to reiterate my strong interest in working for you. Please keep me in mind if a similar position becomes available in the near future.

Again, thank you for the opportunity to interview and best wishes to you and your staff.

Sincerely yours,

Harold Beaumont

cc: Dr. Cliff Stoudt
    Geriatrics

Questions for You, Questions for Them

You've finished your exhaustive research, contacted everyone you've known since kindergarten, compiled a professional-looking and sounding resume, and written brilliant letters to the dozens of companies your research has revealed are perfect matches for your own strengths, interests, and abilities. Unfortunately, all of this preparatory work will be meaningless if you are unable to successfully convince one of those firms to hire you.

If you were able set up an initial meeting at one of these companies, your resume and cover letter obviously piqued someone's interest. Now you have to traverse the last minefield—the job interview itself. It's time to make all that preparation pay off.

This chapter will attempt to put the interview process in perspective, giving you the "inside story" on what to expect and how to handle the questions and circumstances that arise during the course of a normal interview—and even many of those that surface in the bizarre interview situations we have all experienced at some point.

Why Interviews Shouldn't Scare You

Interviews shouldn't scare you. The concept of two (or more) persons meeting to determine if they are right for each other is a relatively logical idea. As important as research, resumes, letters, and phone calls are, they are inherently impersonal. The interview is your chance to really see and feel the company firsthand, so think of it as a positive opportunity, your chance to succeed.

That said, many of you will still be put off by the inherently inquisitive nature of the process. Though many questions *will* be asked, interviews are essentially experiments in chemistry. Are you right for the company? Is the company right for you? Not just on paper—*in the flesh.*

If you decide the company is right for you, your purpose is simple and clear-cut—to convince the interviewer that you are the right person for the job, that you will fit in, and that you will be an asset to the company now and in the future. The interviewer's purpose is equally simple—to decide whether he or she should buy what you're selling.

This chapter will focus on the kinds of questions you are likely to be asked, how to answer them, and the questions you should be ready to ask of the interviewer. By removing the workings of the interview process from the "unknown" category, you will reduce the fear it engenders.

But all the preparation in the world won't completely eliminate your sweaty palms, unless you can convince yourself that the interview is an important, positive life experience from which you will benefit—even if you don't get the job. Approach it with enthusiasm, calm yourself, and let your personality do the rest. You will undoubtedly spend an interesting hour, one that will teach you more about yourself. It's just another step in the learning process you've undertaken.

What to Do First

Start by setting up a calendar on which you can enter and track all your scheduled appointments. When you schedule an interview with a company, ask them how much time you should allow for the appointment. Some require all new applicants to fill out numerous forms and/or complete a battery of intelligence or psychological tests—all before the first interview. If you've only allowed an hour for the interview—and scheduled another at a nearby firm 10 minutes later—the first time you confront a three-hour test series will effectively destroy any schedule.

Some companies, especially if the first interview is very positive, like to keep applicants around to talk to other executives. This process may be planned or, in a lot of cases, a spontaneous decision by an interviewer who likes you and wants you to meet some other key decision makers. Other companies will tend to schedule such a series of second interviews on a separate day. Find out, if you can, how the company you're planning to visit generally operates. Otherwise, a schedule that's too tight will fall apart in no time at all, especially if you've traveled to another city to interview with a number of firms in a short period of time.

If you need to travel out-of-state to interview with a company, be sure to ask if they will be paying some or all of your travel expenses. (It's generally expected that you'll be paying your own way to firms within your home state.) If they don't offer—and you don't ask—presume you're paying the freight.

Even if the company agrees to reimburse you, make sure you have enough money to pay all the expenses yourself. While some may reimburse you immediately, the majority of firms may take from a week to a month to send you an expense check.

Research, Research, and More Research

The research you did to find these companies is nothing compared to the research you need to do now that you're beginning to narrow your search. If you followed our detailed suggestions when you started targeting these firms in the first place, you've already amassed a great deal of information about them. If you didn't do the research *then,* you sure better decide to do it *now.* Study each company as if you were going to be tested on your detailed knowledge of their organization and operations. Here's a complete checklist of the facts you should try to know about each company you plan to visit for a job interview:

The Basics

1. The address of (and directions to) the office you're visiting
2. Headquarters location (if different)
3. Some idea of domestic and international branches
4. Relative size (compared to other similar companies)
5. Annual billings, sales, and/or income (last two years)
6. Subsidiary companies and/or specialized divisions
7. Departments (overall structure)
8. Major accounts, products, or services

The Subtleties

1. History of the firm (specialties, honors, awards, famous names)
2. Names, titles, and backgrounds of top management
3. Existence (and type) of training program
4. Relocation policy
5. Relative salaries (compared to other companies in field or by size)
6. Recent developments concerning the company and its products or services (from your trade magazine and newspaper reading)
7. Everything you can learn about the career, likes, and dislikes of the person(s) interviewing you

The amount of time and work necessary to be this well prepared for an interview is considerable. It will not be accomplished the day before the interview. You may even find some of the information you need is unavailable on short notice.

Is it really so important to do all this? Well, somebody out there is going to. And if you happen to be interviewing for the same job as that other, well-prepared, knowledgeable candidate, who do you think will impress the interviewer more?

As we've already discussed, if you give yourself enough time, most of this information is surprisingly easy to obtain. In addition to the reference sources covered in the Career Resources chapter, the company itself can probably supply you with a great deal of data. A firm's annual report—which all publicly-owned companies must publish yearly for their stockholders—is a virtual treasure trove of information. Write each company and request copies of their last two annual reports. A comparison of sales, income, and other data over this period may enable you to discover some interesting things about their overall financial health and growth potential. Many libraries also have collections of annual reports from major corporations.

Attempting to learn about your interviewer is hard work, the importance of which is underestimated by most applicants (who then, of course, don't bother to do it). Being one of the exceptions may get you a job. Find out if he or she has written any articles that have appeared in the trade press or, even better, books on his or her area(s) of expertise. Referring to these writings during the course of an interview, without making it too obvious a compliment, can be very effective. We all have egos and we all like people to talk about us. The interviewer is no different from the rest of us. You might also check to see if any of your networking contacts worked with him or her at his current (or a previous) company and can help fill you in.

Selection vs. Screening Interviews

The process to which the majority of this chapter is devoted is the actual **selection interview,** usually conducted by the person to whom the new hire will be reporting. But there is another process—the **screening interview**—which many of you may have to survive first.

Screening interviews are usually conducted by a member of the human resources department. Though they may not be empowered to hire, they are in a position to screen out or eliminate those candidates they feel (based on the facts) are not qualified to handle the job. These decisions are not usually made on the basis of personality, appearance, eloquence, persuasiveness, or any other subjective criteria, but rather by clicking off yes or no answers against a checklist of skills. If you don't have the requisite number, you will be eliminated from further consideration. This may seem arbitrary, but it is a realistic and often necessary way for corporations to minimize the time and dollars involved in filling even the lowest jobs on the corporate ladder.

Remember, screening personnel are not looking for reasons to *hire* you; they're trying to find ways to *eliminate* you from the job search pack. Resumes sent blindly to the personnel department will usually be subjected to such screening; you will be eliminated without any personal contact (an excellent reason to construct a superior resume and not send out blind mailings).

If you are contacted, it will most likely be by telephone. When you are responding to such a call, keep these four things in mind: 1) It is an interview, be on your guard; 2) Answer all questions honestly; 3) Be enthusiastic; and 4) Don't offer any more information than you are asked for. Remember, this is another screening step, so don't say anything that will get you screened out before you even get in. You will get the standard questions from the interviewer—his or her attempts to "flesh out" the information included on your resume and/or cover letter. Strictly speaking, they are seeking out any negatives which may exist. If your resume is honest and factual (and it should be), you have no reason to be anxious, because you have nothing to hide.

Don't be nervous—be glad you were called and remember your objective: to get past this screening phase so you can get on to the real interview.

The Day of the Interview

On the day of the interview, wear a conservative (not funereal) business suit— *not* a sports coat, *not* a "nice" blouse and skirt. Shoes should be shined, nails cleaned, hair cut and in place. And no low-cut or tight-fitting clothes.

It's not unusual for resumes and cover letters to head in different directions when a company starts passing them around to a number of executives. If you sent them, both may even be long gone. So bring along extra copies of your resume and your own copy of the cover letter that originally accompanied it.

Whether or not you make them available, we suggest you prepare a neatly-typed list of references (including the name, title, company, address, and phone number of each person). You may want to bring along a copy of your high school or college transcript, especially if it's something to brag about. (Once you get your first job, you'll probably never use it—or be asked for it—again, so enjoy it while you can!)

On Time Means Fifteen Minutes Early

Plan to arrive fifteen minutes before your scheduled appointment. If you're in an unfamiliar city or have a long drive to their offices, allow extra time for the unexpected delays that seem to occur with mind-numbing regularity on important days.

Arriving early will give you some time to check your appearance, catch your breath, check in with the receptionist, learn how to correctly pronounce the interviewer's name, and get yourself organized and battle ready.

Arriving late does not make a sterling first impression. If you are only a few minutes late, it's probably best not to mention it or even excuse yourself. With a little luck, everybody else is behind schedule and no one will notice. However, if you're more than fifteen minutes late, have an honest (or at least serviceable) explanation ready and offer it at your first opportunity. Then drop the subject as quickly as possible and move on to the interview.

The Eyes Have It

When you meet the interviewer, shake hands firmly. People notice handshakes and often form a first impression based solely on them.

Try to maintain eye contact with the interviewer as you talk. This will indicate you're interested in what he or she has to say. Eye contact is important for another reason—it demonstrates to the interviewer that you are confident about yourself and your job skills. That's an important message to send.

Sit straight. Body language is also another important means of conveying confidence.

Should coffee or a soft drink be offered, you may accept (but should do so only if the interviewer is joining you).

Keep your voice at a comfortable level, and try to sound enthusiastic (without imitating Charleen Cheerleader). Be confident and poised and provide direct, accurate, and honest answers to the trickiest questions.

And, as you try to remember all this, just be yourself, and try to act like you're comfortable and almost enjoying this whole process!

Don't Name Drop . . . Conspicuously

A friendly relationship with other company employees may have provided you with valuable information prior to the interview, but don't flaunt such relationships. The interviewer is interested only in how you will relate to him or her and how well he or she surmises you will fit in with the rest of the staff. Name dropping may smack of favoritism. And you are in no position to know who the interviewer's favorite (or least favorite) people are.

On the other hand, if you have established a complex network of professionals through informational interviews, attending trade shows, reading trade magazines, etc., it is perfectly permissible to refer to these people, their companies, conversations you've had, whatever. It may even impress the interviewer with the extensiveness of your preparation.

Fork on the Left, Knife on the Right

Interviews are sometimes conducted over lunch, though this is not usually the case with entry-level people. If it does happen to you, though, try to order something in the middle price range, neither filet mignon nor a cheeseburger.

Do not order alcohol—ever! If your interviewer orders a carafe of wine, politely decline. You may meet another interviewer later who smells the alcohol on your breath, or your interviewer may have a drinking problem. It's just too big a risk to take after you've come so far. Just do your best to maintain your poise, and you'll do fine.

The Importance of Last Impressions

There are some things interviewers will always view with displeasure: street language, complete lack of eye contact, insufficient or vague explanations or answers, a noticeable lack of energy, poor interpersonal skills (i.e., not listening or the basic inability to carry on an intelligent conversation), and a demonstrable lack of motivation.

Every impression may count. And the very *last* impression an interviewer has may outweigh everything else. So, before you allow an interview to end, summarize why you want the job, why you are qualified, and what, in particular, you can offer their company.

Then, take some action. If the interviewer hasn't told you about the rest of the interview process and/or where you stand, ask him or her. Will you be seeing other people that day? If so, ask for some background on anyone else with whom you'll be interviewing. If there are no other meetings that day, what's the next step? When can you expect to hear from them about coming back?

Ask for a business card. This will make sure you get the person's name and title right when you write your follow-up letter. You can staple it to the company file for easy reference as you continue networking. When you return home, file all the business cards, copies of correspondence, and notes from the interview(s) with each company in the appropriate files. Finally, but most importantly, ask yourself which firms you really want to work for and which you are no longer interested in. This will quickly determine how far you want the process at each to develop before you politely tell them to stop considering you for the job.

Immediately send a thank-you letter to each executive you met. These should, of course, be neatly typed business letters, not handwritten notes (unless you are most friendly, indeed, with the interviewer and want to stress the "informal" nature of your note). If you are still interested in pursuing a position at their company, tell them in no uncertain terms. Reiterate why you feel you're the best candidate and tell each of the executives when you hope (expect?) to hear from them.

On the Eighth Day God Created Interviewers

Though most interviews will follow a relatively standard format, there will undoubtedly be a wide disparity in the skills of the interviewers you meet. Many of these executives (with the exception of the human resources staff) will most likely not have extensive interviewing experience, have limited knowledge of interviewing techniques, use them infrequently, be hurried by the other duties, or not even view your interview as critically important.

Rather than studying standardized test results or utilizing professional evaluation skills developed over many years of practice, these nonprofessionals react intuitively—their initial (first five minutes) impressions are often the lasting and over-riding factors they remember. So you must sell yourself—fast.

The best way to do this is to try to achieve a comfort level with your interviewer. Isn't establishing rapport—through words, gestures, appearance common interests, etc.—what you try to do in *any* social situation? It's just trying to know one another better. Against this backdrop, the questions and answers will flow in a more natural way.

The Set Sequence

Irrespective of the competence levels of the interviewer, you can anticipate an interview sequence roughly as follows:

- Greetings
- Social niceties (small talk)
- Purpose of meeting (let's get down to business)
- Broad questions/answers
- Specific questions/ answers
- In-depth discussion of company, job, and opportunity
- Summarizing information given & received
- Possible salary probe (this should only be brought up at a second interview)
- Summary/indication as to next steps

When you look at this sequence closely, it is obvious that once you have gotten past the greeting, social niceties and some explanation of the job (in the "getting down to business" section), the bulk of the interview will be questions—yours and the interviewer's. In this question and answer session, there are not necessarily any right or wrong answers, only good and bad ones.

Be forewarned, however. This sequence is not written in stone, and some interviewers will deliberately **not** follow it. Some interviewers will try to fluster you by asking off-the-wall questions, while others are just eccentric by nature. Be prepared for anything once the interview has started.

It's Time to Play Q & A

You can't control the "chemistry" between you and the interviewer—do you seem to "hit it off" right from the start or never connect at all? Since you can't control such a subjective problem, it pays to focus on what you *can* control—the questions you will be asked, your answers and the questions you had better be prepared to ask.

Not surprisingly, many of the same questions pop up in interview after interview, regardless of company size, type, or location. I have chosen the 14 most common— along with appropriate hints and answers for each—for inclusion in this chapter. Remember: There are no right or wrong answers to these questions, only good and bad ones.

Substance counts more than speed when answering questions. Take your time and make sure that you listen to each question—there is nothing quite as disquieting as a lengthy, intelligent answer that is completely irrelevant to the question asked. You wind up looking like a programmed clone with stock answers to dozens of questions who has, unfortunately, pulled the wrong one out of the grab bag.

Once you have adequately answered a specific question, it is permissible to go beyond it and add more information if doing so adds something to the discussion and/or highlights a particular strength, skill, course, etc. But avoid making lengthy speeches just for the sake of sounding off. Even if the interviewer asks a question that is right up your "power alley", one you could talk about for weeks, keep your answers short. Under two minutes for any answer is a good rule of thumb.

Study the list of questions (and hints) that follow, and prepare at least one solid, concise answer for each. Practice with a friend until your answers to these most-asked questions sound intelligent, professional and, most important, unmemorized and unrehearsed.

"Why do you want to be in this field?"

Using your knowledge and understanding of the particular field, explain why you find the business exciting and where and what role you see yourself playing in it.

"Why do you think you will be successful in this business?"

Using the information from your self-evaluation and the research you did on that particular company, formulate an answer which marries your strengths to their's and to the characteristics of the position for which you're applying.

"Why did you choose our company?"

This is an excellent opportunity to explain the extensive process of education and research you've undertaken. Tell them about your strengths and how you match up with their firm. Emphasize specific things about their company that led you to seek an interview. Be a salesperson—be convincing.

"What can you do for us?"

Construct an answer that essentially lists your strengths, the experience you have which will contribute to your job performance, and any other unique qualifications that will place you at the head of the applicant pack. Use action-oriented words to tell exactly what you think you can do for the company—all your skills mean nothing if you can't use them to benefit the company you are interviewing with. Be careful: This is a question specifically designed to *eliminate* some of that pack. Sell yourself. Be one of the few called back for a second interview.

"What position here interests you?"

If you're interviewing for a specific position, answer accordingly. If you want to make sure you don't close the door on other opportunities of which you might be unaware, you can follow up with your own question: "I'm here to apply for your occupational therapist opening. Is there another position open for which you feel I'm qualified?"

If you've arranged an interview with a company without knowing of any specific openings, use the answer to this question to describe the kind of work you'd like to do and why you're qualified to do it. Avoid a specific job title, since they will tend to vary from firm to firm.

If you're on a first interview with the human resources department, just answer the question. They only want to figure out where to send you.

"What jobs have you held and why did you leave them?"

Or the direct approach: "Have you ever been fired?" Take this opportunity to expand on your resume, rather than precisely answering the question by merely recapping your job experiences. In discussing each job, point out what you liked about it, what factors led to your leaving, and how the next job added to your continuing professional education. If you have been fired, say so. It's very easy to check.

"What are your strengths and weaknesses?"

Or **"What are your hobbies (or outside interests)?"** Both questions can be easily answered using the data you gathered to complete the self-evaluation process. Be wary of being too forthcoming about your glaring faults (nobody expects you to volunteer every weakness and mistake), but do not reply, "I don't have any." They won't believe you and, what's worse, you won't believe you. After all, you did the evaluation—you know it's a lie!

Good answers to these questions are those in which the interviewer can identify benefits for him or herself. For example: "I consider myself to be an excellent planner. I am seldom caught by surprise and I prize myself on being able to anticipate problems and schedule my time to be ahead of the game. I devote a prescribed number of hours each week to this activity. I've noticed that many people just react. If you plan ahead, you should be able to cut off most problems before they arise."

You may consider disarming the interviewer by admitting a weakness, but doing it in such a way as to make it relatively unimportant to the job function. For example: "Higher mathematics has never been my strong suit. Though I am competent enough, I've always envied my friends with a more mathematical bent. In this industry, though, I haven't found this a liability. I'm certainly quick enough in figuring out how close I am to deadlines."

"Do you think your extracurricular activities were worth the time you devoted to them?"

This is a question often asked of entry-level candidates. One possible answer: "Very definitely. As you see from my resume, I have been quite active in the Student Government and French Club. My language fluency allowed me to spend my junior year abroad as an exchange student, and working in a functioning government gave me firsthand knowledge of what can be accomplished with people in the real world. I suspect my marks would have been somewhat higher had I not taken on so many activities outside of school, but I feel the balance they gave me contributed significantly to my overall growth as a person."

"What are your career goals?"

Interviewers are always seeking to probe the motivations of prospective employees. Nowhere is this more apparent than when the area of ambition is discussed. The key answer to this question might be; "Given hard work, company growth, and personal initiative, I'd look forward to being in a top executive position by the time I'm 35. I believe in effort and the risk/reward system—my research on this company has shown me that it operates on the same principles. I would hope it would select its future leaders from those people who displaying such characteristics."

"At some future date would you be willing to relocate?"

Pulling up one's roots is not the easiest thing in the world to do, but it is often a fact of life in the corporate world. If you're serious about your career (and such a move often represents a step up the career ladder), you will probably not mind such a move. Tell the interviewer. If you really *don't* want to move, you may want to say so, too—though I would find out how probable or frequent such relocations would be before closing the door while still in the interview stage.

Keep in mind that as you get older, establish ties in a particular community, marry, have children, etc., you will inevitably feel less jubilation at the thought of moving once a year or even "being out on the road." So take the opportunity to experience new places and experiences while you're young. If you don't, you may never get the chance.

"How did you get along with your last supervisor?"

This question is designed to understand your relationship with (and reaction to) authority. Remember: Companies look for team players, people who will fit in with their hierarchy, their rules, their ways of doing things. An answer might be: "I prefer to work with smart, strong people who know what they want and can express themselves. I learned in the military that in order to accomplish the mission, someone has to be the leader and that person has to be given the authority to lead. Someday I aim to be that leader. I hope then my subordinates will follow me as much and as competently as I'm ready to follow now."

"What are your salary requirements?"

If they are at all interested in you, this question will probably come up, though it is more likely at a second interview. The danger, of course, is that you may price yourself too low or, even worse, right out of a job you want. Since you will have a general idea of industry figures for that position (and may even have an idea of what that company tends to pay new people for the position), why not refer to a range of salaries, such as $25,000 - $30,000?

If the interviewer doesn't bring up salary at all, it's doubtful you're being seriously considered, so you probably don't need to even bring the subject up. (If you know you aren't getting the job or aren't interested in it if offered, you may try to nail down a salary figure in order to be better prepared for the next interview.)

"Tell me about yourself"

Watch out for this one! It's often one of the first questions asked. If you falter here, the rest of the interview could quickly become a downward slide to nowhere. Be prepared, and consider it an opportunity to combine your answers to many of the previous questions into one concise description of who you are, what you want to be, and why that company should take a chance on you. Summarize your resume—briefly—and expand on particular courses or experiences relevant to the firm or position. Do not go on about your hobbies or personal life, where you spent your summer vacation, or anything that is not relevant to securing that job. You may explain how that particular job fits in with your long-range career goals and talk specifically about what attracted you to their company in the first place.

"Do you have any questions?"

It's the last fatal question on our list, often the last one an interviewer throws at you after an hour or two of grilling. Even if the interview has been very long and unusually thorough, you *should* have questions—about the job, the company, even the industry. Unfortunately, by the time this question off-handedly hits the floor, you are already looking forward to leaving and may have absolutely nothing to say.

Preparing yourself for an interview means more than having answers for some of the questions an interviewer may ask. It means having your own set of questions—at least five or six—for the interviewer. The interviewer is trying to find the right person for the job. You're trying to find the right job. So you should be just as curious about him or her and the company as he or she is about you. Be careful with any list of questions prepared ahead of time. Some of them were probably answered during the course of the interview, so to ask that same question at this stage would demonstrate poor listening skills. Listening well is becoming a lost art, and its importance cannot be stressed enough. (See the box on this page for a short list of questions you may consider asking on any interview).

The Not-So-Obvious Questions

Every interviewer is different and, unfortunately, there are no rules saying he or she has to use all or any of the "basic" questions covered above. But we think the odds are against his or her avoiding all of them. Whichever of these he or she includes, be assured most interviewers do like to come up with questions that are "uniquely theirs." It may be just one or a whole series—questions developed over the years that he or she feels help separate the wheat from the chaff.

You can't exactly prepare yourself for questions like, "What would you do if...(fill in the blank with some obscure occurrence)?," "What do you remember about kindergarten?," or "What's your favorite ice cream flavor?" Every interviewer we know has his or her favorites and all of these questions seem to come out of left field. Just stay relaxed, grit your teeth (quietly), and take a few seconds to frame a reasonably intelligent reply.

Your Turn to Ask the Questions

1. What will my typical day be like?
2. What happened to the last person who had this job?
3. Given my attitude and qualifications, how would you estimate my chances for career advancement at your company?
4. Why did you come to work here? What keeps you here?
5. If you were I, would you start here again?
6. How would you characterize the management philosophy of your company?
7. What characteristics do the successful employees at your company have in common?
8. What's the best (and worst) thing about working here?

The Downright Illegal Questions

Some questions are more than inappropriate—they are illegal. The Civil Rights Act of 1964 makes it illegal for a company to discriminate in its hiring on the basis of race, color, religion, sex, or national origin. It also means that any interview questions covering these topics are strictly off-limits. In addition to questions about race and color, what other types of questions can't be asked? Some might surprise you:

- Any questions about marital status, number and ages of dependents, or marriage or child-bearing plans.
- Any questions about your relatives, their addresses, or their place of origin.
- Any questions about your arrest record. If security clearance is required, it can be done after hiring but before you start the job.

A Quick Quiz to Test Your Instincts

After reading the above paragraphs, read through the 10 questions below. Which ones do you think would be legal to ask at a job interview? Answers provided below.

1. Confidentially, what is your race?
2. What kind of work does your spouse do?
3. Are you single, married, or divorced?

4. What is your native language?

5. Who should we notify in case of an emergency?

6. What clubs, societies, or organizations do you belong to?

7. Do you plan to have a family?

8. Do you have any disability?

9. Do you have a good credit record?

10. What is your height and weight?

The answer? Not a single question out of the 10 is legal at a job interview, because all could lead to a discrimination suit. Some of the questions would become legal once you were hired (obviously a company would need to know who to notify in an emergency), but none belong at an interview.

Now that you know what an interviewer can't ask you, what if he or she does? Well, don't lose your cool, and don't point out that the question may be outside the law—the nonprofessional interviewer may not realize such questions are illegal, and such a response might confuse, even anger, him or her.

Instead, whenever any questions are raised that you feel are outside legal boundaries, politely state that you don't understand how the question has bearing on the job opening and ask the interviewer to clarify his or herself. If the interviewer persists, you may be forced to state that you do not feel comfortable answering questions of that nature. Bring up the legal issue as a last resort, but if things reach that stage, you probably don't want to work for that company after all.

Testing and Applications

Though not part of the selection interview itself, job applications, skill tests, and psychological testing are often part of the pre-interview process. You should know something about them.

The job application is essentially a record-keeping exercise—simply the transfer of work experience and educational data from your resume to a printed application forms. Though taking the time to recopy data may seem like a waste of time, some companies simply want the information in a particular order on a standard form. One difference: Applications often require the listing of references and salary levels achieved. Be sure to bring your list of references with you to any interview (so you can transfer the pertinent information), and don't lie about salary history; it's easily checked.

Many companies now use a variety of psychological tests as additional mechanisms to screen out undesirable candidates. Although their accuracy is subject to question, the companies that use them obviously believe they are effective at identifying applicants whose personality makeups would preclude their participating positively in a given work situation, especially those at the extreme ends of the behavior spectrum.

Their usefulness in predicting job accomplishment is considered limited. If you are normal (like the rest of us), you'll have no trouble with these tests and may even find them amusing. Just don't try to outsmart them—you'll just wind up outsmarting yourself.

Stand Up and Be Counted

Your interview is over. Breathe a sigh of relief. Make your notes—you'll want to keep a file on the important things covered for use in your next interview. Some people consider one out of 10 (one job offer for every 10 interviews) a good score—if you're keeping score. We suggest you don't. It's virtually impossible to judge how others are judging you. Just go on to the next interview. Sooner than you think, you'll be hired. For the right job.

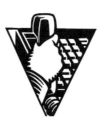

JOB
OPPORTUNITIES
DATABANK

CHAPTER TWENTY-THREE

Job Opportunities Databank

The Job Opportunities Databank contains listings for nearly 350 general medical and surgical hospitals, rehabilitation centers, intermediate and long-term care facilities, and pharmaceutical companies that offer entry-level hiring and/or internships. It is divided into two sections: Entry-Level Job and Internship Listings, which provides full descriptive entries for companies in the United States; and Additional Companies, which includes name, address, and telephone information only for companies that did not respond to our inquiries. For complete details on the information provided in this chapter, please consult "How to Use the Job Opportunities Databank" in the front of this directory.

Entry-Level Job and Internship Listings

Adventist Health Systems/Sunbelt Inc.
2400 Bedford Rd.
Orlando, FL 32803-1489
Phone: (407)897-1919
Fax: (407)897-5521

Business Description: Operator of general medical and surgical hospitals.

Officers: Mardian Jay Blair, President; Calvin Weiss, Sr. VP of Finance.

Benefits: Benefits include medical insurance (80/20 co-pay), vision insurance, dental insurance, tuition assistance, and life insurance.

Application Procedures: Come in for an application or submit a resume to the human resources department at one of the eighteen hospitals that the company operates. Candidates for finance positions must possess a CPA.

▶ **Internships**

Contact: Calvin Weiss, Sr. VP & Finance Officer.

Type: Paid.

Qualifications: Applicants must have a college degree.

A.L. Laboratories, Inc.
1 Executive Dr.
PO Box 1399
Fort Lee, NJ 07024
Phone: (201)947-7774
Fax: (201)947-0912

Business Description: International pharmaceutical company engaged in developing, manufacturing, and marketing branded, value-added generic pharmaceuticals, as well as animal health micronutrients and bulk antibiotics. A.L. Laboratories is currently developing treatments for periodontitis, denture stomatitis, and vaginal yeast infections, as well as for respiratory and systemic diseases in broilers, turkeys, and cattle. For the past several years, the company has been carrying out a capital expenditure program that includes expanding plant capacity, modernizing its laboratories, and upgrading its information systems. At the same time, A.L. Laboratories has reduced its activity in the human nutrition segment.

Officers: William P. Altman, Vice Pres. Pharmaceutical Business Development; Nils Johannesson, Vice Pres. Pharmaceutical Research and Development; Iris D. Daniels, Asst. Sec.; Glenn E. Hess, Secretary; Robert A. Pudlak, VP of Finance & CFO; Jeffrey E. Smith, Exec. VP; John S. Towler, Controller; Thomas E. Wagner, Dir. of Information Systems.

Average Entry-Level Hiring: Hiring levels are expected to increase in the next few years.

Benefits: Benefits include an employee pension plan, a savings plan, tuition assistance, bonuses/incentives, medical insurance, dental insurance, vision insurance, life insurance, short-term disability, long-term disability, paid holidays, two flexible holidays per year, and one to two weeks vacation per year.

Human Resources: Lorraine Catarcil; Patricia Giles.

Application Procedures: Send resume and cover letter to one of the following: Lorraine Catarcil.; Patricia Giles.

▶ **Internships**

Type: The company does not offer an internship program.

Alaska Psychiatric Institute

2900 Providence Dr.
Anchorage, AK 99508
Phone: (907)561-1633

Opportunities: Hires psychiatric nursing assistants with at least a high school diploma and appropriately degreed and certified nurses.

Benefits: Benefits include medical insurance, life insurance, dental insurance, vision insur-

ance, savings plan, profit sharing, and retirement plans.

Human Resources: Gale White.

Application Procedures: Those interested should apply in person. Jim Gordon.

▶ **Internships**

Contact: Jim Gordon, Administrative Assistant.

Type: Offers paid internships. College credit is available. **Number Available Annually:** 1.

Qualifications: Must be a college student.

Allergan Inc.

2525 Dupont Dr.
PO Box 19534
Irvine, CA 92713-9534
Phone: (714)752-4500
Toll-free: 800-347-4500

Business Description: Produces prescription and non-prescription eye and skin care products, including contact lenses and lens care products, ophthalmic surgical products, and pharmaceuticals.

Officers: Edgar J. Cummins, Sr. VP & CFO; Gavin S. Herbert, CEO & Chairman of the Board.

Benefits: Benefits include medical insurance, dental insurance, vision insurance, life insurance, long-term disability, short-term disability, a savings plan, tuition assistance, bonuses/incentives, 10-11 paid holidays and two personal/sick days per year, 10 vacation days after one year, maternity leave, company-sponsored sports teams, a cafeteria, flex time, a smoke-free environment, and training programs.

Human Resources: Randy Starling.

Application Procedures: The company posts available positions in the employment lobby every week. An employment opportunity listing is also published. Additionally, the company accepts unsolicited resumes. Interested candidates should contact Human Resources for more information.

▶ **Internships**

Type: The company offers an internship program.

Qualifications: Must be a college student.

Application Procedure: Interested candidates should contact Human Resources.

Allied Services

PO Box 1103
Scranton, PA 18501
Phone: (717)348-1405

Business Description: Rehabilitation hospitals specializing in physical therapy, speech, and psychological therapy.

Officers: James Brady, President; Tom Parshall, Sr. VP; William Schoen, Vice Chairman of the Board; Jackie Fletcher-Brozena, VP of Operations; Jacqueline Cooney, Asst. VP.

Opportunities: Hires GNs, administrative workers, clinical workers, and social workers.

Benefits: Offers a comprehensive benefit program, including medical insurance, life insurance, dental insurance, and vision insurance.

Application Procedures: Send resume to Human Resources.

▶ Internships

Contact: Francine Kevra, Corporate Education.

Type: Offers unpaid internships for credit to junior college students. **Number Available Annually:** 5.

Application Procedure: Apply to Francine Kevra in the Corporate Education Department.

Alta Bates-Herrick Hospital

2855 Telegraph, Ste. 614
Berkeley, CA 94131
Phone: (510)540-1584
Fax: (510)204-4852

Business Description: Services provided are for acute care, rehabilitation, and mental health, both psychiatric and rehabilitative. There are also two Sportcare outpatient facilities.

Employees: 2,600. The entry level hiring number indicates 40 nursing positions, and 50 non-nursing positions.

Average Entry-Level Hiring: 90.

Opportunities: Physical therapy, speech therapy, occupational therapy, nursing, medical social workers—B.S. degree and California license registration. Radiology technicians, respiratory therapist, radiation oncology—certification required. Clerical and support positions available in business services, accounting, admitting, administration, engineering, medical records, and other specialized areas such as the AIDS clinic.

Human Resources: Mary Martha Beaton; Linda Camezon.

Alternatives Inc.

PO Box 338
Somerville, NJ 08876
Phone: (908)685-1444

Business Description: Chain of physical therapist offices.

Officers: Nancy Good, President.

Opportunities: Hires entry-level part-time staff. Previous experience and a high school diploma are required.

Benefits: Benefits include medical insurance, life insurance, dental insurance, disability insurance, and 401(k).

Human Resources: Steve Kalucki.

Application Procedures: Send resume and cover letter to the attention of

▶ Internships

Contact: Steve Kalucki.

Type: Offers paid and unpaid internships. **Number Available Annually:** 1.

Qualifications: College students majoring in psychology or social work.

According to the U.S. Department of Labor's moderate growth projections . . . the number of positions available for occupational therapists will increase approximately 49 percent between the years 1988 and 2000. This translates to an increase of 10,000 positions.

Source: *The American Journal of Occupational Therapy*

American Health Partners

28 W. 23rd St.
New York, NY 10011
Phone: (212)366-8900
Fax: (212)366-8648

Employees: 98.

Average Entry-Level Hiring: 2-3.

Opportunities: Positions as editorial assistants and research assistants require a college degree, typing and computer skills, knowledge of grammar, good writing skills, and an independent attitude.

Human Resources: Mary Witherall.

▶ **Internships**

Type: The company does not offer an internship program.

American Healthcare Management Inc.

660 American Ave., Ste. 200
King of Prussia, PA 19406
Phone: (215)768-5900

Business Description: Owns and operates hospitals, with emphasis on acute care.

Officers: Bruce J. Colburn, Controller; Brian G. Costello, Vice Pres.; Robert M. Dubbs, VP, Counsel & Sec.; Robert W. Fleming, Jr., Sr. VP; William A. Johnsen, Sr. VP & Finance Officer; Marvin Rushkoff, Chairman of the Board; Thomas M. Sposito, Vice Pres.; Steven Volla, Pres., CEO, CFO & Treasurer.

Opportunities: The company offers minimal entry level positions.

Benefits: Benefits include medical insurance, 401(k), dental insurance, life insurance, long term disability, 12 sick days, two weeks paid vacation.

Human Resources: Brian G. Costello; Jennifer Gordon.

Application Procedures: Send resume and cover letter to the attention of Brian G. Costello. PO Box 1509, King of Prussia, PA 19406.

▶ **Internships**

Type: The company does not offer any internship programs.

American Medical International Inc.

414 N. Camden Dr.
Beverly Hills, CA 90210
Phone: (310)278-6200

Business Description: American Medical International and its affiliates operate about 50 hospitals in the United States. The company is the nation's 3rd largest hospital chain and employs nearly 37,000 at its hospitals.

Officers: Harry J. Gray, CEO & Chairman of the Board; W. Randolph Smith, Sr. VP & CFO.

Application Procedures: Accepts unsolicited resumes. Applications will be mailed to those requesting them by mail and by phone. Apply in person or send resume and cover letter to the attention of Human Resources.

American Medical International Inc.
AMI Brookwood Medical Center

2010 Brookwood Medical Center
Birmingham, AL 35259
Phone: (205)877-1000
Fax: (205)877-2548

Business Description: A complete health care complex. The company supports a core of medical, surgical, and emergency facilities, including a variety of specialized centers—Medical and Surgical Services, Women's Medical Center, Regional Cancer Institute, Center for Mental Health, Business Health Services, Eye Institute, Foot Care Center, DIACON - Diabetes Control Centers, The Center for Health and Fitness, The Occupational Health Center, Home Care, Home Care Plus, and Hospice, Nutrition Counseling, The Center for Rehabilitation, The Family Counseling Center, and Family Health Centers.

Officers: Gregory H. Burfitt, President; Cathy Nazeer, CFO; Paul Pretsch, Sr. VP of Mktg.

Average Entry-Level Hiring: Hiring levels are expected to remain constant over the next year.

Opportunities: Hires accountants, hospital administrators, managers, departmental directors, registered nurses, dieticians, pharmacists, physicians, respiratory therapists, radiology technologists, occupational therapists, sonographers, polysomnographic technicians, medical lab technicians, medical record administrators, product line managers, secretaries, LPNs, PBX operators, receptionists, financial assistants, insurance clerks, dietary aides, patient transporters, cooks, environmental service technicians, security officers, and plant operation maintenance workers.

Benefits: Benefits include life insurance, medical insurance, dental insurance, vision insurance, long-term disability, an employee pension plan, a 401(k) plan, child-care programs, flex time, a smoke-free environment, a cafeteria, tuition assistance, bonuses/incentives, employee assistance program, free and covered employee parking, service award plans, workers compensation, and up to 3 days paid bereavement leave.

Human Resources: Linda Foster; Patti Reese; Marsha Fields.

Application Procedures: Recruits regionally at college campuses in the southeast on college placement days. Recruits at trade shows and professional exhibits, including nursing and allied health professional associations. Recruits through employment agencies, including state employment offices and occupational rehabilitation services. Maintains a job hotline at 205-877-1910. Apply in person at AMI Brookwood Medical Center, Human Resources, 557 Brookwood Blvd., Birmingham, Alabama, between 9:00 A.M. and 3:30 P.M., or send resume and cover letter to the attention of Linda Foster.

▶ Internships

Type: Offers an internship program through the individual medical schools.

American Treatment Centers Inc.
PO Box 667
Lebanon, IN 46052
Phone: (317)482-0991

Business Description: Rehabilitation hospitals for alcohol and drug addiction.

Officers: Richard Shabi, President; Michael Heiniger, Controller; Jon Millan, Dir. of Mktg.; Bobbie Hennessy, VP of Admin.; Bobbie Hennessy, VP of Admin.

Aquatic Rehabilitation Center Inc.
10567 Montgomery Dr.
Cincinnati, OH 45242
Phone: (513)793-5525

Business Description: Physical therapy clinic.

Officers: Stephen Kempf, President.

Arizona State Hospital
2500 E. VanBuren
Phoenix, AZ 85008
Phone: (602)244-1331

Opportunities: Hires appropriately degreed and certified nurses, psychiatric staff, psychologists, and occupational therapists.

Benefits: Benefits include medical insurance, life insurance, dental insurance, vision insurance, savings plan, paid holidays, and disability insurance.

Human Resources: Sue Wilson.

Application Procedures: Those interested

should apply in person. Tonya Prindall, Health Services Personnel Specialist.

▶ Internships

Type: The company does not offer an internship program.

Assured Health Systems Inc.
20 Mall Rd.
Burlington, MA 01803
Phone: (617)273-9966

Business Description: Health care and residential care.

Officers: Ron Geraty, President; Barry Lyons, CFO.

Opportunities: Hires data entry operators and receptionists with a college degree or previous experience.

Benefits: Benefits include life insurance, dental insurance, tuition assistance, child-care programs, elder-care programs, and a 401(k) plan.

Application Procedures: Send a resume for screening.

▶ Internships

Type: The company does not offer an internship program.

> The area of greatest employment growth within the past decade has been that of the small organizations—companies with fewer than 500 employees.
>
> Source: Journal of Career Planning & Employment

Baptist Rehabilitation Institute of Arkansas
9601 Interstate 630, Exit 7
Little Rock, AR 72205-7249
Phone: (501)223-7578

Benefits: Benefits include medical insurance, life insurance, dental insurance, vision insurance, a savings plan, and child or elder care.

▶ Internships

Type: The company offers paid internships to students for college credit in physical therapy, pharmacy, human resources, administration, occupational therapy, and social work areas.

Application Procedure: Send applications to the Vice President of Human Resources.

Barnes Hospital

1 Barnes Hospital Plz.
St. Louis, MO 63110
Phone: (314)362-0701
Fax: (314)362-0708

Employees: 6,000.

Average Entry-Level Hiring: Unknown.

Opportunities: Nurse—two-, three-, or four-year degree. Occupational and physical therapists—bachelor's degree.

Human Resources: Carol Esrock; Wally Kline.

Application Procedures: Call for more information.

Baxter Healthcare Corp.

70 S. Cleveland Ave.
Westerville, OH 43081
Phone: (614)794-1505

Business Description: Surgical and medical instruments and hospital apparel. Mail-order pharmaceuticals.

Officers: Jim Tobin, President; Robert Lambrix, Sr. VP; Ergin Uskup, VP of Intl. Sales; Barbara Morris, Sr. VP.

Opportunities: Hires entry-level physical therapists.

Benefits: Benefits include medical insurance, life insurance, dental insurance, and vision insurance. Also offers savings plan, profit sharing, elder-care programs, and a 401(k) plan.

Human Resources: Colleen Shannon.

Application Procedures: Fill out an application or send a resume to the attention of Colleen Shannon.

▶ Internships

Type: The company does not offer an internship program.

Bergan Mercy Hospital Sisters of Mercy

7500 Mercy Rd.
Omaha, NE 68124
Phone: (402)398-6168
Fax: (402)398-6920

Employees: 2,600.

Average Entry-Level Hiring: 500+ per year.

Opportunities: All positions require Nebraska state licensure or eligibility for licensure. RN/LPN home care— two years of acute care experience. Physical therapist—B.S. in physical therapy from an accredited PT school. Occupational therapist—B.S. in OT, AOTA licensure. Medical technologist—B.S. ASCP registry. Radiology technologist—Completion of 24 month program in radiology from an accredited program, ARRT registered. Radiation therapy technologist—same as RT, including completion of 12 month program in radiation therapy. Pharmacist—B.S. or Doctorate in pharmacy.

Human Resources: Katie Staebell; Gail Hafer.

Berlex Laboratories Inc.

300 Fairfield Rd.
Wayne, NJ 07470
Phone: (201)694-4100

Business Description: Engaged in manufacturing, fabricating and/or processing drugs in pharmaceutical preparations.

Officers: Jorge Engel, CEO & Pres.; Robert Liptrot, Dir. of Sales; Howard Robin, VP of Finance; Edward Walters, Dir. of Info. Systems.

Human Resources: Jack W. Malpass.

Application Procedures: Interested candidates can fill in an application in person on Wednesdays or can submit completed applications to Robin Coleman.

▶ Internships

Type: The company does not offer any internship programs.

Beth Abraham Hospital

612 Allerton Ave.
Bronx, NY 10467
Phone: (212)920-6021
Fax: (212)920-2632

Employees: 950.

Average Entry-Level Hiring: Unknown.

Opportunities: Physician assistants—New York State registration required. Physical therapist, registered nurses, LPNs, occupational therapist—New York State license required. Nursing attendant—New York State certification and completion of 102 hour course for nursing home aide. Registered pharmacist—New York

State registration required. Secretary—typing and word processing skills required, Lotus 1-2-3.

Human Resources: Matt Stollper.

Beth Israel Hospital
70 Parker Ave.
Passaic, NJ 07055
Phone: (201)365-5008
Fax: (201)471-5531

Employees: 900.

Average Entry-Level Hiring: Unknown.

Opportunities: RN—two-, or three-, or four-year degrees. Many other entry-level positions available.

Human Resources: Patricia Wilson.

Application Procedures: Call for more information.

Birchwood Laboratories Inc.
7900 Fuller Rd.
Eden Prairie, MN 55344
Phone: (612)937-7900

Business Description: Engaged in manufacturing, fabricating and/or processing drugs in pharmaceutical preparations. Manufacturer of polishes, waxes, disinfectants, or other sanitation preparations.

Officers: J.A. Hay, President; W.M. Shannon, Dir. of Data Processing; S.M. Souder, Dir. of Mktg.; N. Villwock, Treasurer.

Benefits: Benefits include medical insurance, dental insurance, and life insurance.

Human Resources: J. Manuele.

Application Procedures: Fill out an application or send resume and cover letter to the attention of the Human Resources Department.

▶ Internships

Type: The company does not offer an internship program.

BOC Health Care Inc.
110 Allen Rd.
PO Box 804
Liberty Corner, NJ 07938-0804
Phone: (908)647-9200

Business Description: Manufacturer of medical, surgical, ophthalmic and/or veterinary instruments and apparatus. Engaged in providing health care services or services related to the provision of health care.

Human Resources: Robert C. Hodge.

Application Procedures: Send resume and cover letter to the attention of Teresa Drummond.

▶ Internships

Type: The company does not offer an internship program.

Your next job need not be at another company. Pay attention to the special skills of people newly hired or recently promoted by your current employer. That will give you an indication of what talents are valued so you can upgrade your skills and re-invent your job to make sure it stays relevant to your company's needs.

Source: *Money*

Boehringer Ingelheim Pharmaceuticals Inc.
900 Ridgebury Rd.
Ridgefield, CT 06877
Phone: (203)798-9988

Business Description: Engaged in manufacturing, fabricating and/or processing drugs in pharmaceutical preparations.

Officers: John Babecki, Info. Systems Mgr.; Digby Barrios, President; Werner Gerstenberg, Exec. VP & CFO; A. James Ueberroth, VP of Mktg.

Benefits: Benefits include medical insurance, dental insurance, life insurance, savings plan, free parking, and up to five paid vacation/sick days.

Human Resources: Richard E. Lindstrom.

Application Procedures: The company advertises vacant positions in the newspaper. Interested applicants should complete applications and return them to the human resources department.

▶ Internships

Type: The company does not offer an internship program.

Bon Secours Hospital

1050 NE 125th St.
North Miami, FL 33161
Phone: (305)891-8850

Opportunities: Hires entry-level personnel in all areas. Requirements depend on the position, but may include previous experience and college course work.

Benefits: Benefits include medical insurance, life insurance, dental insurance, vision insurance, tuition assistance, dependent care account, pension plan, and credit union membership.

Human Resources: Mattie Reddick, Recruiting Specialist.

Application Procedures: Send resume and cover letter, fill out an application, and talk to a recruiter.

▶ Internships

Type: The company does not offer any internship programs.

Bournewood Hospital

300 South St.
Brookline, MA 02167
Phone: (617)320-8352

Human Resources: Sandy McInerny.

Braintree Hospital

250 Pond St.
Braintree, MA 02184
Phone: (617)848-5353

Opportunities: Requires at least a bachelor's degree.

Benefits: Benefits include medical insurance, dental insurance, life insurance, and short-term disability.

Application Procedures: Call or apply to a specific department directly or send resume to the attention of Delorese Plate, Recruitment Coordinator.

Bridgeport Hospital

267 Grant St.
Bridgeport, CT 06610
Phone: (203)384-3384
Fax: (203)384-3966

Employees: 2,500.

Average Entry-Level Hiring: Unknown.

Opportunities: Medical technicians, PTs, OTs, nuclear medicine technicians—experience preferred.

Human Resources: Jedd Santos.

Application Procedures: Call for more information.

Bristol Hospital, Inc.

Brewster Rd.
Bristol, CT 06010
Phone: (203)585-3211
Fax: (203)585-3028

Employees: 1,500.

Average Entry-Level Hiring: Unknown.

Human Resources: Mark Rouleau; Sharon Osenkonski.

Application Procedures: Call for current vacancies and requirements.

Burger Physical Therapy and Rehabilitation Agency Inc.

101 E. Natoma St.
Folsom, CA 95630
Phone: (916)985-0112

Opportunities: Hires therapists with a five-year degree and therapist's aides with a two-year degree.

Benefits: Benefits include medical insurance, life insurance, dental insurance, vision insurance, tuition assistance, child-care programs, elder-care programs, and a 401(k) plan.

Human Resources: Jim Harbison.

Application Procedures: Contact Human Resources by phone.

▶ Internships

Type: Offers paid internships for college credit. **Number Available Annually:** 12-15.

Qualifications: Must be a college student to apply.

Application Procedure: Internships are awarded through the colleges.

Burroughs Wellcome Co.

3030 Cornwallis Rd.
Research Triangle Pa., NC 27709
Phone: (919)248-3000

Business Description: Pharmaceutical manufacturer.

Officers: Philip R. Tracy, CEO; Steve D.

Corman, VP of Finance; Tim Rothwell, VP of Mktg.; Glen Weingarth, Human Resources Dir.

Benefits: Benefits include medical insurance, life insurance, dental insurance, vision insurance, child-care programs, and tuition assistance.

Human Resources: Mitchell Spencer.

Application Procedures: Hiring practices vary depending on the position. Contact the Human Resources department for specific information.

▶ **Internships**

Type: The company does not offer an internship program.

Camargo Manor Inc.
7625 Camargo Rd.
Madeira, OH 45243
Phone: (513)561-6210

Business Description: Intermediate care nursing home.

Officers: Tom Cunningham, Dir. of Admin.; Jerry Stanislaw, Controller.

Human Resources: Carol Ochnelle.

▶ **Internships**

Type: The company does not offer an internship program.

Cancer Care Treatment Centers of America
3455 Salt Creek Ln., Ste. 200
Arlington Hts., IL 60005-1090
Phone: (708)342-7300

Business Description: In and out-patient cancer treatment.

Officers: Richard J. Stephenson, President; Roger O'Connor, VP of Mktg.

Cancer Treatment Associates
1100 Grampian Blvd.
Williamsport, PA 17701
Phone: (717)326-8181

Business Description: Operator of cancer treatment hospital.

Officers: Francis Powers, President.

Opportunities: Hires directors, department heads, technicians, NRNs, and LPNs with college degrees and previous experience.

Benefits: Offers various benefits upon hiring.

Human Resources: Kay Hofer; Sandy Mohonski.

Application Procedures: Apply in person or send resume.

Cardinal Hill Hospital
2050 Versailles Rd.
Lexington, KY 40504
Phone: (606)254-5701

Opportunities: Hires entry-level staff in all areas. Requirements depend on specific position.

Benefits: Benefits include medical insurance, life insurance, dental insurance, credit union membership, and a tax shelter annuity.

Human Resources: Leonard Wills, Director.

Application Procedures: Job openings are posted. Send resume or apply in person to Leonard Wills.

▶ **Internships**

Type: Offers unpaid internships. College credit is available. **Number Available Annually:** 2-5.

Qualifications: Must be a college student.

If complacency is bad for your career, thinking into the future will keep you ahead of change. To others, it will seem as if you are moving effortlessly into the better jobs in the successful department or company. In fact, it will be because you worked hard, planned well and prepared yourself.

Source: *Business Monday/Detroit Free Press*

Care Enterprises Inc.
2742 Dow Ave.
Tustin, CA 92680
Phone: (714)544-4443

Business Description: Pharmaceutical wholesaler and nursing services provider.

Officers: John W. Adams, CEO; Gary L. Massimino, Exec. VP.

Benefits: Benefits include medical insurance, life insurance, dental insurance, and 401(k).

Human Resources: Diane Krosner; Jacky Brandon.

Application Procedures: Hires entry-level staff for the following positions: clerical; nurses aides; housekeepers; laundry; and kitchen help. All prospective applicants must have a high school diploma and be able to communicate effectively in English. Send resume and cover letter to the attention of Human Resources.

▶ **Internships**

Type: Offers paid internships. **Number Available Annually:** 2-3.

Qualifications: College graduates.

Whether you are using file cards or a computer, the trick to your job search is developing a discipline to your efforts. As you begin to send out your resume, you should automatically assign yourself a follow-up date. The idea is to realize that you are now marketing a product that you know very well: yourself.

Source: *H&MM*

CareUnit of Colorado
1290 S. Potomac St.
Aurora, CO 80012
Phone: (303)745-2273
Fax: (303)369-9556

Opportunities: Hires entry-level staff in all areas. Requirements vary depending on the position.

Benefits: Benefits include HML insurance plan, 401(k), and vacation days.

Human Resources: Julie Hansberry, Contact.

Application Procedures: Send resume and cover letter to the attention of Personnel or apply in person and fill out an application.

▶ **Internships**

Type: Offers unpaid internships for college credit. **Number Available Annually:** 3.

Qualifications: College students.

Application Procedure: Applications should be sent to the Personnel Department.

Carolina Medicorp, Inc.
Forsyth Memorial Hospital
3333 Sials Creek Pkwy.
Winston-Salem, NC 27103
Phone: (919)718-5420
Toll-free: 800-777-1876
Fax: (919)718-9253

Business Description: Forsyth Memorial Hospital is the second largest hospital in North Carolina with 911 beds.

Employees: 3,800. 2800 at Forsyth Memorial Hospital.

Average Entry-Level Hiring: 500.

Opportunities: Registered nurses—B.S.N. or associate degree, all clinical areas. Allied health—B.S. degree or two-year technical degree. Areas include respiratory, medical technology, physical and occupational therapy, pharmacy, radiology, radiation oncology, and cytotechnology.

Human Resources: Ann Nusser; Diane Poindexter; Manika Stanley; Sophie Pawlak.

Casa Colina Hospital for Rehabilitation
255 E. Bonita Ave.
Pomona, CA 91767
Phone: (714)593-7521

Benefits: Benefits include medical insurance, life insurance, dental insurance, and retirement plans.

Human Resources: George Bays.

Application Procedures: Entry-level positions are available in the dietary and housekeeping areas. Apply in person or send resume and cover letter to the attention of Human Resources.

▶ **Internships**

Contact: George Bays, Recruiter.

Type: Offers paid and college credit internships.

Qualifications: College juniors and seniors.

Charter Care Corp.
24500 Meadow Brook Rd.
Novi, MI 48375
Phone: (313)477-2000

Business Description: Nursing homes.

Officers: Alexander Spiro Jr., President.

Opportunities: Hires entry-level nurses, nursing assistants, and dietary staff. All applicants must be properly certified.

Benefits: Benefits include medical insurance, life insurance, dental insurance, child-care programs, and 401(k).

Application Procedures: Fill out an application. Resumes are not necessary.

▶ **Internships**

Type: Offers paid internships to college students and professionals. To apply, contact the president of the company. **Number Available Annually:** 1.

Charter Hospital of Long Beach

6060 Paramount Blvd.
Long Beach, CA 90805
Phone: (310)220-1000

Opportunities: Entry-level positions require previous experience and a college degree.

Benefits: Benefits include medical insurance, life insurance, dental insurance, vision insurance, tuition assistance, and profit sharing.

Application Procedures: Contact the human resources department by phone or in person and submit a resume.

▶ **Internships**

Type: Internships are available to college-level juniors and seniors. **Number Available Annually:** Six.

Children's Hospital

8301 Dodge St.
Omaha, NE 68114
Phone: (402)390-8834
Fax: (402)390-8755

Employees: 570.

Average Entry-Level Hiring: 75.

Opportunities: RN, pharmacist—Nebraska license, accredited graduate. Radiology technician—ART registered. Medical technologists—bachelor's degree, ASCP registered. Respiratory therapist—registered or registry eligible.

Human Resources: Sarah Minarick.

Children's Hospital of Orange County

455 S. Main St.
Orange, CA 92668
Phone: (714)997-3000

Opportunities: The company hires entry level staff for clerical positions who have previous experience.

Benefits: Benefits include medical insurance, dental insurance, vision insurance, and a retirement plan.

Human Resources: Nora Rodriguez.

Application Procedures: Applicants should go to the personnel department in person to apply.

▶ **Internships**

Type: The company offers paid internships and internships for college credit. The application procedures vary according to positions. Contact the company for more information.

Ciba-Geigy Corp.
Ciba-Geigy Pharmaceutical Div.

556 Morris Ave.
Summit, NJ 07901
Phone: (908)277-5000

Business Description: Engaged in manufacturing, fabricating and/or processing drugs in pharmaceutical preparations.

Officers: Frank Lasaracina, Controller; William Sheldon, Dir. of Mktg.; Doug Watson, President.

Human Resources: Paul Sartori.

▶ **Internships**

Type: Contact the company for more information.

Colmery-O'Neil Department of Veterans Affairs Medical Center

2200 Gage Blvd.
Topeka, KS 66622
Phone: (913)272-3111
Fax: (913)271-4309

Employees: 1,120.

Average Entry-Level Hiring: 20.

Opportunities: The following positions require a college degree: medical technologist, vocational rehabilitation specialist, pharmacist, physical therapist, occupational therapist, dietician, physician assistant, and social work associate.

Psychologist—Ph.D. required. Social worker—M.S.W. required. Registered nurse—must be a graduate of a professional nursing program or have a bachelor's degree. Nurse anesthetist—must be a graduate of a school of professional nursing and anesthesia. LPN, PTA, OTA—specialized education required.

Human Resources: Christine Myers; Wanda Lyon.

Columbia Health Systems Inc.

2025 E. Newport Rd.
Milwaukee, WI 53211
Phone: (414)961-3300

Business Description: Operators of medical clinics and nursing homes.

Officers: John Sculler, President.

J ob-seekers long have looked to health care as one of their most dependable sources of openings. That's not going to change any time soon, especially as the number of people age 75 and over climbs sharply in the 1990s.

Source: *Business Week*

Columbia Hospital Corp.

777 Main St.
Fort Worth, TX 76102
Phone: (817)878-7700

Officers: Darla Mason, Contact.

Communi-Care/Pro-Rehab Inc.

PO Box 2808
Boone, NC 28607
Phone: (704)264-5987
Toll-free: 800-284-4001
Fax: (704)264-1151

Business Description: Provides speech-language pathology services, physical therapy, and occupational therapy to nursing homes and hospitals. Corporate offices are in North Carolina, with therapists working in central and eastern states. They also serve corporate accounts with fee-for-service, direct billing, or combination contracts.

Officers: Dr. Kenneth A. Hubbard, President; Ms. Lynn R. Hubbard, M.A., Exec. VP.

Benefits: Benefits include medical insurance, short-term disability, sick days, reimbursement for professional licenses, jury duty leave, travel expenses, tuition assistance, a 401(k) plan, stock option plan, and referral bonuses.

Application Procedures: Send resume to the State recruiter's office.

▶ Internships

Type: Offers internships for speech pathologists in each individual location.

Community Hospitals Indianapolis Three Hospital Network

1500 N. Ritter Ave.
Indianapolis, IN 46219
Phone: (317)355-5483
Fax: (317)351-7726

Business Description: Operates a network of three hospitals.

Employees: 6,000. Employee figure represents a total from all three hospitals.

Average Entry-Level Hiring: Unknown.

Opportunities: Hires registered nurses with an associate's degree; physical or occupational therapists and medical technicians with a bachelor's degree; laboratory technicians with an associate's degree; and physical therapy assistants, speech pathologists, nurse anesthetists, nuclear medicine technicians, respiratory therapists, and pharmacists with the required certification.

Human Resources: Jim Bennett, East; Sarah Code, Nurse Recruiter; Erin Farrell, North; Kay Vohs, South.

Application Procedures: Call for more information; North—(317)841-5326; South—(317)887-7280.

Community Lifecare Enterprises

PO Box 20130
Springfield, IL 62708-0130
Phone: (217)523-9368

Business Description: Operator of skilled nursing care facilities other than hospitals. Operator of nursing or personal care facilities that require a lesser degree of care than skilled or intermediate care facilities.

Human Resources: Gary Engelmann.

Application Procedures: Send resume and cover letter to the attention of Gary Engelmann.

Comprehensive Care Corp.

16305 Swingley Ridge Dr., Ste. 100
Chesterfield, MO 63017
Phone: (314)537-1288

Opportunities: Hires entry-level staff in all areas. Requirements vary depending on the position.

Benefits: Benefits include medical insurance, life insurance, dental insurance, vision insurance, savings plan, profit sharing, and 401(k).

Human Resources: Mrs. Chris Margolis; Steve Toth.

Application Procedures: Apply in person, call, or send resume and cover letter to the attention of Steve Toth.

▶ Internships

Type: The company does not offer an internship program.

Concord Hospital

250 Pleasant St.
Concord, NH 03301
Phone: (603)225-2711

Employees: 1,200.

Average Entry-Level Hiring: Unknown.

Opportunities: RNs and physical and occupational therapists.

Human Resources: Jacqui McGettigan.

Application Procedures: Call for more information.

Connecticut Valley Hospital

Silver St.
Middletown, CT 06457
Phone: (203)344-2666

Officers: Regina Jones, Contact.

Opportunities: Hires nurses with training, psychologists with a bachelor's degree, and social workers with a bachelor's degree who have passed the social work examination.

Benefits: Benefits include medical insurance, life insurance, dental insurance, tuition assistance, child-care programs, elder-care programs, personal and vacation leave, and deferred compensation.

Application Procedures: Positions advertised in classifieds. Send resume and cover letter to the attention of Regina Jones.

▶ Internships

Type: Offers paid and unpaid internships to college students of rehabilitative services, psychology, and social work. **Number Available Annually:** 6.

Application Procedure: Psychology internships are listed in the American Psychological Association Journal. Can apply to the Director of Psychology.

Continental Medical Systems Inc.

600 Wilson Ln.
PO Box 715
Mechanicsburg, PA 17055
Phone: (717)790-8300
Fax: (717)766-8277

Business Description: Provides comprehensive medical rehabilitation programs and services. Offers community-based rehabilitation programs and services for patients suffering from strokes and other neurological disorders, orthopedic problems, head injuries, spinal cord injuries, work-related disabilities, and multiple trauma.

Officers: Kenneth F. Barber, Exec. VP & Chief Development Officer; John Bauer, VP & Controller; Roger Breed, VP of Corp. Communications; Richard W. Fiske, VP of Development; Brad E. Hollinger, Sr. VP; David A. Jones, Vice Pres.; Kevin L. Krause, VP of Corp. Development; Dennis L. Lehman, Sr. VP & CFO; Lisa L. MacLean, VP of Mktg.; Stephen G. Marcus, VP of Development; Susan McBroom, Vice Pres.; Anthony F. Misitano, Sr. VP; Kenneth L. Moore, VP & Treasurer; Robert A. Ortenzio, Pres. & COO; Rocco A. Ortenzio, CEO & Chairman of the Board; Scott Romberger, VP & Corp. Controller; Joseph P. Smith, Sr. VP; Deborah M. Welsh, Esq., Vice Pres.

Opportunities: Hires physiatrists, physical therapists, occupational therapists, speech pathologists, RNs, physician specialists, aides, and other medical personnel. These positions require healthcare experience, preferably in the rehabilitation field. Also hires marketing directors, assistants, and administrative support staff.

Benefits: Benefits include medical insurance, dental insurance, life insurance, long-term disability, vision insurance, 401(k), smoke-free environment, and tuition assistance. Also offers a stock purchase plan, paid holidays, sick days, maternity leave, and paid vacations.

Human Resources: Gwen Kissinger; Rodney R. Olsen.

Application Procedures: Recruits nationally at college campuses. Faxed resumes are accepted. Call (717)766-8277. Send resume and cover letter to the attention of the Director of Recruitment. Gwen Kissinger.

▶ **Internships**

Type: Offers an internship program.

Application Procedure: Send applications to the Director of Recruitment.

Thirty years after the Equal Pay Act was passed, women are still earning only 70 cents for every dollar a man makes.

Source: *Working Women*

Cook County Hospital
749 S. Winchester
Chicago, IL 60612
Phone: (312)633-7571

Employees: 6,000.

Average Entry-Level Hiring: 50 per year.

Opportunities: RN—associate, diploma or bachelor's degree required. Many other entry-level positions are typically available.

Application Procedures: Contact the Human Resources Department for more information.

Coreance Inc.
350 Broadway
Boulder, CO 80303
Phone: (303)494-3108

Business Description: Rehabilitation center.

Officers: Joe Costello, President.

CPC St. Johns River Hospital
6300 Beach Blvd.
Jacksonville, FL 32216
Phone: (904)724-9202

Opportunities: Hires entry-level personnel in

---

all areas. Requirements vary depending on the position.

Benefits: Benefits include medical insurance, life insurance, dental insurance, and 401(k).

Human Resources: Priscilla McReynolds.

Application Procedures: Apply in person or send resume and cover letter to the attention of Priscilla McReynolds.

▶ **Internships**

Contact: Priscilla McReynolds.

Type: Offers unpaid internships for college credit.

Application Procedure: Send resume and cover to contact person.

Craig Hospital
3425 S. Clarkson St.
Englewood, CO 80110
Phone: (303)789-8000

Business Description: Operator of specialty hospitals.

Officers: Ron Branish, Controller; Marlene Casini, Dir. of Mktg.; Dennis O'Malley, President.

Opportunities: Applicants must take a drug screen test and a physical examination.

Benefits: Benefits include health care and life insurance, dental insurance, and long-term disability.

Human Resources: Kevin McVeigh.

Application Procedures: Fill out an application in Human Resources.

▶ **Internships**

Type: The company does not offer an internship program.

De Paul Hospital
4143 S. 13th St.
Milwaukee, WI 53221
Phone: (414)281-4400

Business Description: Operator of specialized outpatient facilities.

Officers: Thomas Bozewicz, President; David Oines, CFO; Aenone M. Rosario, Dir. of Mktg.

Opportunities: Applicants must take a physical examination as well as a drug test.

Benefits: Benefits include dental insurance,

medical insurance, long-term disability, short-term disability, and pension plan.

Human Resources: Herbert Steffes.

Application Procedures: Interested candidates should forward applications to the human resources department. Advertises in the classified section of newspapers.

▶ **Internships**

Type: The company does not offer an internship program.

Deaconess Hospital of Cleveland

4229 Pearl Rd.
Cleveland, OH 44109
Phone: (216)459-6300

Business Description: Operator of general medical and surgical hospitals.

Officers: Howard Friedlander, Sr. VP & Finance Officer; Thomas C. Gagen, CEO; Martha Kalin, VP of Mktg.; Miles Visker, Dir. of Info. Systems.

Opportunities: Applicants must take a physical examination.

Benefits: Benefits include dental insurance, medical insurance, vision insurance, long-term disability, paid holidays, paid vacations, maternity leave, pension plan, and tuition assistance.

Human Resources: Amy Clark.

Application Procedures: Applications can be filled out on site. Advertises in the newspaper. The company often promotes from within. Interested candidates should contact the Personnel Department.

▶ **Internships**

Type: The company does not offer internships.

Deaton Hospital and Medical Center of Christ Lutheran Church

611 S. Charles St.
Baltimore, MD 21230
Phone: (410)547-8500

Opportunities: Hires in such areas as food service, housekeeping, security, and nursing. Nursing positions include health care aides and nurses (degrees are required).

Benefits: Benefits include medical insurance, life insurance, disability, personal/sick days,

vacation days, an employee assistance program, 401(k), tuition assistance, and free parking.

Human Resources: Julie Jones, Personnel Recruiter.

Application Procedures: Those interested should apply in person, by phone, or send resume to Julie Jones, Personnel Recruiter.

▶ **Internships**

Contact: Julie Jones, Personnel Recruiter.

Type: Offers summer internships. **Number Available Annually:** 10-20.

Qualifications: Nurses who are between their third and fourth year of school.

L ike your appearance, your attitude can deteriorate from bad habits you develop. Just as you can let the heels of your shoes run down, you can let your attitude run down. And, like your shoes, your attitude can reach a point of where it is so run down that you might as well throw it away and start fresh.

Source: Business Monday/Detroit Free Press

Delaware Curative Workshop

1600 Washington St.
Wilmington, DE 19802
Phone: (302)656-2521

Opportunities: Hires entry-level custodial staff, clerical staff, and clinical technicians. Requirements vary depending upon the position.

Benefits: Benefits include medical insurance, life insurance, savings plan, disability insurance, and 401(k).

Human Resources: Mr. Andreola.

Application Procedures: Send resume and cover letter.

▶ **Internships**

Type: Offers unpaid internships for college credit. **Number Available Annually:** 6.

Qualifications: College students.

Application Procedure: Internships are arranged through the universities.

Department of Veterans Affairs Medical Center

Shreveport Hwy.
Alexandria, LA 71301
Phone: (318)473-0010

Employees: 978.

Average Entry-Level Hiring: 15-20.

Opportunities: Nurses—bachelor's degree in nursing, graduation from a three-year diploma program in nursing, or graduation from associate degree program in a school of professional nursing or comparable education. Pharmacist—bachelor's degree in pharmacy, one-year of internship, and licensed to practice pharmacy. Physical therapist—bachelor's degree in physical therapy and one-year of professional physical therapy experience or graduate education in appropriate field.

Human Resources: Hilda S. McBride; Cora C. Chauppette, Pharmacist.

Detroit Osteopathic Hospital Corp.

PO Box 5153
Southfield, MI 48086
Phone: (313)746-4300

Business Description: Osteopathic hospital.

Officers: Thomas Caulfield, President; Jacqueline Primeau, VP of Finance; Bob Blair, Dir. of Mktg.; Franklin Joseph, Manager.

Opportunities: Hires in various areas, such as nursing, physical therapy, social work, accounting, and computer systems. A college degree is required.

Benefits: Benefits include medical insurance, dental insurance, life insurance, vacation days, vision insurance, and annuities.

Human Resources: Franklin Joseph.

Application Procedures: Applicants should contact Franklin Joseph by mail only. No unsolicited resumes are accepted.

▶ **Internships**

Type: The company does not offer an internship program.

Dover Nursing Center

PO Box 635
Dover, DE 19901
Phone: (302)734-5953

Opportunities: Hires entry-level nurses and nurses aides. Applicants must be certified.

Benefits: Benefits include medical insurance.

Application Procedures: Applications are kept on file until a position opens.

▶ **Internships**

Type: The company does not offer any internship programs.

Drake Center Inc.

151 W. Galbraith Rd.
Cincinnati, OH 45216
Phone: (513)948-2500

Business Description: Physical rehabilitation center.

Officers: Earl Gilreath, CEO.

Opportunities: Hires entry-level clinical and non-clinical staff. A college degree is required.

Benefits: Benefits include medical insurance, life insurance, dental insurance, vision insurance, and savings plan.

Human Resources: Sherry Torbeck, Contact.

Application Procedures: Apply in person and fill out an application or send resume and cover letter to Sherry Torbeck.

▶ **Internships**

Type: Offers paid and unpaid internships in nursing, physical therapy, and occupational therapy. **Number Available Annually:** 5-10.

Qualifications: College students.

Application Procedure: A waiver is signed by the students' educational program, and the department head handles the procedure from there.

DRCA Medical Corp.

3 Riverway
Houston, TX 77056
Phone: (713)439-7511

Business Description: Physical rehabilitation services.

Officers: Jose E. Kauachi, Pres. & Treasurer; Siraj Q. Jiwani, CFO; Preston Myers Jr., VP of Business Development; Albert J. Tenorio Jr., VP of Operations.

Opportunities: Requires a college degree or previous experience.

Benefits: Benefits include medical insurance,

life insurance, dental insurance, tuition assistance, and a 401(k) plan.

Application Procedures: Apply in person, contact by phone, or send resume to Human Resources.

Drexler and Associates
9002 Meridian St.
Indianapolis, IN 46260
Phone: (317)573-4445

Business Description: Hearing and speech clinics.

Officers: Patricia Chun, Dir. of Industrial Relations; Geraldine B. Drexler, Dir. of Industrial Relations.

Opportunities: The Company hires entry level positions in all areas. The requirements vary depending on the position.

Benefits: Benefits include medical insurance and life insurance.

Application Procedures: Applications for positions can be made to the president of the company. Candidates should send resumes to the Company.

▶ Internships

Type: The Company does not offer any internships.

Duke University Medical Center
Box 40001
Durham, NC 27706
Phone: (919)684-2015
Fax: (919)681-7926

Opportunities: RN—associate or bachelor's degree. Various other allied health positions available.

Application Procedures: Call the employment office for more information.

Edgewood Children's Center
1801 Vicente St.
San Francisco, CA 94116
Phone: (415)681-3211

Officers: Edi Hoffman, Contact.

Opportunities: Hires entry-level kitchen and maintenance staff, clerical staff, and counseling staff. Counseling positions required a bachelor's degree and some previous experience.

Benefits: Benefits include medical insurance, dental insurance, and 401(k).

Application Procedures: Send resume and cover letter to the attention of Edi Hoffman.

▶ Internships

Contact: Edi Hoffman.

Type: Offers unpaid internships for college credit. **Number Available Annually:** 10.

Qualifications: College students.

Application Procedure: Contact Edi Hoffman for application information.

A myriad of possibilities for volunteer service are available in the United States and abroad, ranging from community service to education to development projects. . . In addition to the personal rewards volunteer service offers, volunteering can actually be a step toward a future career goal.

Source: *Journal of Career Planning & Employment*

Englewood Hospital
350 Engle St.
Englewood, NJ 07631
Phone: (201)894-3490
Fax: (201)894-4791

Employees: 2,500.

Average Entry-Level Hiring: Unknown.

Opportunities: No information on specific opportunities available.

Evangelical Health Systems
2025 Windsor Dr.
Oak Brook, IL 60521
Phone: (708)572-9393
Fax: (708)572-9139

Business Description: Owns and operates a chain of hospitals and outpatient clinics.

Officers: Steven Heck, Dir. of Info. Systems; John G. King, CEO & Pres.; Richard Risk, Exec. VP of Mktg.; William Wheeler, VP of Finance.

Opportunities: Drug screening is required of all employees.

Human Resources: Ms. Harriett Fram.

Application Procedures: Interested candidates should forward resume or fill out application on site. Company advertises in newspaper. Ms. Harriett Fram.

▶ **Internships**

Type: The company may offer internships at certain facilities. Interested applicants should contact the particular facility in which they are interested.

F. Edward Hebert Hospital

1 Sanctuary Dr.
New Orleans, LA 70114
Phone: (504)363-2200

Opportunities: Hires physical therapists and occupational therapists with previous experience. Some entry-level positions require no experience.

Benefits: Benefits include medical insurance, life insurance, dental insurance, vision insurance, tuition assistance, long and short-term disability, and a 401(k) plan.

Application Procedures: Prefers applicants apply to the Human Resources Department for jobs that are listed.

▶ **Internships**

Type: Offers internships for college credit.

Fairbanks Hospital, Inc.

8102 Clearvista Pkwy.
Indianapolis, IN 46256
Phone: (317)849-8222

Opportunities: Entry-level positions available for secretarial, accounting, dietary, and housekeeping staff. All positions require at least a high school degree. Dietary and housekeeping positions require previous experience. Accounting positions require related college course work.

Benefits: Benefits include medical insurance, dental insurance, pension plan, flexible spending plan, and tuition assistance.

Human Resources: Sharon Baker.

Application Procedures: Send resume and cover letter or apply in person to Sharon Baker.

Fairfax Hospital

3300 Gallows Rd.
Falls Church, VA 22046
Phone: (703)698-3298
Toll-free: 800-234-4405
Fax: (703)698-3448

Employees: 3,500.

Average Entry-Level Hiring: Varies.

Opportunities: RNs, physical therapists, medical technicians, and pharmacists.

Application Procedures: Call for more information.

Fairfield Hills Hospital

PO Box 5525
Newtown, CT 06470
Phone: (203)426-2531

Opportunities: Hires entry-level staff in all areas. Depending on the position, previous experience, college course work, and/or a college degree may be required.

Benefits: Benefits include medical insurance, life insurance, dental insurance, savings plan, and child-care programs.

Application Procedures: Send resume and cover letter and an application to the director or head of the department of interest.

▶ **Internships**

Contact: Robin Plamondon.

Type: Offers paid and unpaid internships in psychology. **Number Available Annually:** 8.

Application Procedure: Students must be referred from their school. Applications should be sent to contact.

First Hospital Corp.

240 Corporate Blvd.
Norfolk, VA 23502
Phone: (804)459-5100

Opportunities: Hires mostly for clerical positions with previous experience.

Benefits: Benefits include a health plan, life insurance, and a 401(k) plan.

Human Resources: Karen Benson; Chris Culley.

Application Procedures: Fill out an application or send a resume to Chris Culley or Karen Benson.

Flambeau Medical Center

98 Sherry Ave., Box 310
Park Falls, WI 54552
Phone: (715)762-2484
Fax: (715)762-4257

Employees: 70.

Average Entry-Level Hiring: 10.

Opportunities: RN—three-, or four-year degree. Physical therapist—four-year degree. Anesthetist CRNE—two-year degree after nursing.

Human Resources: Judy Reese.

Forbes Health System Healthmark

500 Finley St.
Pittsburgh, PA 15206
Phone: (412)665-3841
Fax: (412)665-3852

Employees: 2,700.

Average Entry-Level Hiring: Unknown.

Opportunities: Registered nurses (all specialities), physical therapist, occupational therapist, radiology technicians—no requirements specified.

Human Resources: Davida Brown; Anne Marie Grzybek; Mary Jane Krosoff.

Franciscan Health System

1 MacIntyre Dr.
Aston, PA 19014
Phone: (215)358-3950
Fax: (215)358-4207

Business Description: Operator of general medical and surgical hospitals.

Officers: Ronald R. Aldrich, CEO & Pres.; Ellen Barron, VP of Mktg.; Robert H. Davis, VP of Info. Systems; Donald A. Westerman, Sr. VP.

Benefits: Benefits include medical insurance, dental insurance, vision insurance, life insurance, flexible benefits plan, stock option plan, pension plan, and vacation days.

Human Resources: James O. Wilson.

Application Procedures: Interested candidates should fill out applications on site and send resume and cover letter to the attention of the Manager of Human Resources.

▶ **Internships**

Type: The company offers summer internships for college credit in accounting.

Qualifications: Applicants for summer internships must be college students.

Application Procedure: Applications for summer internships should be sent to the manager of human resources.

Fulton State Hospital

600 E. 5th St.
Fulton, MO 65251-1798
Phone: (314)592-4100
Fax: (314)592-3000

Employees: 1,200.

Average Entry-Level Hiring: Unknown.

Opportunities: RN—associate or bachelor's degree in nursing. Physical therapist, occupational therapist—bachelor's degree preferred.

Application Procedures: Contact personnel for more information.

To make yourself more attractive to international employers, you might start with simple things: brushing up on your foreign languages or even learning a new one; seizing opportunities to travel abroad, whether for business or pleasure; cultivating overseas friends; or just reading widely about other cultures.

Source: *Money*

Genesis Health Ventures

148 W. State St.
Kennett Square, PA 19348
Phone: (215)444-6350

Business Description: Operator of skilled nursing care facilities other than hospitals.

Application Procedures: Interested candidates should forward resumes to Mary Ann in the Human Resource Department.

▶ **Internships**

Type: The company does not offer any internship programs.

Geriatric and Medical Centers Inc.

5601 Chestnut St.
Philadelphia, PA 19139
Phone: (215)476-2250

Business Description: Engaged in providing such miscellaneous local transportation as ambulances, vanpools or chauffeured limousines. Wholesaler of medical, dental, surgical, X-ray or hospital equipment and supplies. Operator of skilled nursing care facilities other than hospitals. Operator of intermediate care facilities.

Officers: Robert F. Carfagno, Sr. VP & CFO; Daniel Veloric, Pres. & Chairman of the Board.

Human Resources: James J. Wankmiller.

Application Procedures: Interested candidates should submit completed applications and resumes to the Human Resources Department.

▶ **Internships**

Type: The company does not offer any internship programs.

Glaxo Inc.

5 Moore Dr.
Research Triangle Park, NC 27709
Phone: (919)248-2100

Business Description: A research based company whose corporate purpose is the discovery, development, manufacturing and marketing of safe, effective medicines of the highest quality, including anti-ulcerants, commodity antibiotics, and fine chemicals. The company is Glaxo Holdings' largest subsidiary.

Officers: Dr. E. Mario, CEO; Dr. C.A. Sanders.

Benefits: The company offers a full benefits package for full-time employees including medical insurance, and paid vacations and holidays.

Human Resources: Steve Sons.

Application Procedures: Places newspaper advertisements for certain openings. Additionally the company advertises vacant positions on its Jobline. Send resume and cover letter to the attention of to the Human Resources Department.

▶ **Internships**

Type: The company offers a paid summer internship program.

Qualifications: Internships are offered to graduating high school and college students.

Glenbeigh Hospital of Cleveland

18120 Puritas Ave.
Cleveland, OH 44135
Phone: (216)476-0222

Opportunities: Hires for openings in housekeeping, dietary, and counseling departments. Some positions require previous experience, others require some college course work or college degree.

Benefits: Benefits include medical insurance, life insurance, vision insurance, savings plan, tuition assistance, and profit sharing.

Human Resources: Chris Mohnickey.

Application Procedures: Apply in person or send resume and cover letter to the attention of Chris Mohnickey.

▶ **Internships**

Type: The hospital offers unpaid internships. **Number Available Annually:** 3.

Qualifications: Applicants must be college juniors or seniors.

Application Procedure: Apply in person or contact the personnel department by phone.

Good Neighbor Services Inc.

2177 Youngman Ave.
St. Paul, MN 55116
Phone: (612)698-6544

Opportunities: Hires entry-level staff in nursing, housekeeping, social work, therapeutic recreation, and dietary aides. Previous experience required; college degree required for therapeutic recreation and social work staff.

Benefits: Benefits include medical insurance, dental insurance, vision insurance, and 401(k).

Application Procedures: Apply in person or send resume and cover letter.

▶ **Internships**

Type: The company does not offer an internship program.

Grady Memorial Hospital

PO Box 26208
Atlanta, GA 30035-3801
Phone: (404)616-1900
Fax: (404)616-6033

Human Resources: Carolyn Hughes.

Great Lakes Rehabilitation Hospital

22401 Foster Winter Dr.
Southfield, MI 48075
Phone: (313)569-1500

Opportunities: Hires entry-level staff in all areas. A college degree is required.

Benefits: Benefits include medical insurance, life insurance, dental insurance, and 401(k).

Application Procedures: Only accepts applications for specific job openings. Send resume and cover letter to the attention of Heather Miller.

▶ Internships

Contact: Heather Miller.

Type: Offers unpaid internships for college credit. **Number Available Annually:** 3.

Qualifications: College seniors.

Greenery Rehabilitation Group Inc.

400 Centre St.
Newton, MA 02158
Phone: (617)244-4744

Business Description: A provider of rehabilitation services for persons with head injuries. The company also operates skilled and intermediate care facilities for geriatric and medically demanding patients. Also, the company has established a close working relationship with the National Head Injury Foundation and its affiliated state chapters.

Officers: Steven C. Adams, VP of Mktg.; Pelino Campea, CFO; George M. Ferencik, Pres. & COO; Gerald M. Martin, CEO & Chairman of the Board.

Benefits: Benefits include medical insurance, 401(k), dental insurance, vacation days, and child care.

Human Resources: James M. Young.

Application Procedures: Send resume and cover letter to the attention of department in which applicant is making application.

▶ Internships

Type: The company does not offer any internship programs.

Greenville Health Corp. Pain Therapy Centers

100 Mallard St.
Greenville, SC 29601
Phone: (803)455-8257

Opportunities: Entry-level positions offered in all areas. Requires a master's degree for social therapy and certification for occupational therapy.

Benefits: Benefits include medical insurance, life insurance, dental insurance, a savings plan, tuition assistance, a 401(k) plan, child or elder care.

Application Procedures: Apply in person or send resume to the Personnel Department.

▶ Internships

Type: Offers paid internships for college credit to graduate students.

Application Procedure: Apply in person to the Personnel Department.

The two-year college has emerged as one of the nation's primary job-training institutions, providing education for **allied health**, high-technology, business, and other fields.

Source: *Journal of Career Planning & Employment*

Greenville Hospital System

701 Grove Rd.
Greenville, SC 29605
Phone: (803)455-8976
Fax: (803)455-5959

Employees: 5,600. The entry level hiring numbers indicate positions in different areas; administration, nursing, laboratory, and other allied health areas.

Average Entry-Level Hiring: 331-395.

Opportunities: Registered nurses in all clinical areas, medical technologists, occupational and physical therapists. Administrative—master's degree.

Human Resources: Robin Stelling, Nurse; Cheryl Dyer, Professional/Allied Health.

Hallmark Healthcare Inc.

300 Galleria Pkwy., Ste. 650
PO Box 723049
Atlanta, GA 30339-0049
Phone: (404)933-5500
Fax: (404)933-1886

Business Description: Operator of specialty hospitals.

Officers: J.T. McAfee, CEO & Pres.

Human Resources: Betsy Kennedy.

Application Procedures: Contact the company for more information.

Your future in the world of work will depend at least in part on your ability to express yourself in groups. One thing you can do in the near future is sign up for a class in public speaking. There you can get practice and guidance in speaking in front of a group.

Source: *Business Monday/Detroit Free Press*

Hamot Health Systems Inc.

100 State St.
Erie, PA 16507
Phone: (814)870-7000

Opportunities: May require some previous experience, a college degree, or some college coursework depending on position.

Benefits: Benefits include medical insurance, life insurance, dental insurance, vision insurance, savings investment plan, tuition assistance, and profit sharing.

Application Procedures: Apply in person.

▶ Internships

Type: Offers unpaid internships to college students. **Number Available Annually:** 200.

Application Procedure: Apply through school.

Health & Hospital Services

1715 114th Ave. SE, Ste. 10
Bellevue, WA 98004
Phone: (206)454-8068
Fax: (206)453-5152

Business Description: Operator of general

medical and surgical hospitals. Provider of management services.

Officers: Hermann Goeppele, VP of Finance; Monica Herran, President; H.W. Kriz, VP of Mktg.

Benefits: Benefits include King County Medical Insurance, employee pension plan, and long-term disability.

Human Resources: Scott Houston.

Application Procedures: Interested applicants should forward resumes and/or application to Scott Houston.

▶ Internships

Type: The company does not typically offer any internship programs.

Health Care and Retirement Corp.

1 SeaGate Ave.
Toledo, OH 43604
Phone: (419)247-5023

Benefits: Benefits include medical insurance, life insurance, dental insurance, and 401(k).

Human Resources: Chuck Hall.

Application Procedures: Send resume and cover letter.

▶ Internships

Type: Offers internships of various types depending on the department.

Application Procedure: Contact Human Resources, if interested.

Health-Care Compare

750 Riverpoint
West Sacramento, CA 95605
Phone: (916)374-4600

Business Description: Provides cost containment programs for workers' compensation and group health insurance. The company offers its programs in Arizona, California, New Mexico, and Texas, and plans to expand into Florida, Michigan, and Oregon. Revenues are derived from charging insurance carriers or employers a percentage of the amount they saved by participating in the company's programs. Currently, the company derives most of its revenues from its workers' compensation cost containment program, but it plans to expand its group health cost containment program. The company's healthcare provider network consists of approximately 26,700 hospitals, physicians, clinics, ambulance companies, physical therapists, and other providers. The company's claims processing system was jointly developed by itself and Electronic Data Systems Corporation. The two companies will also jointly develop and market products and services derived from OUCH's database.

Officers: Terry Borchers, VP of Mktg. & Sales; Clark H. Cameron, VP & General Counsel; James W. Cameron, Jr., CEO & Chairman of the Board; Kelly L. Cook, Exec. VP of Operations; John Dodgshon, Dir. of Info. Systems; David A. Edelstein, CFO; Roger Favero, Vice Pres.; W. Robert Keen, President; Edward L. Lammerding, Secretary.

Benefits: Benefits include stock option plans for key employees and an employee stock ownership plan. Also offers dental insurance, medical insurance, and a 401(k) plan.

Human Resources: M. Wilbourn.

Application Procedures: Applications are accepted for advertised positions only. Send resume and cover letter to the attention of M. Wilbourn.

▶ **Internships**

Type: The company does not offer an internship program.

Health Management Associates Inc.
5811 Pelican Bay Blvd., Ste. 500
Naples, FL 33963
Phone: (813)598-3175
Fax: (813)597-5794

Business Description: Operator of general medical and surgical hospitals. Operator of psychiatric hospitals.

Officers: Kelly Curry, Sr. VP & Finance Officer; Earl Holland, Exec. VP of Mktg.; Jim Jordan, Dir. of Info. Systems; William J. Schoen, CEO & Pres.

Benefits: Benefits include 401(k), dental insurance, tuition assistance, health insurance, paid vacation days, sick days, and holidays.

Human Resources: Fred Drow.

Application Procedures: Send resume and cover letter to the attention of Fred Drow.

▶ **Internships**

Type: The company does not offer any internship programs.

Health Midwest
2302 E. Meyer Blvd.
Kansas City, MO 64132
Phone: (816)276-9297

Opportunities: Hires analysts, clerical workers, and medical assistants.

Human Resources: Caryn Lowe.

Health Resources Inc.
15770 N. Dallas Pkwy., 5th Fl.
Dallas, TX 75248
Phone: (214)233-3900

Business Description: Operator of skilled nursing care facilities other than hospitals.

Officers: Robert L. Griffis, CEO & Pres.; Jeff Hands, Info. Systems Mgr.; Henry L. Richbourg, Jr., Sr. VP of Mktg.; Joseph R. Rzepka, CFO.

Human Resources: JoAnn Cowger.

Health South Rehab Inc.
15406 Manchester Rd.
Ellisville, MO 63011
Phone: (314)821-5300

Opportunities: Hires entry-level personnel in all areas. Requirements vary depending on the position being applied for.

Benefits: Benefits include medical insurance, life insurance, savings plan, and 401(k).

Human Resources: Colleen Shick, Contact.

Application Procedures: Send resume and cover letter to the attention of Delores White.

▶ **Internships**

Type: The company does not offer any internship programs.

Healthcare International Inc.
912 S. Capital of Texas Hwy., 4th Fl.
Austin, TX 78746
Phone: (512)346-4300

Business Description: Operator of general medical and surgical hospitals. Operator of psychiatric hospitals.

Officers: James L. Fariss Jr., CEO & Chairman

of the Board; Michael Heeley, VP of Mktg.; Elliott H. Weir, Exec. VP of Finance.

Application Procedures: Contact the company for more information.

▶ **Internships**

Type: Offers an internship program. Contact the company for more information.

W hat is underway in the 1990s is more than a massive corporate restructuring or a one-time adjustment. It's an overhaul of the U.S. labor force, a sea of change in the kinds of jobs and the type of work that will be available. Workers in this new era will have to be more flexible, more willing to move cross-country for a job, more willing to go back to school. Today's college graduate can expect 12 to 13 jobs in three to four different careers over her or his lifetime.

Source: *USA Today*

Healthfocus Inc.

301 W. Milam Rd.
Wharton, TX 77488
Phone: (409)532-4810

Business Description: Provides speech and physical therapy.

Officers: Danny Francis, President; Dennis Buchanan, Vice Pres.

Opportunities: Hires general staff with at least a high school diploma and licensed therapists.

Benefits: Benefits include medical insurance, life insurance, dental insurance, savings investment plan, accidental death insurance, a 401(k) plan, and a cafeteria plan.

Application Procedures: Apply in person to the Personnel Department.

▶ **Internships**

Type: Offers an internship program to applicants with a high school diploma or a license.

HealthSouth Rehabilitation Corp.

2 Perimeter Pk. S., Ste. 224W
Birmingham, AL 35243
Phone: (205)967-7116

Business Description: Specialized rehabilitation company with 31 outpatient facilities. In 1989, these facilities admitted 42,000 patients and handled 430,000 visits. The company also operates 13 inpatient facilities.

Officers: Aaron Beam, Jr., Sr. VP & CFO; Thomas W. Carman, Sr. VP; William T. Owens, Vice Pres.; Richard M. Scrushy, CEO, Pres. & Chairman of the Board.

Human Resources: Brandon O. Hale.

Application Procedures: Interested candidates should submit a completed application, a resume or both to the Human Resources Department. Brancon O. Hale.

▶ **Internships**

Type: The company offers paid internships.

Qualifications: Internships are available to college graduates.

Application Procedure: Interested candidates should contact the Human Resources Department.

HealthTrust Inc.

4525 Harding Rd.
Nashville, TN 37205
Phone: (615)383-4444

Business Description: HealthTrust is one of the largest hospital management companies in the U.S. It owns and operates more than 80 acute-care hospitals. Healthtrust's facilities are located in 21 southern and western states; 40 are the only providers of acute-care services in their communities. The hospitals generally provide a full range of inpatient and outpatient health care services, including medical/surgical, obstetrics and pediatric care, pharmacies, laboratories, and other support facilities and emergency care. Some of the company's facilities include Selma Medical Center, Selma, Alabama; Encino Hospital, Encino, California; Palm Beach Regional Hospital, Lake Worth, Florida; Edward White Hospital, St. Petersburg, Florida; Medical Center of Baton Rouge, Baton Rouge, Louisiana; Brownwood Regional Hospital, Brownwood, Texas; Diagnostic Center Hospital and Sun Belt Regional Medical Center, Houston, Texas;

Bayshore Medical Center, Pasadena, Texas; Northern Virginia Doctors Hospital, Arlington, Virginia. The company also operates facilities in joint venture with other corporations.

Officers: Michael A. Koban, Jr., VP & Treasurer; R. Clayton McWhorter, CEO & Chairman of the Board.

Benefits: Benefits include an employee pension plan, an employee stock ownership plan, and bonuses/incentives.

Human Resources: Tom Neill.

Application Procedures: Send resume and cover letter to the attention of Carolyn Schneider, Executive Director.

▶ Internships

Type: The company does not offer any internship programs.

Healthwin Hospital

20531 Darden Rd.
South Bend, IN 46634
Phone: (219)272-0100

Opportunities: Hires secretaries with experience, speech therapists, and respiratory therapists. Also hires licensed LPNs and RNs. Requirements vary but may include previous experience or a college degree.

Benefits: Benefits include medical insurance, life insurance, dental insurance, and vision insurance. Also offers savings plan, tuition assistance, a retirement plan, and paid vacations.

Human Resources: Lee Ann Goble, Human Services Director.

Application Procedures: Contact Lee Ann Goble, Personnel Department.

Hebrew Rehabilitation Center for Aged

1200 Centre St.
Roslindale, MA 02131
Phone: (617)325-8000

Opportunities: Hires degreed occupational, physical, and recreational therapists.

Benefits: Benefits include medical insurance, life insurance, dental insurance, and 401(k).

Human Resources: Rachel Boyer.

Application Procedures: Send resume and cover letter in attention to the personnel department or apply in person.

▶ Internships

Type: Offers paid and unpaid internships. College credit is available. **Number Available Annually:** 20.

Qualifications: College students.

Application Procedure: Fill out an application or send resume.

Helian Health Group Inc.

9600 Blue Larkspur
Monterey, CA 93940
Phone: (408)646-9000

Business Description: Provides outpatient related medical services.

Officers: Thomas D. Wilson, CEO; Donald C. Blanding, Treasurer; J. Spencer Davis, VP of Intl. Sales; Andrew W. Miller, VP of Operations.

Hennepin County Medical Center

701 Park Ave.
Minneapolis, MN 55415
Phone: (612)347-2277
Fax: (612)347-3377

Employees: 2,000.

Average Entry-Level Hiring: Nurses—109; physical therapists—50.

Opportunities: RNs and physical therapists.

Human Resources: Annette Stech.

Application Procedures: Call for more information.

Hill Crest Hospital

6869 5th Ave. S.
Birmingham, AL 35212
Phone: (205)833-9000

Benefits: Benefits include medical insurance, life insurance, dental insurance, and vacation days.

Application Procedures: Accepts unsolicited resumes; send resume and cover letter to the attention of Human Resource Department or apply in person. Hires entry-level staff in all areas. Prospective employees must have a college degree.

▶ **Internships**

Type: Offers unpaid internships. **Number Available Annually:** varies.

Qualifications: College or high school students.

A powerful combination of workers who equip themselves to be competitive and employers who provide them with challenging jobs can help businesses stay on top. But to mesh these elements managers must give employees a voice in their jobs and enable workers to develop new skills throughout their careers. Workers must get as much schooling as possible, demand broader duties on the job, and take on more responsibility for the company's success.

Source: Business Week

Hillhaven Corp.
1148 Broadway Plaza
Tacoma, WA 98402
Phone: (206)572-4901

Business Description: Engaged in the operation of retail drug stores. Operator of skilled nursing care facilities other than hospitals.

Officers: Richard K. Eamer, CEO & Chairman of the Board; Robert F. Pacquer, Sr. VP & CFO.

Benefits: Benefits vary depending upon position but may include health insurance and/or paid vacation.

Application Procedures: Interested candidates should forward resumes to Vicki Harey.

▶ **Internships**

Type: The company does not offer any internship programs.

Hoechst-Roussel Pharmaceuticals Inc.
Rte. 202-206 N.
Somerville, NJ 08876
Phone: (908)231-2000

Business Description: Engaged in manufacturing, fabricating and/or processing drugs in pharmaceutical preparations.

Officers: Hubert E. Huckle, Chairman of the Board; Gerald McMurtry, Exec. VP of Mktg. & Sales; Anthony Tursi, VP of Finance.

Benefits: Benefits include health care and life insurance, dental insurance, tuition assistance, and a 401(k) plan.

Human Resources: Rob Slone.

Application Procedures: Send resume and cover letter to the attention of Human Resources.

Horizon Healthcare Corp.
6001 Indian School Rd. NE, Ste. 530
Albuquerque, NM 87110
Phone: (505)881-4961

Business Description: Provides long-term health care. The company has 52 long-term care centers and retirement facilities in eight states.

Officers: Klemett L. Belt, Exec. VP & CFO; Neal M. Elliott, CEO, Pres. & Chairman of the Board; Charles H. Gonzales, VP of Government Programs; Michael A. Jeffries, Sr. VP of Operations; William C. Mitchell, VP of Operations Western Div.; Randi S. Nathanson, VP, General Counsel & Sec.; Mark W. Ohlendorf, VP of Finance; Ernest A. Schofield, VP & Controller; Jeffrey A. Shepard, VP of Operations Eastern Div.

Human Resources: Rod Panyek.

▶ **Internships**

Type: Offers an internship program.

Qualifications: Administrators-in-training.

Hospital Corporation of America
1 Park Plaza
Nashville, TN 37202
Phone: (615)327-9551

Business Description: A Nashville-based health care company that either owns or manages hospitals, psychiatric units, and other medical facilities in the United States. In 1989, the company and Doheny Development Corp. embarked on a joint venture to produce a 200,000 square-foot medical mart facility in Dallas, Texas.

Officers: Thomas F. Frist, Jr., CEO, Pres. & Chairman of the Board; Roger E. Mick, Exec. VP & CFO.

Benefits: Offers a full benefits package to full-time employees.

Application Procedures: Accepts walk-in applicants between 8:30 and 4:00. Send resume and cover letter to the attention of the Staffing Assistant, Human Resources, PO Box 550, 1 Park Plaza, Nashville, TN 37202.

▶ **Internships**

Contact: Judy Collier.

Type: Offers paid internships in legal, clerical, and data-processing areas.

Qualifications: Internship applicants must be at least through their second year of college.

Application Procedure: Send applications to the attention of Judy Collier or to Human Resources.

Howard University Hospital
400 Byrant St.
Washington, DC 20059
Phone: (202)806-7714
Fax: (202)483-6693

Employees: 2,000.

Average Entry-Level Hiring: Unknown.

Opportunities: Nurses, M.S.W.s, respiratory therapists, physical and occupational therapists—requirements not specified.

Application Procedures: Contact Employment Services for information.

Humana Medical Plan Inc.
3400 Lakeside Dr.
Miramar, FL 33027
Phone: (305)621-4222

Business Description: Engaged in providing health care services or services related to the provision of health care.

Officers: Ronald J. Berding, Dir. of Engineering; Robert Wieckert, Dir. of Sales; Thomas C. Wyss, Admin. Mgr.

Benefits: Benefits include insurance plans, savings plans, a basic retirement plan, health care programs, and dental insurance.

Human Resources: Jennifer Pottinger; Ann Befley.

Application Procedures: Accepts walk-in applicants. Maintains a job hotline at (305)626-5700. Send resume and cover letter to the attention of Ann Befley.

▶ **Internships**

Type: Offers an internship program.

Ingalls Memorial Hospital and Health System
1 Ingalls Dr.
Harvey, IL 60426
Phone: (708)333-0737
Fax: (708)333-2300

Employees: 2,500.

Average Entry-Level Hiring: Unknown.

Opportunities: Nurse—associate or bachelor's degree or state work permit. Physical therapists—bachelor's degree required.

Application Procedures: All applicants must have a resume. Contact the Personnel Office for more information.

Inova Health Systems Inc.
8001 Braddock Rd.
Springfield, VA 22151
Phone: (703)321-4286

Business Description: A health care network based in northern Virginia. The company owns and operates general medical hospitals.

Officers: Knox Singleton, President.

Benefits: Benefits include tuition assistance, tax deferred annuities, life insurance, medical insurance, dental insurance, and paid vacation and holidays.

Application Procedures: Send resume and cover letter to the attention of Personnel Department or submit a completed application to the company.

▶ **Internships**

Type: Offers informal summer positions.

Integrated Health Services Inc.
11011 McCormick Rd.
Hunt Valley, MD 21031
Phone: (410)584-7050

Business Description: Operates nursing homes and retirement hotels.

Officers: Robert Elkins, CEO; Steven Drury, CFO.

Opportunities: Hires entry-level clerical, accounts payable, and administrative staff. College degree and previous experience required.

Benefits: Benefits include medical insurance, life insurance, dental insurance, vision insurance, profit sharing, and 401(k).

Application Procedures: Send resume and cover letter to the attention of Personnel.

▶ **Internships**

Type: The company does not offer an internship program.

Students with the luxury of a couple of years until graduation should start plotting for that first job and snagging some experience *now*. But with many employers reluctant to pay even the modest salary of an internship, getting actual business experience is increasingly difficult. One strategy: Try a so-called externship, typically a one-week, unpaid stint at a company that provides a snapshot of various careers and a chance to network with insiders. Externships can be particularly useful for liberal-arts majors without a clear career track.

Source: *U.S. News and World Report*

Intermountain Health Care Inc.
36 S. State St., 20th Fl., Ste. 2200
Salt Lake City, UT 84111
Phone: (801)533-8282
Fax: (801)531-9789

Business Description: Engaged in the operation of establishments that provide general or specialized medicine or surgery by medical doctors. Operator of general medical and surgical hospitals. Operator of psychiatric hospitals. Operator of specialty hospitals.

Officers: Scott Parker, President.

Benefits: Benefits include health care and life insurance, dental insurance, a savings plan after one year, and tuition assistance after 6 months.

Human Resources: Lonnie Deet.

Application Procedures: Maintains a job hotline at (801)533-3654. Applications accepted for openings only. Send resume and cover letter to the attention of to the Human Resource Specialist.

IOLAB Corp.
500 Iolab Dr.
Claremont, CA 91711
Phone: (714)624-2020
Fax: (714)399-1425

Business Description: Manufacturer of ophthalmic pharmaceuticals, intraocular lenses, and microsurgical equipment.

Officers: Bob Darretta, President; Don Duffy, VP & Controller; John Gilbert, VP of Mktg.

Average Entry-Level Hiring: The company expects hiring levels to increase over the next few years.

Opportunities: Positions typically available at IOLAB include scientific managers, cost accountants, master production schedulers, mechanical engineers, pharmaceutical scientists, AS400 computer programmer analysts, pharmaceutical lab technicians, CAD/CAM-UGII technicians, pharmaceutical product managers, marketing analysts, secretaries, equipment mechanics, and intraocular lens production workers/operators.

Benefits: Benefits include dental insurance, life insurance, medical insurance, savings plan, long-term disability, short-term disability, an employee pension plan, an employee stock ownership plan, a 401(k) plan, a smoke-free environment, a subsidized cafeteria, vacation, sick time, holidays, and tuition assistance.

Human Resources: Paul E. Krueger, Ph.D.; Stephanie McCarthy.

Application Procedures: Recruits at college campuses nationwide for positions in the pharmaceutical sciences, and in southern California for other positions. Also uses professional association networking and tele-recruits from member directories. Phone calls not accepted. Faxed resumes are accepted. Send resume and cover letter to the attention of Stephanie McCarthy.

▶ **Internships**

Type: Offers an informal internship program.

Jewish Hospitals Inc.
3200 Burnett Ave.
Cincinnati, OH 45229
Phone: (513)569-2000

Opportunities: Entry-level opportunities available in foodservice, clerical, and housekeeping positions. Requires a high school GED.

Benefits: Benefits include medical insurance,

life insurance, dental insurance, savings investment plan, tuition assistance, disability benefits, military leave, child or elder care.

Human Resources: Betty Barnet, Personnel Contact; Theresa Murphy, Personnel Contact.

Application Procedures: Send resumes and applications to the attention of Theresa Murphy.

▶ Internships

Type: Offers unpaid internships for college credit to senior students.

Application Procedure: Contact the specific department offering the internship.

Kentfield Rehabilitation Hospital

PO Box 338
Kentfield, CA 94914-0338
Phone: (415)456-9680

Opportunities: Hires entry-level personnel in all areas. Previous experience is required for rehabilitation positions. Some college course work is required for all positions.

Benefits: Benefits include medical insurance, life insurance, dental insurance, vision insurance, profit sharing, and 401(k).

Application Procedures: Call, fill out application, and/or send resume and samples to Human Resources.

▶ Internships

Type: Offers college credit internships in physical and occupational therapy. **Number Available Annually:** 4.

Qualifications: College students.

Application Procedure: To apply, the internship must be approved by the director of the sponsoring school's department. Applications should be sent to Derrick in Human Resources.

Laguna Honda Hospital and Rehabilitation Center

375 Laguna Honda Blvd.
San Francisco, CA 94116
Phone: (415)664-1580

Opportunities: Hires entry-level clerical staff. Previous experience required.

Benefits: Benefits include medical insurance, life insurance, dental insurance, and tuition assistance.

Application Procedures: Applications are processed through the civil service.

▶ Internships

Type: Offers unpaid internships. **Number Available Annually:** 4.

Qualifications: College students.

Application Procedure: Applications are not handled at the hospital. Apply through the state civil service office.

Living Centers of America

15415 Katy Fwy.
Houston, TX 77094
Phone: (713)578-4700

Business Description: Operator of skilled nursing care facilities other than hospitals.

Officers: Stan Brezenk, Controller; Floyd Rhoades, President; Dorthy Wiley, Dir. of Mktg.; Lee Williams, VP of Finance.

Benefits: Benefits include medical insurance, dental insurance, 401(k), life insurance, traveler's insurance, three days bereavement, one half sick day a month, two weeks vacation after first year, three weeks vacation after five years, and free parking.

Human Resources: K. Muthu Muthuswamy.

Application Procedures: The center advertises in local papers. Send a resume to the attention of Theresa Tucker.

▶ Internships

Type: Offers an internship program.

Loma Linda University Medical Center

24887 Taylor St., Box 2000
Loma Linda, CA 92354
Phone: (714)824-4330
Toll-free: 800-722-2770
Fax: (714)824-4058

Employees: 5,000.

Average Entry-Level Hiring: 200-300.

Opportunities: Pharmacists—requires California State Board of Pharmacy license; both full-time and part-time, day and evening positions available. Respiratory therapist—California license required and graduate of two-year AMA approved school. Medical technologist—California license required. Occupational therapist—B.S. degree in OT, member of AOTA. Physical therapist—B.S. degree in Physical Therapy and California license. Registered Nurse Radiologic technologist—valid certificate in General Diagnostic Radiological Technology issued by the State of California Department of Health.

Human Resources: Elmerissa; Tom Hudson.

Application Procedures: Send resume and cover letter. For information regarding other available positions call the job line at (714)824-4330.

Employment for recreational therapists is expected to grow much faster than average, chiefly because of anticipated growth in the need for long-term care, rehabilitation, and services for the developmentally disabled. Job prospects should be favorable for those with a strong clinical background.

Source: *Occupational Outlook Quarterly*

Lutheran Hospital—La Crosse
1910 S. Ave.
La Crosse, WI 54601
Phone: (608)785-0530
Fax: (608)785-2181

Employees: 2,300.

Average Entry-Level Hiring: 200.

Opportunities: Physical and occupational therapists, medical lab technicians, and medical records staff.

Human Resources: Judy Eddy.

Application Procedures: Call for more information.

Maine Department of Human Services
State House, Station 11
Augusta, ME 04333
Phone: (207)289-2736
Fax: (207)626-5555

Opportunities: Hires entry-level staff for the central office: clerical, professional, technical, nursing, data entry, and case workers.

Benefits: Benefits include medical insurance, life insurance, and dental insurance.

Application Procedures: Applications can be filled out in person. Contact the Bureau of Human Resources, Maine State Personnel Office.

▶ **Internships**

Type: The company does not offer an internship program.

Manor Care Inc.
10750 Columbia Pike
Silver Spring, MD 20901
Phone: (301)681-9400

Business Description: Holding company with interests in the healthcare and hospitality industries.

Officers: Stewart Bainnum, Jr., CEO, Pres. & Chairman of the Board; Joseph Buckley, Sr. VP Information Resources and Development; James A. MacCutcheon, Sr. VP of Finance & Treasurer.

Human Resources: Roberta McCall; Charles A. Shields.

Application Procedures: The company publicizes job vacancies through its Job Hotline, 1-800-648-2041. Interested applicants should forward resumes to the Employment Office. Roberta McCall.

Marianjoy Rehabilitation Hospital and Clinics
26 W. 171 Roosevelt Rd.
Wheaton, IL 60187
Phone: (708)462-4000

Opportunities: The company hires entry-level staff in many areas. Most positions require a college degree.

Benefits: Benefits include medical insurance, life insurance, dental insurance, a pension plan, and disability.

Human Resources: Marilyn Mather.

Application Procedures: Available positions are typically advertised in the newspaper. Interested applicants should contact the company recruiter, forward resumes to the company, or apply in person.

▶ **Internships**

Type: The company does not offer any internship programs.

Massachusetts Respiratory Hospital

2001 Washington St.
Braintree, MA 02184
Phone: (617)848-2600

Benefits: Benefits include medical insurance, dental insurance, life insurance, vision insurance, savings plan, and tuition assistance.

Human Resources: David Glacier, Director, Human Relations.

Application Procedures: Call, apply in person, or send resume with samples. Those interested should fill out an application and turn it in to any human resources agent.

▶ Internships

Contact: David Glacier, Director, Human Relations.

Type: Offers internships for college credit.

Qualifications: College students.

McNeil Pharmaceutical

Welsh & McKean Roads
Spring House, PA 19477
Phone: (215)628-5000

Business Description: Engaged in manufacturing, fabricating and/or processing drugs in pharmaceutical preparations.

Officers: M.D. Casey, President; T.E. Nystrom, VP of Finance; J.C. Vaughan, VP of Sales; C.E. Williams, VP of Product Development.

Benefits: Benefits include tuition assistance, medical insurance, dental insurance, vision insurance, and life insurance.

Human Resources: M.G. Judge.

Application Procedures: Maintains a job hotline at (215)628-7840. Send resume and cover letter to the company.

▶ Internships

Type: Offers an internship program.

Medical Center Hospital of Vermont

University of Vermont
111 Colchester Ave.
Burlington, VT 05401
Phone: (802)656-2825
Fax: (802)656-2792

Business Description: MCHV is a teaching hospital with 500 beds.

Employees: 3,000.

Average Entry-Level Hiring: Unknown.

Opportunities: Registered nurses, medical-surgical/maternal-child; medical, radiology, and nuclear medicine technologists; physical, radiation, occupational, and respiratory therapists; respiratory technicians; pharmacists; dieticians; health record analysts—no requirements specified.

Application Procedures: Contact Human Resources for information.

Medical College of Georgia

Personnel Div./Employment Section
1120 15th St.
Augusta, GA 30912-8100
Phone: (706)721-3081
Fax: (706)721-7192

Employees: 6,000.

Average Entry-Level Hiring: 200.

Opportunities: Registered nurses, LPNs (all areas), physical therapists, occupational therapists, respiratory therapists, medical technologists, medical secretaries/transcriptionists—no requirements specified.

Human Resources: Mary Haygan.

Application Procedures: Call for more information.

Medical University of South Carolina

State Institution
171 Ashley Ave.
Charleston, SC 29425-1035
Phone: (803)792-2071
Fax: (816)792-9533

Business Description: The MUSC Medical Center is made up of the Medical University Hospital, the Children's Hospital, the Storm Eye Institute, the Institute of Psychiatry, all outpatient clinics, and the Charleston Memorial Hospital. The mission of the MUSC Medical Center includes teaching students and physicians, the provision of tertiary care, and human research. Research programs are ongoing and staff is needed to support the research projects. There are 572 beds in the teaching hospital, which will soon have 600 beds. All patients will soon be in single bedrooms and there will be 50 intensive care beds.

Employees: 7,700.

Average Entry-Level Hiring: 800-1000.

Opportunities: There is a job vacancy listing published annually which identifies hard-to-fill vacancies, these are always available. Another listing, published weekly, includes clerical openings, some patient care aide, and administrative and managerial openings. Call for listing(s).

Human Resources: Jean W. Turner; Kathy Leitch; Nancy Adams, Nursing.

According to the Bureau of Labor Statistics, the rapid growth of women entering the workforce—about 2.3% per year from 1975 to 1990—is expected to slow, growing at a rate of 1.6% per year in the next fifteen years. By 2005, minorities are expected to account for more than 25% of all working people in the US, with the fastest growth occurring among Hispanics, who will make up over 11% of the workforce by 2005.

Source: *Forbes*

Mediplex Group Inc.
15 Walnut St.
Wellesley, MA 02181
Phone: (617)446-6900

Business Description: Owns and operates skilled care facilities and rehabilitation centers.

Officers: Abraham D. Gosman, CEO; Frederick R. Leathers, CFO; William J. Hartigan, Sr. VP; Daniel J. Kane, COO; Susan R. Scavone, VP of Human Resources.

Opportunities: Hires entry-level staff in all areas. Applicants must be 18 years of age or older.

Benefits: Benefits include medical insurance, life insurance, dental insurance, disability insurance, and 401(k).

Human Resources: Judith Carden.

Application Procedures: Send resume in attention to the human resources department.

▶ Internships

Type: An internship program is currently being developed for college students. Contact the human resources department at the specific facility of interest.

Mediplex Rehab-Camden Institute of Brain Injury Rehabilitation Research and Training
3 Cooper Plaza, Ste. 518
Camden, NJ 08103
Phone: (609)342-7600

Business Description: A rehabilitation treatment center that includes vocational training and special education programs. The facility serves those who have survived a traumatic brain injury.

▶ Internships

Contact: Peter Dunn, Training Coordinator.

Type: Offers paid programs for preprofessional research aides, allied health trainees, graduate interns, and postdoctoral fellows.

Duties: Preprofessional research aides assist in experiential work-study programs; allied health trainees get supervised experience in physical therapy, occupational therapy, respiratory care, speech-language pathology, therapeutic recreation, and nursing. Graduate interns work with school counseling, vocational services, and job placement; and postdoctoral fellows get supervised experience in psychotherapy, neuropsychology, and rehabilitation practices.

Qualifications: Preprofessional research aides should be college seniors or recent college graduates; allied health trainees should be enrolled in allied health programs; graduate internships should be advanced graduate students; and postdoctoral fellows should be licensed psychologists, have a doctorate in a field of psychology, and have finished a predoctoral clinical internship.

Memorial Health Services
2801 Atlantic Ave.
Long Beach, CA 90801
Phone: (310)595-2000
Fax: (310)595-2539

Business Description: Memorial Health Services owns and operates surgical and trauma hospitals and skilled nursing care facilities.

Officers: Richard Graniere, VP of Finance; Dick Williams, President.

Benefits: Benefits include medical insurance, dental insurance, vision insurance, a credit union, and tuition assistance.

Application Procedures: Maintains a job hotline for nursing at (310)933-3399 and for other positions at (310)933-2482. Accepts walk-in applicants. Send resume and cover letter to the attention of Human Resources.

▶ **Internships**

Type: The company is not offering any internships at this time.

Memorial Hospital of South Bend and Memorial Health System

615 N. Michigan St.
South Bend, IN 46601
Phone: (219)284-7407
Fax: (219)284-7445

Employees: 240.

Average Entry-Level Hiring: Unknown.

Opportunities: RN—license and two-, three- or four-year degree required. Physical and occupational therapists—bachelor's degree.

Human Resources: Sue Long.

Application Procedures: Call for more information.

Memorial Medical Center

3625 University Blvd.
Jacksonville, FL 32216
Phone: (904)399-6666

Opportunities: Hires entry-level staff for medical records work, dietary work, and clerical positions.

Benefits: Benefits include medical insurance, life insurance, dental insurance, optional life insurance, long-term disability, and flexible spending accounts.

Application Procedures: Fill out application at the Human Resources Department. The department can be reached at (904) 399-6700.

▶ **Internships**

Type: Offers internships for college credit in occupational therapy areas.

Application Procedure: Apply to the Human Resources Department.

Memorial Regional Rehabilitation Center

3599 University Blvd. S.
Jacksonville, FL 32216
Phone: (904)399-6819

Opportunities: Hires degreed physical therapists, speech therapists, and occupational therapists.

Benefits: Benefits include medical insurance, life insurance, dental insurance, vision insurance, savings plan, tuition assistance, and child-care programs.

Human Resources: Brenda Worpham.

Application Procedures: Applications can be filled out on site. Attach copies of all degrees and licenses to the application. Send resume and cover letter.

▶ **Internships**

Type: Offers paid and unpaid internships. **Number Available Annually:** 1-5.

Qualifications: College graduates.

Application Procedure: Internships are arranged through the schools.

Mercy Hospital

2215 Truxton Ave.
Box 119
Bakersfield, CA 93302
Phone: (805)632-5580
Fax: (805)861-9727

Employees: 1,500.

Average Entry-Level Hiring: 200.

Opportunities: Nurses—two-, three-, or four-year degrees. Physical therapist—master's degree. Technicians require an academic education.

Human Resources: Smoki Francisco, Nursing.

Mercy Hospital Medical Center

6th & University
Des Moines, IA 50314
Phone: (515)247-3100
Fax: (515)298-8831

Employees: 4,200.

Average Entry-Level Hiring: Unknown.

Opportunities: RN—associate or bachelor's degree. Social workers—M.S.W. required. Occupational therapists—bachelor's degree required. Physician assistants—state licensure required.

Application Procedures: Contact personnel for more information.

Mercy Services for Aging

34605 12 Mile Rd.
Farmington Hills, MI 48331
Phone: (313)489-6180

Opportunities: Hires entry-level secretarial, clerical, accounting, and human resources staff.

Benefits: Benefits include medical insurance, life insurance, dental insurance, child-care programs, and 401(k).

Application Procedures: Apply in person or send resume and cover letter to the attention of Employment Manager.

▶ **Internships**

Type: Offers paid internships. **Number Available Annually:** 6.

Qualifications: College students.

Application Procedure: Apply in person.

Every resume should pass the "so what?" test. It's not enough to simply list your accomplishments. You need to demonstrate the impact of your actions on your department or the company at large. Beverly Robsham, president of Robsham & Associates, an outplacement firm in Boston, MA, advocates the "PAR" approach when delineating accomplishments: "Specify the *problem*, the *actions* you took, and the *results* for the company."

Source: *Working Woman*

Meridian Healthcare Inc.

515 Fairmount Ave.
Towson, MD 21286
Phone: (410)296-1000

Business Description: Services: Skilled nursing care facility.

Officers: Edward Burchell, CEO; Wallace E. Boston Jr., VP of Finance; Linda Miller, Dir. of Mktg.; Kenneth Goad, Dir. of Systems; Michael Cunningham, Human Resources Dir.

Opportunities: The company hires entry-level

staff in administrative and finance areas. Requirements vary according to the position but previous experience is helpful.

Benefits: Benefits include medical insurance, life insurance, dental insurance, savings plan, tuition assistance, child-care programs, 401(k), and an additional retirement plan.

Human Resources: Peggy Flores.

Application Procedures: Send resume and cover letter to the attention of Mike Cunningham.

▶ **Internships**

Type: The company does not offer any internship programs.

Merrell Dow Pharmaceuticals Inc.

2110 E. Galbarith
Cincinnati, OH 45215
Phone: (513)948-9111

Business Description: Engaged in manufacturing, fabricating and/or processing drugs in pharmaceutical preparations.

Officers: Gerald Blaine, Controller; M.J. Randall, Dir. of Info. Systems; D.B. Sharrock, Pres. & COO.

Human Resources: J.L. Aitken.

▶ **Internships**

Type: The company offers paid internships.

Qualifications: High school and/or college students.

Application Procedure: Interested candidates should send a resume to the attention of the Human Resources department.

Methodist Evangelical Hospital

315 E. Broadway
Louisville, KY 40202
Phone: (502)629-6000

Business Description: Owns and operates Norton, Kosair Children's, and Methodist Evangelical hospitals in Louisville, Kentucky.

Officers: Rodney Wolford, President.

Benefits: Benefits include employee assistance program and child-care programs.

Application Procedures: Interested applicants can fill out an application in person. Send resume and cover letter to the attention of

Human Resources Department, PO Box 35070, Louisville, KY 40232.

▶ Internships

Type: The company does not offer any internship programs.

Methodist Hospital

8303 Dodge St.
Omaha, NE 68114
Phone: (402)390-8827
Fax: (402)390-8722

Employees: 2,333. The number of entry level employees hired reflects 70 people hired for medical positions and 25 people hired for non-medical positions.

Average Entry-Level Hiring: 95.

Opportunities: RN (all areas), physical therapy, pharmacy, radiologic technologist, nuclear medicine technicians, radiation therapy, respiratory therapy technicians—Nebraska licensure and accredited graduate.

Human Resources: Jeannie Fields, medical recruiter; Tracy Stabbe, Clerical; Joan Hilts, Entry-level; Kelli Green, Business.

Methodist Hospital of Indiana Inc.

1701 N. Senate Blvd.
Indianapolis, IN 46202
Phone: (317)929-2000

Opportunities: Hires entry-level staff in most areas. Requirements vary depending on the position.

Benefits: Benefits include medical insurance, life insurance, dental insurance, savings plan, tuition assistance, and profit sharing.

Human Resources: Judy McGraw, Contact.

Application Procedures: Apply in person and fill out an application. Submit the application to the department of interest.

▶ Internships

Type: The company does not offer an internship program.

MetroHealth Medical Center

2500 MetroHealth Dr.
Cleveland, OH 44109
Phone: (216)459-4134
Fax: (216)459-5234

Employees: 6,000.

Average Entry-Level Hiring: Unknown.

Opportunities: Registered nurse—associate degree or diploma required, B.S.N. preferred. Physical therapist, occupational therapist, clinical dietitian, and pharmacist—bachelor's degree and state licensure. Medical technologist—B.S. in chemistry or biology, or NRCC or ASCP certification. Respiratory therapist—associate degree. X-ray technician—associate degree or certification.

Human Resources: Shelley Thompson.

Meyer Rehabilitation Institute University of Nebraska Medical Center

600 S. 42nd St.
Omaha, NE 68198-5450
Phone: (402)559-6430
Fax: (402)559-5737

Business Description: The facility works with people with developmental disabilities or other chronic handicaps.

▶ Internships

Contact: Erlene Steele, Education Coordinator.

Type: Offers five paid traineeships and three paid postdoctoral fellowships. **Applications Received:** 20.

Duties: Trainees participate in meetings and treatment sessions with such departments as occupational therapy, physical therapy, special education, psychology, speech pathology, nutrition, and nursing. Postdoctoral fellows perform various duties in such departments as nursing, nutrition, psychology, speech pathology, and rehabilitative and genetic medicine.

Qualifications: Trainees should either have or be working toward a master's degree.

Michigan Hand Rehabilitation Center Inc.

23750 Elmira St.
Redford, MI 48239
Phone: (313)538-9005

Opportunities: Candidates for certified therapists require college degrees.

Benefits: The company offers medical, dental, and optical insurance for employees.

Application Procedures: Applicants should send resume to the assistant director.

▶ **Internships**

Type: The company offers unpaid internships and internships for college credit. The number available fluctuates depending on the number of applicants.

Michigan Health Care Corp.
7430 2nd Ave.
Detroit, MI 48202
Phone: (313)874-9100

Opportunities: Require previous experience.

Benefits: Benefits include medical insurance, life insurance, dental insurance, vision insurance, savings investment plan, and tuition assistance.

Human Resources: Linda Wheeler.

Application Procedures: Applications can be filled out on site between 9:30 and 4:30. Interested applicants should send a resume and any other additional information or contact the Personnel Department by phone.

Trade and professional associations are good sources of information about jobs in your target field. Look for associations in *The Encyclopedia of Associations.*

Source: *Executive Female*

Michigan Sports and Orthopedic Physical Therapy Center
28800 Ryan Rd., Ste. 110
Warren, MI 48092
Phone: (313)558-3600

Officers: David Crowley.

Opportunities: Hires degreed physical therapists, physical therapy assistants, and experienced office help.

Benefits: Benefits are discussed at the time of the interview.

Application Procedures: Send resume and cover letter.

▶ **Internships**

Type: Offers unpaid internships for college credit. **Number Available Annually:** 3.

Qualifications: College students enrolled in physical therapy classes at Wayne State University and Macomb County Community College.

Mid-America Health Centers
120 S. Market St., Ste.320
Wichita, KS 67202
Phone: (316)262-4206

▶ **Internships**

Type: The company does not offer an internship program.

Mid-America Rehabilitation Hospital
5701 W. 110th St.
Overland Park, KS 66211
Phone: (913)491-2400

Opportunities: Hires entry-level housekeeping and dietary staff with previous experience.

Benefits: Benefits include medical insurance, life insurance, dental insurance, vision insurance, profit sharing, and 401(k).

Human Resources: Lisa Hachenberg.

Application Procedures: Fill out an application and send resume and cover letter to the attention of Lisa Hachenberg.

▶ **Internships**

Contact: Lisa Hachenberg.

Type: Offers unpaid internships for college credit in physical therapy.

Qualifications: College graduates.

Application Procedure: Send application or resume to Lisa Hachenberg.

Miles Inc. Pharmaceutical Div.
400 Morgan Ln.
West Haven, CT 06516
Phone: (203)937-2000
Fax: (203)934-8553

Business Description: Engaged in manufacturing, fabricating and/or processing drugs in pharmaceutical preparations.

Officers: J.A. Akers, VP of Finance; G.B. Rosenberg, Dir. of Mktg.; R. Scott, Dir. of Data Processing; H.K. Wallrabe, President.

Benefits: Benefits include medical insurance, dental insurance, and 401(k).

Human Resources: D.A. Matley.

Application Procedures: Interested candidates should forward resumes to human resources and wait to be contacted for an interview.

▶ **Internships**

Type: The company does not offer an internship program.

Milford Memorial Hospital Inc.

PO Box 199
Milford, DE 19963
Phone: (302)422-3311

Business Description: Operator of general medical and surgical hospitals.

Officers: L.G. Davis, CEO; R.H. Dougherty, CFO; Jack Price, Dir. of Info. Systems; Donna Streletzky, Director.

Benefits: Benefits include medical insurance, dental insurance, life insurance, taxable annuities, and accidental death and dismemberment insurance.

Human Resources: John W. Kafader, Jr.

Application Procedures: The company advertises for specific job openings. Interested candidates should contact the human resources department.

▶ **Internships**

Type: The company offers a limited internship program. Positions are typically unpaid. Interested candidates should contact the human resources department.

Qualifications: Requirements for internships vary.

Miller Medical Group PC

1633 Church St.
Nashville, TN 37206
Phone: (615)340-8500

Business Description: Outpatient clinic.

Officers: Mike Law, Dir. of Industrial Relations; Larry Lance, CFO; Patty Czarnik, Dir. of Mktg.; Suzanne Brinkley, Dir. of Info. Systems.

Opportunities: Hires entry-level clerical staff with previous experience.

Benefits: Benefits include medical insurance, life insurance, dental insurance, and retirement plans.

Human Resources: Martha Underwood.

Application Procedures: Send resume and cover letter to the attention of Martha Underwood.

▶ **Internships**

Type: This company does not offer an internship program.

> To gain more control over your career, develop strong communications skills, both listening and talking. This means understanding and being able to translate what corporate goals are, and being able to talk to management. Actively solicit feedback.
>
> Source: *Dallas Morning News*

Mississippi Baptist Medical Center

1225 N. State St.
Jackson, MS 39202-2002
Phone: (601)968-1296
Toll-free: 800-844-1084
Fax: (601)968-4137

Employees: 3,000.

Average Entry-Level Hiring: Unknown.

Opportunities: Radiologic technologists, physical therapists, and other allied health professionals.

Application Procedures: Contact the Human Resources Department for more information.

Montebello Rehabilitation Hospital-University of Maryland Medical System

2201 Argonne Dr.
Baltimore, MD 21218
Phone: (410)554-5200

Opportunities: Hires both professional and non-professional positions for entry-level staff.

Benefits: Benefits include medical insurance, life insurance, dental insurance, vision insurance, savings plan, child-care programs, and elder-care programs.

Human Resources: Shirley Jenkins.

Application Procedures: Send application or resume to the attention of the Human Resources Department.

Mount Auburn Hospital

330 Mt. Auburn St.
Cambridge, MA 02238
Phone: (617)499-5066
Fax: (617)499-5584

Employees: 1,800.

Opportunities: RN—certified, two- or four-year degree, must pass Massachusetts board. Laboratory technician, respiratory therapy—four year degree. No other requirements specified.

Application Procedures: Contact the company for more information.

Mount Sinai Hospital

500 Blue Hills Ave.
Hartford, CT 06112
Phone: (203)242-4431
Toll-free: 800-882-6602
Fax: (203)286-4629

Human Resources: Colette Austin.

MSC Corp.

3800 Frederick Ave.
Baltimore, MD 21229

Business Description: Owns and manages intermediate care facilities.

Officers: Lovell Jones, President.

Muro Pharmaceutical Inc.

890 East St.
Tewksbury, MA 01876
Phone: (508)851-5981

Business Description: Engaged in manufacturing, fabricating and/or processing drugs in pharmaceutical preparations.

Benefits: Offers full benefits for full-time employees, including a 401(k) plan.

Human Resources: Marilyn Komulainen.

Application Procedures: Send resume and cover letter to the attention of the Human Resources Department.

▶ **Internships**

Type: The company does not offer an internship program.

Muscatatuck State Developmental Center

PO Box 77
Butlerville, IN 47223
Phone: (812)346-4401
Fax: (812)346-6308

Employees: 1,350.

Average Entry-Level Hiring: Unknown.

Opportunities: Nurse IV—possession of a valid license to practice nursing in the state of Indiana as an RN. Charge nurse—one year of full-time paid professional experience in psychiatric, developmental disability, or geriatric nursing; possession of a valid license to practice nursing in the state of Indiana as an RN; an accredited bachelor's degree in nursing may substitute for the required experience. Behavior clinician III—one year of full-time paid professional experience in the performance of psychological services, which includes diagnostic interviewing, report preparation, interpretation of test results, and/or treatment of emotional disorders; a master's degree in psychology, educational psychology, guidance and counseling, tests and measurements, or psychometry required; internship training at the doctoral level or doctoral coursework in any of the above areas may substitute for the required experience with a maximum substitution of one year. Mental Health Administrator III— two years of full-time paid professional work experience in the provision of therapeutic patient services for the mentally ill or mentally retarded; a bachelor's degree in business administration, nursing, mental health technology, psychology, social work, education, vocational rehabilitation, speech pathology and audiology, or one of the adjunctive therapies (music, recreation, physical, occupational, or industrial) required; accredited graduate training in any of the above areas may substitute for the required experience with a maximum substitution of two years. Audiologist III—licensure as an audiologist by the Indiana Board of Examiners on Speech Pathology and Audiology required. Dietitian IV—registration as a dietitian or proof of eligibility for admission to the Dietitian Registration Examination; must successfully pass the Dietitian's Registration Examination of the Commission on Dietetic Registration prior to the granting of permanent status. Psychologist I—current certification as a psychologist by the Indiana State Psychology Board, proof must accompany application.

Psychiatric attendant V—two years of full-time paid work experience; a high school diploma may substitute for the required experience.

Human Resources: Julie Broome Nursing; Patricia Spanagel Dietitians.

Application Procedures: All applicants must be certified to an eligible list by filing a State Application PD/100 with Indiana State Personnel Department, Indianapolis, IN; and be available for Jennings County, #40.

Nanticoke Memorial Hospital

801 Middleford Rd.
Seaford, DE 19973
Phone: (302)629-6611

Business Description: Operator of general medical and surgical hospitals.

Officers: Douglas J. Connell, VP of Finance; E.H. Hancock, President; Donald Pinner, Vice Pres. Management.

Benefits: Benefits include medical insurance, and optional dental insurance and vision insurance.

Human Resources: William Fay.

Application Procedures: Interested candidates should forward resumes to the human resources department.

▶ **Internships**

Type: The company does not offer any internship programs.

National HealthCorp L.P.

PO Box 1398
Murfreesboro, TN 37133
Phone: (615)890-2020

Business Description: Engaged in the operation of apartment buildings. Operator of skilled nursing care facilities other than hospitals. Operator of nursing or personal care facilities that require a lesser degree of care than skilled or intermediate care facilities.

Officers: W. Andrew Adams, President; Charlotte A. Swafford, Treasurer.

Benefits: Benefits include medical insurance, dental insurance, vision insurance, 401(k), and stock option plan.

Application Procedures: Interested candidates should forward resumes to the company. The company advertises for vacant physical

therapy, occupational therapy, and speech pathology positions.

▶ **Internships**

Type: The company offers a Dietetic and Administrative Training Program to interns. Applicants should contact Tish Freeman.

Qualifications: Interested candidates must have a college degree or must submit a transcript for consideration.

In a survey produced by the American Dental Association's Bureau of Economic and Behavioral Research, 66.7 percent of dentists in 1990 reported employing one or more dental hygienists—the highest percentage on record and an increase of 13.1 percent since 1983.

Source: *JADA*

National Heritage Inc.

11350 N. Meridian St., Ste. 200
Carmel, IN 46032
Phone: (317)580-8585

Officers: Karen Wagner, Contact.

National Medical Care Inc.

1601 Trapelo Rd.
Waltham, MA 02154
Phone: (617)466-9850

Business Description: Operator of nursing or personal care facilities that require a lesser degree of care than skilled or intermediate care facilities. Engaged in the operation of establishments providing home health care services.

Officers: Robert Armstrong, VP & Controller; Constantine L. Hampers, CEO & Chairman of the Board.

Benefits: The company offers a flexible compensation package including medical insurance and a 401(k).

Application Procedures: The company advertises for specific positions. Interested candidates should forward resumes to the human resources department.

▶ **Internships**

Type: The company does not offer any internship programs.

National Medical Enterprises Inc.
2700 Colorado Ave.
Santa Monica, CA 90404
Phone: (310)998-8000

Business Description: One of the largest health care service companies in the United States, owning and operating over 500 acute-care, psychiatric, and rehabilitation hospitals, and long-term care and substance abuse treatment facilities. Also operates internationally.

Officers: Richard K. Eamer, CEO & Chairman of the Board; Taylor R. Jenson, Exec. VP & CFO.

Benefits: Benefits include medical insurance, dental insurance, vision insurance, and a retirement plan.

Human Resources: Alan R. Ewalt.

Application Procedures: Send resume and cover letter to the attention of Human Resources Department.

▶ **Internships**

Type: The company offers clerical, office, and administrative internships.

Qualifications: Requirements vary but may include previous experience or a college degree.

National Pharmacies Inc.
491 Edward H. Ross Dr.
Elmwood Park, NJ 07407
Phone: (201)794-1001

Business Description: Engaged in manufacturing, fabricating and/or processing drugs in pharmaceutical preparations.

Officers: Martin Wygod, CEO.

Benefits: The company offers a full benefit plan to full-time employees.

Human Resources: Celest Puch.

Application Procedures: The company prefers in-person applications, but accepts resumes as well. Applications and resumes are kept on file for six months. Interested candidates should direct their submissions to the Human Resource Department.

▶ **Internships**

Type: The company occasionally offers internships to college students. Interested candidates should contact the Human Resource Department for more information.

National Rehabilitation Centers
PO Box 2549
Brentwood, TN 37024
Phone: (615)377-2937

Business Description: Operator of specialized outpatient facilities.

Benefits: Benefits include medical insurance, dental insurance, and life insurance.

Human Resources: Linda Boggess.

Application Procedures: Send resume and cover letter to the attention of Pam Feinstein.

▶ **Internships**

Contact: Marianne Blackwell.

Type: Offers an internship program for physical therapists, occupational therapists, speech and language pathologists.

Qualifications: Education and experience is helpful.

Application Procedure: Send applications to the attention of Marianne Blackwell.

NeuroCare Inc.
1001 Galaxy Way
Concord, CA 94520
Phone: (510)686-5500

Business Description: Acute head injury rehabilitation hospital.

Officers: Michael Grishman, President.

Opportunities: Hires entry-level clinicians and physical therapists with college degrees.

Benefits: Benefits include medical insurance, 401(k), and paid vacation.

Human Resources: Erin Krajewski; Sharon Schofield.

Application Procedures: Call to schedule an appointment. Phone: (510)682-9000.

▶ **Internships**

Contact: James Cole, Personnel Dept.

Type: Paid internships are available for college credit. **Number Available Annually:** 2.

Qualifications: Internships are available to college graduates.

Application Procedure: Call to schedule an appointment between 8:00 and 12:00 am.

NeuroCare of Orange County Inc.

6 Jenner St.
Irvine, CA 92718
Phone: (714)453-1000

Business Description: Offices of physical rehabilitation therapists.

New England Rehabilitation Hospital

2 Rehabilitation Way
Woburn, MA 01801
Phone: (617)935-5050

Opportunities: Hires entry-level staff. Must be a licensed physical therapist.

Benefits: Benefits include medical insurance, life insurance, dental insurance, auto insurance, and household insurance.

Application Procedures: Posts job listings. Depending upon the position, call or send resume and cover letter to the attention of Head of Occupational Therapy, Nursing, or Physical Therapy.

▶ Internships

Type: The company does not offer an internship program.

New England Rehabilitation Hospital

13 Charles St.
Portland, ME 04102
Phone: (207)775-4000

Opportunities: Hires entry-level staff in food service, housekeeping, clerical, rehabilitation, and AIDS areas. A high school diploma is required.

Benefits: Benefits include medical insurance, life insurance, dental insurance, tuition assistance, and child-care programs.

Human Resources: Candice Kalvert.

Application Procedures: Call to schedule an appointment or apply in person from 8 a.m. to 8 p.m.

▶ Internships

Contact: Candice Kalvert, Asst. VP of Human Resources.

Type: Offers paid and unpaid internships. **Number Available Annually:** Under 5.

Qualifications: College students.

Application Procedure: Letter of entrance must be handed in with application.

The US Congress's Office of Technology Assessment estimated in 1990 that US companies spent $30 billion to $40 billion annually on training, mostly in programs for executives, salespeople, and technical workers.

Source: *Business Week*

New Life Treatment Centers Inc.

570 Glenneyre St.
Laguna Beach, CA 92651
Phone: (714)494-8383

Opportunities: Hires entry-level dietary and support staff. Previous experience and/or a college degree may be required.

Benefits: Benefits include medical insurance, life insurance, dental insurance, vision insurance, 401(k), and disability insurance.

Application Procedures: Call, apply in person and fill out an application, or send resume and cover letter to Human Resources.

▶ Internships

Type: The company does not offer any internship programs.

New Medico Associates Inc.

470 Atlantic Ave., 7th Fl.
Boston, MA 02210
Phone: (617)426-4100
Fax: (617)426-3030

Business Description: Operator of nursing or personal care facilities that require a lesser degree of care than skilled or intermediate care facilities. Operator of general medical and surgical hospitals. Operator of specialized outpatient facilities.

Officers: Jeffery Goldshine, President.

Opportunities: Hires nurses, nurses aides and therapists.

Human Resources: Paul Marsh; Steve Richelson.

Application Procedures: Send resume and cover letter to the attention of Jerry Freedman.

▶ **Internships**

Type: The company does not offer an internship program.

New Medico Neurologic Center of Michigan

3003 W. Grand River
Howell, MI 48843
Phone: (517)546-4210

Opportunities: The center hires nurses with previous experience and a college degree.

Benefits: Benefits include medical insurance, dental insurance, vision insurance, and tuition assistance.

Human Resources: Kim Martin-Smith.

Application Procedures: Contact the personnel department, unsolicited resumes will not be accepted.

Newport Hospital

11 Friendship St.
Newport, RI 02840
Phone: (401)846-6400

Business Description: Operator of general medical and surgical hospitals.

Officers: R.J. Healey, CEO & Pres.; Sandra F. King, Dir. of Mktg. & Sales; J. Onorato, CFO; Dale Silva, VP of Data Processing.

Benefits: Benefits include medical insurance, dental insurance, and vision insurance for full-time employees. Part-time employees who work less than 32 hours a week receive partial benefits.

Human Resources: Shirley Miller.

Application Procedures: Interested candidates should complete and return applications to the human resources department.

▶ **Internships**

Type: The company offers an internship program. Interested candidates should contact human resources for more information.

Norrell Health Care Inc.

3535 Piedmont Rd., NE
Atlanta, GA 30305
Phone: (404)240-3000

Business Description: Intermediate care nursing homes.

Benefits: Some benefits provided depending on employment status.

Human Resources: Linda Arnold; Deborah Thomas, Director of Corporate Recruiting.

Application Procedures: Apply in person or contact by phone.

North Broward Hospital District

303 SE 17th St.
Fort Lauderdale, FL 33316
Phone: 800-222-4337

Employees: 5,500.

Average Entry-Level Hiring: Unknown.

Opportunities: Positions for all allied health professionals, pharmacists, and medical technologists are available; no requirements specified.

Application Procedures: Contact Human Resources for information.

North Colorado Medical Center

1801 16th St.
Greeley, CO 80631
Phone: (303)352-4121

Business Description: Operator of general medical and surgical hospitals.

Officers: Vicki Baier, Mktg. Mgr.; Troy Bailey, Info. Systems Mgr.; Richard Stenner, President; Dale Weyerts, Vice Pres.

Benefits: Benefits include life insurance, medical insurance, dental insurance.

Human Resources: Ken Nickerson.

Application Procedures: Interested applicants should forward resumes for specific job openings to the human resources department. Vacancies are posted on the company's job hotline: (303)350-6565.

▶ **Internships**

Type: The company does not offer an internship program.

North Louisiana Rehabilitation Hospital

1401 Ezell St.
Ruston, LA 71270
Phone: (318)251-3126

Opportunities: Hires entry-level nursing staff. College degree and nursing license required.

Benefits: Benefits include medical insurance, life insurance, dental insurance, vision insurance, savings plan, tuition assistance, and profit sharing.

Application Procedures: Send resume and cover letter to the attention of Personnel. For other positions, contact Job Service.

▶ **Internships**

Type: Offers unpaid internships.

Qualifications: Graduate students.

Application Procedure: Application procedure is processed through the sponsoring institution.

Northern Virginia Doctors Hospital Corp.

601 S. Carling Springs
Arlington, VA 22204
Phone: (703)671-1200

Opportunities: Hires entry-level staff in many areas, including psychiatric units, pharmacy, physical therapy, dietary, housekeeping, material management, business office, and switchboard. Requirements vary depending on the position.

Benefits: Benefits include medical insurance, life insurance, dental insurance, savings plan, and 401(k).

Application Procedures: Apply in person or send resume and cover letter to the attention of Human Resources.

▶ **Internships**

Type: Offers unpaid internships for college credit in the physical therapy, laboratory, and imaging departments. **Number Available Annually:** 36-48.

Qualifications: College students.

Application Procedure: Call for application information.

Northwest Community Hospital

800 W. Central Rd.
Arlington Heights, IL 60005
Phone: (708)259-1000
Fax: (708)506-4395

Employees: 2,500.

Average Entry-Level Hiring: Unknown.

Opportunities: RN—two-, three-, or four-year degree. Many other entry-level positions are available.

Human Resources: Karolynn Kuecher, Nursing.

Application Procedures: Call for more information.

The methods advocated by W. Edwards Deming and other such quality gurus are more about changes in organization and attitude than about the statistical control charts they are often associated with. Two recent books about Deming: *Deming Management at Work*, by Mary Walton, and *The Man Who Discovered Quality: How W. Edwards Deming Brought the Quality Revolution to America—the Stories of Ford, Xerox, and GM*, by Andrea Gabor.

Source: *The New York Times Book Review*

NovaCare Inc.

1016 W. 9th Ave.
King of Prussia, PA 19406
Phone: (215)992-7200

Business Description: Provides physical therapy, occupational therapy, and speech/language pathology services to the nursing home industries under 3100 contracts with 1780 facilities in 32 states.

Officers: John H. Foster, CEO & Chairman of the Board; C. Arnold Renschler, M.D., Pres. & COO.

Benefits: Benefits include: medical insurance, dental insurance, 401(k), day care benefits, and a flexible spending program.

Human Resources: Arthur A. Price, Ph.D.

Application Procedures: Interested candidates should forward resumes to Marianne Barker or the Human Resources Department. Applications will be held on file for one year.

▶ **Internships**

Type: The company offers summer internships in accounting.

Qualifications: Must be a college student.

Application Procedure: Interested candidates should contact the Human Resources Department.

Nu-Med Inc.

PO Box 18260
Encino, CA 91416-8260
Phone: (818)990-2000

Business Description: Operator of psychiatric hospitals. Operator of specialty hospitals.

Officers: Stuart Bruck, VP of Mktg.; Yoram Dor, Exec. VP & CFO; Maurice Lewitt, CEO & Chairman of the Board.

Benefits: The company offers benefits to full-time employees only.

Human Resources: Carol Shardt.

Application Procedures: Interested applicants should forward resumes to the company. Resumes will remain on file for two years.

▶ **Internships**

Type: The company does not offer any internship programs.

Occupational Medical Corporation of America Inc.

9811 Bigge St.
Oakland, CA 94603
Phone: (510)569-9766

Business Description: Employment-related health care and preventive medical services.

Officers: Don R. Livingston, Chairman of the Board; Alfonso S. Reyes Jr., VP of Finance.

Opportunities: Hires entry-level staff in all areas. A college degree is required.

Benefits: Benefits include medical insurance, dental insurance, vision insurance, 401(k), and vacation days.

Application Procedures: Apply in person and fill out an application or send resume and cover letter. Contact the head of the department of interest.

▶ **Internships**

Type: Offers unpaid internships for medical

assistants. Each program is six weeks in length.
Number Available Annually: 2.

Application Procedure: Students should apply through their school.

Omnilife Systems Inc.

1207 N. High St.
Columbus, OH 43201
Phone: (614)299-3100

Business Description: Intermediate care nursing homes.

Officers: Robert Banasik, President.

Opportunities: Hires entry-level staff with previous experience.

Benefits: Benefits include medical insurance and life insurance.

Human Resources: Terri Ruhwedel, Contact.

Application Procedures: Apply in person with Terri Ruhwedel. If you want to work at a specific facility, apply at that location.

▶ **Internships**

Type: This company does not offer an internship program.

Orange Park Medical Center

2001 Kingsley Ave.
Orange Park, FL 32073
Phone: (904)276-8500

Business Description: Operator of general medical and surgical hospitals.

Officers: John Corbett, CFO; Lee Ledbetter, CEO; Margaret Wright, Dir. of Mktg.

Benefits: Offers insurance options, vacation and sick leave, and a savings plan.

Human Resources: Dave Venter.

Application Procedures: Accepts walk-in applicants. Maintains a job hotline. Send resume and cover letter to the attention of the Human Resources Department.

▶ **Internships**

Type: The company does not offer an internship program.

Orlando Regional Healthcare System

1414 S. Kuhl Ave.
Orlando, FL 32806
Phone: (407)841-5186
Fax: (407)237-6374

Employees: 5,000.

Average Entry-Level Hiring: Unknown.

Opportunities: RN—two-, three-, or four-year degree required. Other positions are also available.

Application Procedures: Call Personnel for more information.

Ortho Pharmaceutical Corp.

Rte. 202
PO Box 300
Raritan, NJ 08869
Phone: (908)524-0400

Business Description: Engaged in manufacturing, fabricating and/or processing drugs in pharmaceutical preparations.

Benefits: The company offers full benefits.

Application Procedures: Send resume and cover letter to the attention of Recruiting Department. The company provides a job information line.

▶ **Internships**

Type: The company offers internships in many different areas.

Qualifications: Requirements vary, but may include college degrees or previous experience.

Application Procedure: Interested applicants should contact the department they wish to intern in.

Pacific Sports Medicine

3315 S. 23rd St.
Tacoma, WA 98405
Phone: (206)572-8326

Officers: Francis Corey-Boulet, Contact.

Pain Management Centers

8060 Montgomery Rd., Ste. 101
Cincinnati, OH 45236
Phone: (513)791-8038

Opportunities: Hires degreed physical therapists.

Benefits: Benefits include medical insurance, life insurance, and 401(k).

Application Procedures: Send resume and cover letter to the attention of Jeffry Spain, Medical Director.

▶ **Internships**

Type: The company does not offer an internship program.

> **"Eighty** percent of the initial impression you make is nonverbal," asserts Jennifer Maxwell Morris, a New York-based image consultant, quoting a University of Minnesota study. Some interview tips: walk tall, enter the room briskly while making eye contact with the person you're going to speak to, keep your head up, square your shoulders and keep your hand ready for a firm handshake that involves the whole hand but does not pump.
>
> Source: *Working Woman*

Palo Alto Medical Foundation Urgent Care Center Inc.

300 Homer St.
Palo Alto, CA 94301
Phone: (415)853-2958

Opportunities: Hires entry-level clerical staff. High school diploma required.

Benefits: Benefits include medical insurance, life insurance, dental insurance, and 401(k).

Application Procedures: Send resume and cover letter to the attention of Human Resources Department.

▶ **Internships**

Contact: Lou Shaw, Nurse Training Coord.

Type: Offers paid and college credit internships.

Application Procedure: Call Nurse Training Coordinator.

Palo Alto Veterans Administration Medical Center

3801 Miranda Ave.
Palo Alto, CA 94304
Phone: (415)858-3951
Fax: (415)852-3318

Employees: 2,500.

Average Entry-Level Hiring: Unknown.

Opportunities: Many opportunities are available, including positions in nursing, physical therapy, rehabilitation, and as clerks.

Human Resources: Amy Lee, Nursing.

Application Procedures: Call for more information.

H. Wayne Huizenga co-founded Waste Management, Inc., now the world's largest handler of waste materials, then started a bottled-water business that he sold to concentrate on creating Blockbuster Entertainment. He counsels budding entrepreneurs to plan their products around logical, foreseeable developments.

Source: *Forbes*

Parc Place
5116 E. Thomas Rd.
Phoenix, AZ 85018
Phone: (602)840-4774

Opportunities: The company requires either a college degree or two years previous experience in a related field. Positions include administration, nursing, human resources, secretarial, bachelor's degree counselors, and master's degree therapists.

Benefits: Benefits include medical insurance, profit sharing, dental insurance, paid vacations, sick days, and holidays.

Human Resources: Colleen Wilson.

Application Procedures: Applicants can send resumes to the human resources department or make contact by telephone.

▶ Internships

Contact: Mimi Rodriguez, Program Coordinator.

Type: The company does offer internships that fluctuate in compensation depending on the intern's qualifications. The company typically awards four internships per year.

PersonaCare Inc.
2 E. Read St.
Baltimore, MD 21202
Phone: (410)539-5700

Business Description: Operator of health care facilities.

Officers: Tim Smick, President.

Benefits: Benefits include medical insurance, life insurance, dental insurance, vision insurance, child-care programs, and 401(k).

Application Procedures: Entry-level positions available in accounts payable, accounts receivable, or as a receptionist. Send resume and cover letter.

▶ Internships

Type: The company does not offer an internship program.

Piedmont Hospital Inc.
1968 Peachtree Rd. NW
Atlanta, GA 30309
Phone: (404)350-2222
Fax: (404)605-5000

Business Description: Operator of general medical and surgical hospitals.

Officers: Candice Allen, Dir. of Mktg.; Nancy Shifflet, Controller; Hulett D. Sumlin, Director.

Benefits: Benefits include medical insurance, life insurance, dental insurance, long-term disabilities, a health club, and a credit union.

Human Resources: Joan Kraft.

Application Procedures: The company prefers completed applications to resumes, but will accept either one.

▶ Internships

Type: The company offers a nursing internship program.

Pinecrest State School
PO Box 5191
Pineville, LA 71361-5191
Phone: (318)641-2162
Fax: (318)641-2007

Employees: 20.

Average Entry-Level Hiring: 3-6.

Opportunities: Speech pathologist—must possess or be eligible to obtain a Louisiana license to practice, restricted license will be accepted.

Certificate of professional competence granted by the American Speech and Hearing Association and a master's degree are required. Occupational therapist—current Louisiana Occupational Therapist license or permit. Psychological associate—master's degree in psychology required.

Human Resources: Frank La Vallie, speech pathology, occupational therapy; Don Cross, Psychological Associate.

Plus One Fitness Clinic Inc.

200 Liberty St.
New York, NY 10281
Phone: (212)945-2525

Opportunities: Hire entry-level positions for all areas, except management. Must have a college degree.

Benefits: Offers medical benefits.

Human Resources: Kelly Collins.

Application Procedures: Send resume to the attention of the Senior Management Team.

▶ **Internships**

Contact: Joe Basante, Dir. of Training.

Type: Offers paid internship program. **Number Available Annually:** 1-2.

Application Procedure: Send application to Joe Basante, Director of Training.

Preferred Homecare of America Inc.

150 N.W. 168th St., 2nd Fl.
North Miami Beach, FL 33169
Phone: (305)653-0000
Fax: (305)823-3750

Business Description: Operator of skilled nursing care facilities other than hospitals.

Officers: Jeanette Fernandez, Dir. of Info. Systems; Carlos Herrera, President; Michael S. Samach, CFO; Suzan M. Sattler, VP of Mktg. & Sales.

Human Resources: Linda Burgess.

▶ **Internships**

Type: The company does not offer an internship program.

The Presbyterian Hospital

Columbia Presbyterian Medical Center
New York, NY 10032-3784
Phone: (212)305-1956
Fax: (212)305-2012

Employees: 8,000.

Average Entry-Level Hiring: 450.

Opportunities: Registered nurse—associate degree or B.S.N. eligible for New York State license. Physician assistant—B.S. degree, minimum New York State license. Laboratory technologist, pharmacist—B.S. degree, eligible for New York State license. Physical therapist, occupational therapist—B.A. or B.S. degree, eligible for New York State license. Radiation therapy technician, radiology technician, respiratory technician—associate degree, eligible for New York State license. Social worker—M.S.W. required, and CSW eligible.

Human Resources: Letty Mintz, Nursing; Jo Ann Olson.

Prince County Hospital

259 Beattie Ave.
Summerside, PE, Canada C1N 2A9
Phone: (902)436-9131
Fax: (902)436-1501

Employees: 450.

Average Entry-Level Hiring: 12-15.

Opportunities: Registered nurses, licensed nursing assistants, laboratory technologists, respiratory therapists, pharmacists, ultrasound technologists, physiotherapists—requirements not specified.

Human Resources: Nancy Darling.

Application Procedures: Send resume to the Personnel Department or call for more information.

Pro-Rehab Inc.

PO Box 2420
Boone, NC 28607
Phone: (704)265-0050

Business Description: Services: On-line data retrieval service designed for home users of personal computers.

Officers: Ross Glatzer, CEO; Hyde Perce, VP of Finance.

Opportunities: Hires entry-level staff for occupational therapist, occupational therapist assistant, speech therapist, and speech therapist assistant positions.

Benefits: Benefits include medical insurance, life insurance, dental insurance, vision insurance, and 401(k).

Human Resources: Don O'Uryan.

Application Procedures: Call recruiter to discuss location and send resume and cover letter.

▶ Internships

Contact: Moreen Mazur, Internship Coordinator.

Type: Offers unpaid internships for college credit. **Number Available Annually:** Varies.

Qualifications: College seniors.

PAs work in a team with physicians, nurses, and other health professionals. They are in great demand in all areas. Nationally there were seven jobs for each graduate in 1990. The Department of Labor has placed PAs on its top 15 list for career growth through the year 2000.

Source: *Healthcare Careers*

Providence Ambulatory Health Care Foundation Inc.

469 Angell St.
Providence, RI 02906
Phone: (401)861-6300

Officers: Olive Richy, Contact.

Providence Hospital

1550 Varnum St. NE
Washington, DC 20017
Phone: (202)269-7925
Fax: (202)269-7492

Employees: 1,800.

Average Entry-Level Hiring: Nurses-20.

Opportunities: RNs—associate or bachelor's degree. Other titles contracted out.

Human Resources: Carol Lieberman, Nursing.

Application Procedures: Send a letter of recommendation with applications. Call for more information.

Ramsay Health Care, Inc. Cumberland Hospital

3425 Melrose Rd.
Fayetteville, NC 28304
Phone: (919)485-7181
Fax: (919)485-8465

Business Description: Cumberland Hospital is a private, 175-bed psychiatric/chemical dependency treatment hospital offering inpatient and outpatient services to all age groups.

Employees: 300. The number of entry level people reflects 25 RNs and 5 M.S.W.s hired.

Average Entry-Level Hiring: 30.

Opportunities: RNs—psychiatric background preferred but not required. Social workers—M.S.W. required. Chemical dependency counselors—state certification required. Occupational therapists, COTAs, and recreation therapists—state registration required. Physician assistant—state licensure required.

Human Resources: Robert Reylea.

Ramsey Health Care

639 Loyola Ave., Ste. 1400
New Orleans, LA 70113
Phone: (504)525-2505

Business Description: Operator of psychiatric hospitals. Operator of specialty hospitals.

Benefits: Benefits include medical insurance, dental insurance, 401(k), sick days, a stock plan, paid holidays, paid vacation, and short-term disability insurance.

Human Resources: Barbara Molyneux.

Application Procedures: Send resume and cover letter to the attention of Pamela Neil.

▶ Internships

Type: The company does not offer any internship programs.

Ranchos Los Amigos Medical Center

7601 E. Imperial Hwy.
Downey, CA 90242
Phone: (310)940-7111
Fax: (310)803-3486

Employees: 2,500.

Average Entry-Level Hiring: Unknown.

Opportunities: RN, physical therapist, occupational therapist—bachelor's degree.

Application Procedures: Contact Human Resources for more information.

Rehab Systems Co.
3607 Rosemont Ave.
Camp Hill, PA 17011
Phone: (717)761-8350

Officers: Nancy Stover, Contact.

Rehab Works Inc.
503 S. Greenwood Ave.
Clearwater, FL 34616
Phone: (813)442-6450

Opportunities: Hires physical therapists and will hire office workers through referrals.

Benefits: Benefits include medical insurance, life insurance, long-term disability insurance, and a 401(k) plan.

Application Procedures: Apply through recruiting office.

RehabCare Corp.
112 S. Hanley
Clayton, MO 63105
Phone: (314)537-1288
Toll-free: 800-677-1238

Opportunities: Hires degreed and licensed physical therapists and occupational therapists.

Benefits: Benefits include medical insurance, dental insurance, vision insurance, and 401(k).

Human Resources: Shawn Maloney, Director of Human Resources.

Application Procedures: Does not accept unsolicited resumes. For information, contact Shawn Maloney.

▶ Internships

Type: Offers unpaid internships in physical therapy, occupational therapy, and affiliated occupations.

Qualifications: College students.

Application Procedure: Internships should be arranged through the sponsoring institution, which is then responsible for contacting the coordinator of the company's internship program.

Rehabilitation Hospital of Baton Rouge
8595 United Plaza Blvd.
Baton Rouge, LA 70809
Phone: (504)927-0567

Opportunities: The company hires entry-level therapists who have the required educational levels and are appropriately licensed.

Benefits: Benefits include medical insurance, life insurance, dental insurance, vision insurance, an 401(k) after six months, and a stock option plan.

Human Resources: Dana Peague.

Application Procedures: Interested candidates should forward resumes to the company.

▶ Internships

Type: The company offers unpaid internships and internships for college credits to college seniors. Applicants must go through a screening process. Approximately 10 internships are awarded each year.

Between positions job-seekers do best when they create a daily schedule, establishing structure for what will be done each day. Setting non-job goals to attain achievements outside job-related activities helps maintain self-confidence. Flexibility is essential; a willingness to consider alternatives can lead to opportunities in new fields and offer a chance to explore something new.

Source: *Working Woman*

Rehabilitation Institute of Chicago
345 E. Superior St.
Chicago, IL 60611
Phone: (312)908-6000

Opportunities: Job applicants must meet job criteria. May require a college degree, previous experience, or some college course work.

Benefits: Benefits include medical insurance, dental insurance, life insurance, vision insurance, long-term disability, tuition assistance, and child-care programs.

Application Procedures: Contact by phone to inquire about positions available and send a resume.

Rehabilitation Institute of Michigan
261 Mack Blvd.
Detroit, MI 48201
Phone: (313)745-1203

Opportunities: Requirements for employment vary but may include a high school diploma and/or previous work experience.

Benefits: Benefits include medical insurance, life insurance, dental insurance, vision insurance, savings plan, tuition assistance, and child-care programs.

Human Resources: Pam Biske.

Application Procedures: Prospective applicants with a high school diploma and previous work experience will be considered. The company keeps applications on file for six months. Interested applicants should submit an application to the Human Resource Department.

▶ **Internships**

Type: The company offers paid internships in physical therapy.

Qualifications: College students.

Application Procedure: Applications should be forwarded to the college recruiting staff.

Reproductive Health Services
100 N. Euclid
St. Louis, MO 63108
Phone: (314)367-0300

Opportunities: Hires entry-level counseling staff. A college degree is required.

Benefits: Benefits include medical insurance, life insurance, dental insurance, and tax exempt annuities.

Application Procedures: Send resume and cover letter to the attention of Jodi S.

▶ **Internships**

Contact: Jodi S.

Type: Offers unpaid internships for college credit.

Qualifications: College graduates.

Res-Care Inc.
Res-Care Health Services Div.
1300 Embassy Sq.
Louisville, KY 40299
Phone: (502)491-3464

Business Description: Operator of residential care facilities in which medical care is not a major element, such as drug or alcoholism rehabilitation centers, orphanages, halfway houses or homes for the aged, destitute or physically or mentally handicapped.

Officers: Terry Brownson, President.

Application Procedures: Interested applicants should forward resumes to Carol Webb. Positions vary and are advertised when there are job vacancies.

▶ **Internships**

Type: The company does not offer any internship programs.

Response Technologies Inc.
2001 Charlotte Ave., Ste. 100
Nashville, TN 37203
Phone: (615)320-7300

Business Description: Outpatient cancer treatment and research firm.

A.H. Robins Company Inc.
PO Box 26609
Richmond, VA 23261-6609
Phone: (804)257-2000

Business Description: Manufacturer and marketer of pharmaceuticals.

Officers: John R. Considine, Treasurer; Steven Gootzeit, VP of Mktg.; John R. Stafford, CEO & Pres.

Benefits: The company offers benefit packages based on the position. Benefits include a savings plan and insurance.

Human Resources: Thomas Scanniello.

Application Procedures: The company posts job vacancies on its job line: (804)257-2600. Interested applicants should forward resumes to the attention of the name stated on the message.

▶ **Internships**

Type: The company does not offer any internship programs.

Rocky Mountain Rehabilitation Institute
900 Potomac St.
Aurora, CO 80011
Phone: (303)367-1166

Opportunities: Hires nurses, custodial workers, and physical therapists.

Benefits: Benefits include medical insurance, life insurance, dental insurance, vision insurance, savings plan, and a credit union.

Human Resources: Lauri Wilkes.

▶ **Internships**

Type: Offers an internship program.

Roger Williams Medical Center

825 Chalkstone Ave.
Providence, RI 02908
Phone: (401)456-2288
Fax: (401)456-2029

Employees: 1,500.

Average Entry-Level Hiring: Unknown.

Opportunities: RN—two-, three- or four-year degree required. No other requirements specified.

Human Resources: Rosemary G. Barber.

Roosevelt Warm Springs Institute for Rehabilitation

PO Box 1000
Warm Springs, GA 31830
Phone: (706)655-5001

Opportunities: Hires entry-level staff in all areas.

Benefits: Benefits include medical insurance, life insurance, dental insurance, savings plan, and legal insurance.

Human Resources: Kay Garett.

Application Procedures: Fill out Merrit System application and send resume and cover letter.

▶ **Internships**

Contact: Kay Garett, Personnel Dept.

Type: Offers unpaid internships for college credit in physical therapy, nursing, and counseling. **Number Available Annually:** Varies.

Qualifications: College students.

Rorer Pharmaceutical Corp.

500 Arcola
Collegeville, PA 19426
Phone: (215)628-6000

Business Description: Engaged in manufac-

turing, fabricating and/or processing drugs in pharmaceutical preparations.

Officers: Daniel J. Paracka, CFO; Randy Thurman, President.

Benefits: Benefits include dental insurance, vision insurance, 401(k), savings plan, HMO's, short and long-term disability, and retirement plans.

Application Procedures: Interested applicants should forward resumes or completed applications to the company.

▶ **Internships**

Type: The company offers internships in the corporate and the manufacturing divisions.

Top Traits of Superior Leaders

1. Honest
2. Competent
3. Forward-looking
4. Inspiring
5. Intelligent
6. Fair-minded
7. Broad-minded
8. Courageous
9. Straightforward
10. Imaginative

Source: *Business Credit*

Rotary Rehabilitation Hospital

1874 Pleasant Ave.
PO Box 7008
Mobile, AL 36670
Phone: (205)431-3400

Application Procedures: For application information contact the Personnel Department at (205) 431-4920.

St. David's Health Care System Inc.

PO Box 4039
Austin, TX 78765
Phone: (512)476-7111

Opportunities: Hires applicants with some previous experience or a college degree. At least some college course work is required.

Benefits: Benefits include medical insurance, life insurance, dental insurance, vision insurance, savings investment plan, tuition assistance, and child or elder care.

Application Procedures: Maintains a job hotline at (512)397-4000. Can apply by contacting St. David's by phone.

According to Mack Hanan, author of *Tomorrow's Competition: The Next Generation of Growth Strategies*, in the new order of global business, success will depend on alliances that strengthen the customer, thus securing a company's value in the marketplace. In his book Hanan offers advice on how to compete on value rather than price or performance, how to drive markets, and how to "sell without selling" by co-managing customer operations. The goal is to prosper in a new world where "competition is cooperative, and 3 suppliers are obsolete."

St. John's Hospital
800 E. Carpenter St.
Springfield, IL 62769
Phone: (217)544-6464
Fax: (217)525-5601

Employees: 3,600.

Average Entry-Level Hiring: Unknown.

Opportunities: Registered nurse—bachelor's degree or state permit required. Physical therapist, occupational therapist—bachelor's degree required.

Human Resources: Joan Stennard; Tracie Sayre.

Application Procedures: Call for more information.

St. John's Mercy Medical Center
615 S. New Ballas Rd.
St. Louis, MO 63141
Phone: (314)569-6110
Fax: (314)569-6218

Employees: 4,006.

Average Entry-Level Hiring: 500.

Opportunities: Registered nurses, professionals, management, technicians, clerical, service—educational and skill requirements will vary depending on individual positions.

Human Resources: Mary Jo Lehmann RN, Nursing; Sandi Pingleton; Karen Lucash; Donna Aumiller.

St. John's Regional Medical Center
2727 McClelland Blvd.
Joplin, MO 64804
Phone: (417)625-2003
Fax: (417)625-2896

Employees: 506.

Average Entry-Level Hiring: 300.

Opportunities: Nurses—license certified and at least two years of education. Pharmacy, medical technicians, occupational and respiratory therapists—bachelor's degree required.

Human Resources: Howard Smith.

▶ **Internships**

Type: Offers an internship program. Offered on a case by case program.

St. Joseph Medical Center
3600 E. Harry St.
Wichita, KS 67218
Phone: (316)689-4839
Fax: (316)689-6338

Employees: 2,400.

Average Entry-Level Hiring: 20—Health. 20—Non-Health.

Opportunities: RN—two-, three-, or four-year degrees. Physical and occupational therapists—bachelor's degree required.

Human Resources: Dan Urenda.

St. Joseph Mercy Hospitals of Macomb
17001 19 Mile Rd.
Mt. Clemens, MI 48044
Phone: (313)263-2801
Fax: (313)263-2803

Employees: 2,000.

Average Entry-Level Hiring: 20-30.

Opportunities: Registered nurse, LPN, nurse

assistant, nurse technician in critical care (ER, ICU, CCU, Telemetry), neurology/family practice, oncology, psychiatric services, physical medicine and rehabilitation, orthopedics, pediatrics, surgical services, and women's health; nursery, labor and delivery, and gynecology. Nurse assistant—six months experience in acute care. Nurse technician—completion of medical/surgical rotation in accredited nursing school. Surgical technician—LPN or completion of accredited surgical tech program. Medical technologist—bachelor's degree and ASCP certification. Histology technologist—accredited program in histology. Occupational and physical therapists—bachelor's degree. Physical therapy assistant—associate degree. Radiology technologist—approved school of radiologic technology, American Registry of Radiologic Technologists. Nuclear medicine technologist—accredited Nuclear Medicine Technology program, ARRT or NMTCB. Ultrasound technologist—registered diagnostic medical sonographer and ARRT. Computer tomography technologist—approved school of Radiologic Technology. Respiratory therapist—two-year respiratory therapist program, RRT preferred. Respiratory technician—six months training in approved respiratory therapy program, CRTT preferred.

Human Resources: Diana Palmeri; Virginia Kastner.

▶ **Internships**

Type: Available in some areas.

St. Luke's Metrohealth Medical Center

11311 Shaker Blvd.
Cleveland, OH 44104-9989
Phone: (216)368-7445
Fax: (216)368-7457

Employees: 2,000.

Average Entry-Level Hiring: Unknown.

Opportunities: RN—associate or bachelor's degree. Occupational therapist—bachelor's degree.

Human Resources: Charlotte Stein.

Application Procedures: Call for more information.

St. Michael's Hospital

30 Bond St.
Toronto, ON, Canada M5B 1W8
Phone: (416)360-4000
Fax: (416)867-7488

Employees: 2,400.

Average Entry-Level Hiring: Unknown.

Opportunities: RN—a two-, three-, or four-year degree is required. Other positions available.

Application Procedures: Call the employment coordinator in human resources at (416)867-7401 for more information.

Schering-Plough Corp.

1 Giralda Farms
PO Box 1000
Madison, NJ 07940-1000
Phone: (201)822-7000

Business Description: Develops, manufactures, and markets prescription and over-the-counter medicines and drugs, veterinary medicines and products, cosmetics, and other personal care products.

Officers: Harold R. Hiser Jr., Exec. VP of Finance; Robert P. Luciano, CEO & Chairman of the Board.

Benefits: Benefits include a management recognition plan. Training programs include personal development courses as a part of the management training program. Schering-Plough identifies employees with management potential and provides them with such courses as assertiveness training, problem solving, decision making, and communications. The company also offers medical insurance and dental insurance.

Application Procedures: The company advertises vacant positions in the classified ads, and also accepts unsolicited resumes. Interested candidates should forward resumes to the attention of the Human Resources Department.

▶ **Internships**

Type: The company does not offer any internship programs.

Scottsdale Memorial Health Systems Inc.

3621 Wells Fargo Ave.
Scottsdale, AZ 85251
Phone: (602)481-4500

Opportunities: The company requires that

applicants have some college course work to be eligible for entry-level positions in clerical as well as professional areas.

Benefits: Benefits include 401(k), medical insurance, child-care programs, life insurance, dental insurance, vision insurance, savings plan, and elder-care programs,

Application Procedures: Company accepts applications at the personnel office or resumes by mail.

Squeezed by foreign competition and a slowing economy, employers are increasingly shunning fixed raises in favor of pay plans where employees can enrich themselves only by enriching the company. From hourly workers to managers in pin stripes, those who boost earnings, productivity, or other results prosper. Those who turn in a lackluster performance take home less.

Source: *US News & World Report*

G.D. Searle & Co.
5200 Old Orchard Rd.
Skokie, IL 60077
Phone: (708)982-7000
Fax: (708)982-1480

Business Description: Develops, manufactures, and markets pharmaceuticals for the cardiovascular system, the central nervous system, and the gastrointestinal tract, as well as oral contraceptives, low-calorie sweeteners, anti-inflammatory drugs, and anti-infective drugs. Research and development laboratories are located in Skokie, Illinois; Chesterfield, Missouri; Belgium; India; Japan; and England. Manufacturing facilities are located in Augusta, Georgia; Mt. Prospect, Illinois; Caguas, Puerto Rico; Australia; Belgium; Canada; France; Germany; India; Japan; Korea; Mexico; Pakistan; South Africa; Spain; England; and Venezuela.

Officers: Richard U. Deschutter, Exec. VP; Sheldon Gilgore, M.D., CEO, Pres. & Chairman of the Board.

Benefits: Benefits include medical insurance, dental insurance, vision insurance, an employee pension plan, a 401(k) plan, and short- and long-term disability.

Application Procedures: Places newspaper

advertisements for certain openings and accepts unsolicited resumes. Send resume and cover letter to the attention of Human Resources Department, 4901 Searle Park Rd., Skokie, IL 60077.

▶ Internships

Type: Offers an internship program.

Shaughnessy-Kaplan Rehabilitation Hospital
Dove Ave.
Salem, MA 01970
Phone: (508)741-1200

Opportunities: Hires entry-level dietary and housekeeping staff, unit service aides, and home health aides. Previous experience is required.

Benefits: Benefits include medical insurance, life insurance, dental insurance, savings plan, flexible spending, homeowner's insurance, auto insurance, and disability insurance.

Application Procedures: Posts openings at job office. Apply in person or send resume and cover letter to Central Human Resource Centre or Employment Office.

▶ Internships

Contact: Elaine Antell, Director, Human Relations.

Type: Offers unpaid internships for college credit. **Number Available Annually:** 25.

Qualifications: College juniors or seniors. The sponsoring institution must have a contract with the hospital in order for a student to qualify for the internship.

Shepherd Spinal Center
2020 Peachtree Rd. NW
Atlanta, GA 30309
Phone: (404)352-2020

Opportunities: Hires therapists in all areas. Requires a college degree.

Benefits: Benefits include medical insurance, life insurance, dental insurance, and savings plan.

Human Resources: Betsy Fox; Doris O'Neal.

Application Procedures: Apply in person or send resume to the attention of Human Resources.

▶ Internships

Type: Offers unpaid internships for college credit to senior students.

Application Procedure: Send resume and cover letter to the attention of Human Resources.

Shipley Manor

2723 Shipley Rd.
Wilmington, DE 19810
Phone: (302)479-0111

Opportunities: Hires for dietary and nursing positions. Employees receive on-the-job training.

Benefits: Benefits include medical insurance, life insurance, dental insurance, vision insurance, a 401(k) plan, and a credit union.

Human Resources: Kim Pepe.

Application Procedures: Apply for positions of interest. Applications are kept on file.

▶ Internships

Type: The company does not offer an internship program.

Sierra Tucson Companies Inc.

16500 N. Lago del Oro Pkwy.
Tucson, AZ 85737
Phone: (602)624-4000
Fax: (602)792-2916

Business Description: Sierra Tucson is a 126-bed residential center for the treatment of adults with addictions and mental, emotional and behavioral disorders. In December 1989, Sierra Tucson opened a 65-bed treatment clinic in West Germany. The facility is located in Garmish-Partenkirchen in the State of Bavaria, approximately 60 miles south of Munich.

Officers: William T. O'Donnell, Pres. & Chairman of the Board; Judy Scheib McCaleb, VP of Mktg.; John H. Schmitz, Exec. VP & CFO.

Benefits: Benefits include medical insurance, dental insurance, and vision insurance.

Human Resources: C. Diane Baker.

Application Procedures: The company accepts resumes and keeps them on file for one year. Interested candidates should forward resumes to the attention of Human Resources.

▶ Internships

Type: The company offers unpaid internships to college students that relate to the student's degree. Interested applicants should forward resumes to the attention of Human Resources.

Sinai Health Care System

6767 W. Outer Dr.
Detroit, MI 48235
Phone: (313)493-6800

Opportunities: Hires entry-level applicants for housekeeping, dietary work, and patient transportation. Prefers previous work experience, but it is not mandatory.

Benefits: Benefits include life insurance, dental insurance, and a pension plan.

Application Procedures: Interested applicants should send resumes to the Personnel Department. The department can be reached at (313) 493-6162. All resumes will be kept on file for six months.

▶ Internships

Type: The company occasionally offers unpaid internships for college credit.

Application Procedure: Send resume to the attention of the Employment Office.

SmithKline & French Laboratories

1 Franklin Plaza
Box 7929
Philadelphia, PA 19101
Phone: (215)751-4000

Business Description: Engaged in manufacturing, fabricating and/or processing drugs in pharmaceutical preparations.

Benefits: Benefits include medical insurance, dental insurance, employee pension plan.

Human Resources: G.R. Partridge.

Application Procedures: The company accepts unsolicited resumes with cover letters. Resumes should be forwarded to the attention of the Employment Administrator.

▶ **Internships**

Type: The company offers an internship program.

Average teachers' salaries rose only 3.6 percent during the 1991-92 school year, their smallest increase in 27 years, according to the American Federation of Teachers. Physical therapists, pharmacists and nurses, by contrast, enjoyed raises of up to 7.3 percent.

Source: *U.S. News & World Report*

SmithKline Beecham Corp.

PO Box 7929
Philadelphia, PA 19101
Phone: (215)751-4000
Fax: (215)751-3400

Business Description: Pharmaceutical operations are headquartered in Philadelphia, Pennsylvania. The company also operates a research center in Upper Merion, Pennsylvania; a Consumer Brands operation, which develops and produces over-the-counter health products, is headquartered in Pittsburgh, Pennsylvania; Animal Health operations, located in West Chester, Pennsylvania; clinical laboratories operations, headquartered in King of Prussia, Pennsylvania; and 26 other laboratories in the U.S.

Officers: Robert Bauman, CEO & Chairman of the Board; K.N. Kermes, Exec. VP of Finance.

Benefits: Benefits include an employee pension plan, medical insurance, and dental insurance.

Application Procedures: The company accepts unsolicited resumes. Interested candidates should forward resumes to the Employment Administrator.

▶ **Internships**

Type: The company offers an internship program.

Somatix Therapy Corp.

850 Marina Village Pkwy.
Alameda, CA 94501
Phone: (510)748-3000

Business Description: Operator of medical laboratories.

Human Resources: J. Monahan.

Application Procedures: Send resume and cover letter to the attention of Cecilia in Human Resources.

▶ **Internships**

Type: The company does not typically offer internships, but might consider applications if company had a specific need. Interested candidates should contact the Human Resources Department.

South County Hospital

100 Kenyon Ave.
Wakefield, RI 02879
Phone: (401)782-8000

Business Description: Operator of general medical and surgical hospitals.

Officers: D.J. Mazzarelli, President; Philip E. Trecy, Sr. VP.

Benefits: Offers full medical and dental benefits.

Human Resources: Ralph L. Misto Jr.

Application Procedures: Accepts unsolicited resumes. Advertises in classified. Applications and/or resumes kept on file for one year.

▶ **Internships**

Type: The company does not offer an internship program.

Southboro Medical Group Inc.

24 Newton St.
Southborough, MA 01772
Phone: (508)481-5500

Opportunities: Hires entry-level data entry and reception staff and file clerks. Previous experience and high school diploma required.

Benefits: Benefits include medical insurance, life insurance, tuition assistance, and disability insurance.

Human Resources: Linda Avedisian.

Application Procedures: Send resume and cover letter.

▶ **Internships**

Type: Offers unpaid internships for college credit. **Number Available Annually:** 3.

Qualifications: Medical assistant program students.

Application Procedure: Awarded through training programs.

Southern Baptist Hospital

2700 Napoleon Ave.
New Orleans, LA 70115
Phone: (504)897-5841
Toll-free: 800-627-4724
Fax: (504)897-4449

Employees: 1,400.

Average Entry-Level Hiring: Unknown.

Opportunities: RNs, physical therapists, and allied health professionals.

Application Procedures: Contact the Human Resources Department for more information.

Sparks Regional Medical Center

1311 S. I St.
Fort Smith, AR 72901
Phone: (501)441-4000
Fax: (501)441-5397

Employees: 1,700.

Average Entry-Level Hiring: Unknown.

Opportunities: Registered nurse—associate or bachelor's degree required. Experience preferred but not required. Also hires pharmacists, dieticians, and other allied health professionals.

Application Procedures: Contact the Human Resources Department for more information.

Spaulding Rehabilitation Hospital

125 Nashua St.
Boston, MA 02114
Phone: (617)720-6400

Benefits: Benefits include medical insurance, life insurance, dental insurance, and a savings plan.

Human Resources: Robin Coruso.

Application Procedures: Hires entry-level staff in environmental services, clerical, and food service. Prospective applicants should have previous experience. Send resume and cover letter to the attention of Robin Coruso.

▶ Internships

Contact: Robin Coruso, Human Resources.

Type: Unpaid internships are available for college credit.

Qualifications: College students.

Spine and Sports Medicine Institute of Northern California Inc.

2525 Stanwell
Concord, CA 94520
Phone: (510)686-5400

Officers: Kathy Rosenberg, Contact.

Sport Clinic of Greater Milwaukee Inc.

2250 N. 122nd St.
Wauwatosa, WI 53226
Phone: (414)453-8616

Opportunities: Hires office personnel and physical therapy aides with a high school diploma.

Benefits: Benefits include medical insurance, life insurance, and a pension plan.

Human Resources: Joy Snedeker.

Application Procedures: Call or send resume to Joy Snedeker for office personnel jobs or Yolanda Powers for physical therapy aide positions.

▶ Internships

Contact: John Crowe.

Type: Offers unpaid internships. College credit is available. **Number Available Annually:** 4.

Qualifications: College students who have reached junior status.

Application Procedure: Send resume to John Crowe.

Spring Grove Hospital Center

Wade Ave.
PO Box 3235
Catonsville, MD 21228
Phone: (410)455-6000

Opportunities: Hires beginning nurses and nurses aides. Does not hire at the entry level for technical positions. Some college course work and/or a college degree is required.

Benefits: Benefits include medical insurance, life insurance, dental insurance, vision insurance, and tuition assistance.

Human Resources: Mrs. Thomas.

Application Procedures: Apply in person or send resume and cover letter. All applicants must take the state exam.

▶ Internships

Type: The company does not offer any internship programs.

Membership in a cross-departmental problem-solving group provides a greater understanding of other business units and a broader perspective on issues. You'll need this broader perspective, because lateral moves will be increasingly common in any organization, and may play a part in your job search. "Middle managers must look sideways—not just up—if they want to increase their marketability in the 1990s," notes Beverly Robsham, president of Robsham & Associates, an outplacement firm in Boston, MA. On your resume be sure to mention any cross-departmental activities you've undertaken.

Source: *Working Woman*

Springfield Hospital Center
6655 Sykesville Rd.
Sykesville, MD 21784
Phone: (410)795-2100

Opportunities: Offers entry-level positions in dietary work, housekeeping, and as nursing assistants. All positions require a high school diploma.

Benefits: Benefits include medical insurance, life insurance, dental insurance, and a savings plan.

Application Procedures: Apply in person to the Personnel Department.

▶ Internships

Type: Offers a college internship program.

Application Procedure: Interested candidates should apply in person to the Personnel Department.

Springfield Municipal Hospital
1400 State St.
Springfield, MA 01109
Phone: (413)787-6700

Application Procedures: Hires only through the Civil Service Personnel Department at the Springfield City Hall.

Steris Laboratories
620 N. 51st Ave.
Phoenix, AZ 85043
Phone: (602)278-1400

Business Description: Engaged in manufacturing bulk organic or inorganic medicinal chemicals and derivatives, and/or processing bulk botanical drugs and herbs. Engaged in manufacturing, fabricating and/or processing drugs in pharmaceutical preparations.

Officers: Mike Blank, VP of Mktg.; James McGee, President; Thomas Spence, Dir. of Info. Systems; Robert Sullivan, VP of Finance.

Benefits: The company offers full medical and dental benefits.

Human Resources: Ron Crowe.

Application Procedures: The company accepts solicited and unsolicited resumes. The company advertises vacant positions through the classified ads. Submitted resumes are kept on file for six months and should be sent to the attention of the Human Resources Department.

▶ Internships

Type: Internships are offered through the Regulatory Affairs Department.

Sterling Drug Inc.
Winthrop Pharmaceuticals Div.
90 Park Ave.
New York, NY 10016
Phone: (212)907-2000

Business Description: Engaged in manufacturing, fabricating and/or processing drugs in pharmaceutical preparations.

Officers: Steven N. Martini, Controller; Harry Shoff, President.

Benefits: Benefits include medical insurance, dental insurance, vision insurance.

Human Resources: John G. Barry.

Application Procedures: The company accepts solicited and unsolicited resumes and keeps them on file for six months. Interested candidates should forward resumes to the attention of the Human Resources department.

▶ **Internships**

Type: The company does not offer any internship programs.

Stockton Developmental Center

510 E. Magnolia St.
Stockton, CA 95202
Phone: (209)948-7335
Fax: (209)948-7646

Business Description: All clients served are developmentally disabled. The majority are adults. The youngest age served is fourteen.

Employees: 900.

Average Entry-Level Hiring: Approximately 10 percent turnover annually.

Opportunities: Physician, surgeon, clinical, educational, and counseling psychologists, psychiatric social workers (M.S.W.), physical therapists, occupational therapists, recreational therapists, music therapists, registered nurses, psychiatric technicians, and pharmacists.

Human Resources: Thomas P. Thompson.

Stormont-Vail Regional Medical Center

1500 W. 10th
Topeka, KS 66604
Phone: (913)354-6153
Fax: (913)354-5889

Employees: 1,850.

Average Entry-Level Hiring: 64.

Opportunities: Typically hires 40 entry-level nurses per year, two physical therapists, two occupational therapists, ten respiratory therapists, one social service worker, three radiologists, three medical technicians, and three pharmacists.

Human Resources: Laurie Florence; Betty Hadison.

Summit Care Corp.

2600 W. Magnolia Blvd.
Burbank, CA 91505
Phone: (818)841-8750

Opportunities: Corporate office offers no entry-level positions. Hospitals offer some entry-level. College degree required.

Benefits: Benefits include medical insurance, life insurance, dental insurance, vision insurance, long-term disability, and a 401(k) plan for full-time employees.

Application Procedures: Call or send a resume to the personnel director of each specific department.

Summit Health Ltd.

2600 W. Magnolia Blvd.
PO Box 2100
Burbank, CA 91505-2100
Phone: (818)841-8750

Business Description: An integrated healthcare company operating hospitals, nursing centers, and other health-related facilities in Arizona, California, Iowa, and Texas.

Officers: Donald J. Amaral, Pres. & COO; Don Freeberg, CEO, Pres. & Chairman of the Board; Frank S. Osen, Sr. VP & General Counsel; William C. Scott, Sr. VP; Randolph H. Speer, Sr. VP & CFO.

Benefits: Benefits include medical insurance, dental insurance, vision insurance, life insurance, employee pension plan, and long and short-term disability.

Human Resources: David Rubardt.

Application Procedures: The company accepts solicited and unsolicited resumes. Interested candidates should forward resumes and cover letters to Sue Heinberd.

▶ **Internships**

Type: The company does not offer any internship programs.

Sun Health Corp.

13180 N. 103rd Dr.
Sun City, AZ 85351
Phone: (602)977-7211

Business Description: Owner and operator of general hospitals.

Officers: Leelan W. Peterson, CEO; Gary Turner, Sr. VP; George Perez, COO; Phillip J. Hanson, VP of Human Resources.

Opportunities: Hires entry-level staff in housekeeping and transportation. Previous experience is required.

Benefits: Benefits include medical insurance, life insurance, dental insurance, vision insurance, savings plan, tuition assistance, and child-care programs.

Human Resources: Shirley Cowaldin.

Application Procedures: Maintains a job hotline at (602)974-7984. Apply for posted openings in person.

▶ **Internships**

Type: The company does not offer an internship program.

Companies are foregoing the old five-year plan method of strategic planning for a new, everyday outlook: strategic thinking. This describes what a company does in becoming smart, targeted, and nimble enough to prosper in an era of constant change. The key words for the 1990s are focus and flexibility.

Source: *Fortune*

Syntex Corp.
3401 Hillview Ave.
Palo Alto, CA 94304
Phone: (415)855-5050

Business Description: Involved in the research, development, manufacturing and marketing of human and animal pharmaceutical products and medical diagnostic systems.

Officers: Paul E. Freiman, CEO, Pres. & Chairman of the Board; Thomas L. Gutshall, Exec. VP; Richard P. Powers, Sr. VP & CFO.

Benefits: The company offers a full medical, dental and vision health plan.

Human Resources: Andrew Oravets; Paulette Stepp.

Application Procedures: The company advertises vacant positions through classified ads. The company also accepts unsolicited resumes with cover letters. Interested candidates should forward submissions directly to the employment office.

▶ **Internships**

Type: Offers a summer internship program.
Application Deadline: March.

T2 Clinical Fasting Center of Dallas Inc.
7777 Forest Ln.
Dallas, TX 75230
Phone: (214)661-8000

Opportunities: The Company hires entry level staff in physician and clerical positions. The requirements vary depending upon the position.

Benefits: The Company offers medical and life insurance.

Human Resources: Janet Crepts.

Application Procedures: Applicants should forward resumes to or telephone Janet Crepts at Dallas Diagnostic to apply for positions.

▶ **Internships**

Type: The Company does not offer any internship programs.

Tewksbury Hospital
East St.
Tewksbury, MA 01876
Phone: (508)851-7321

TheraTx Inc.
15030 Ave. of Science
San Diego, CA 92128
Phone: (619)674-1414

Business Description: Physical rehabilitation center.

Officers: Robert L. Gremore, President; Donald R. Myll, VP of Finance; Kip Hallman, VP of Business Development.

TME Inc.
333 N. Sam Houston
Houston, TX 77056
Phone: (713)439-7511

Business Description: Outpatient diagnostic clinic.

Officers: Cherrill Farnsworth, CEO; Stephen Jackson, Exec. VP; William L. Birch, Dir. of Systems; Elizabeth Flores, Human Resources Dir.

Opportunities: Hires clerical workers for entry-level positions.

Benefits: Benefits include medical insurance, life insurance, dental insurance, a 401(k) plan, and disability benefits.

Human Resources: Pamela Castael.

Application Procedures: Send resume to apply.

Tri-State Regional Rehabilitation Hospital

4100 Covert Ave.
Evansville, IN 47715
Phone: (812)476-9983

Opportunities: The Company requires college degrees for all positions. The positions include nursing, social services, optical therapist, speech therapist, and must be able to prove certification when necessary.

Benefits: The Company offers medical insurance, life insurance, dental insurance, savings plan, tuition assistance, profit sharing, long-term disability, paid holidays, vacation and sick days, and a 401K plan.

Human Resources: Sue Nolte.

Application Procedures: Application for a position can be made through phone contact, in person, or by forwarding a resume to human resources.

▶ Internships

Type: The Company does not offer internships.

Unicare Health Facilities Inc.

105 W. Michigan St.
Milwaukee, WI 53203
Phone: (414)278-7799

Opportunities: Hires entry-level clerks and secretarial staff. Previous experience and a high school diploma are required.

Benefits: Benefits include medical insurance.

Human Resources: Nancy Lehninger.

Application Procedures: Send resume and cover letter to the attention of Trish Shult.

▶ Internships

Contact: Trish Shult.

Type: Offers paid internships. Number Available Annually: 2.

Qualifications: College students.

UniHealth America

4100 W. Alameda Ave.
Burbank, CA 91505
Phone: (818)566-6300

Business Description: Operator of general medical and surgical hospitals.

Officers: Paul Alcala, Dir. of Info. Systems; Eric S. Benveniste, Sr. VP & CFO; Paul A. Teslow, President.

Benefits: Benefits include medical insurance, dental insurance, 401(k), and short and long-term disability insurance.

Application Procedures: The company advertises vacant positions in newspapers and accepts solicited and unsolicited resumes. The company keeps applications on file for six months to a year. Applicants should direct submissions to Mojaly Juarez.

▶ Internships

Type: The company offers an internship program.

Package designers benefit from tough times, when the high cost of introducing products and the fight for shelf space at stores is encouraging many manufacturers to turn from new product development to spicing up old packaging for a boost in sales. It's less risky to put money behind known brands rather than newcomers, and some see the redesigning trend as part of a larger effort to buff up brand identities. But companies that fail to introduce new products may hurt themselves in the long run once the economy turns around and they have little in the pipeline.

Source: USA Today

United Health Inc.

105 W. Michigan St.
Milwaukee, WI 53203
Phone: (414)271-9696
Fax: (414)274-2709

Business Description: Operator of skilled nursing care facilities other than hospitals. Operator of intermediate care facilities.

Officers: Robert Abramowski, CFO; Richard Herman, Dir. of Mktg.; Guy W. Smith, President.

Benefits: Benefits include medical insurance, dental insurance, and 401(k).

Human Resources: William Wagner.

Application Procedures: The company

accepts solicited and unsolicited resumes. Interested candidates should direct submissions to Connie Champnoise.

▶ **Internships**

Type: The company does not offer any internship programs.

United Medical Corp.

56 Haddon Ave.
PO Box 200
Haddonfield, NJ 08033
Phone: (609)354-2200

Business Description: United Medical Corporation is comprised of five operating divisions. Three of these divisions provide healthcare services; one develops computerized submissions of pharmaceutical companies' new drug applications to the Food & Drug Administration; and one is a manufacturer of motorized treadmills.

Officers: John Aglialoro, CEO & Chairman of the Board; Joan Carter, Pres. & COO; Arthur W. Hicks, Jr., VP & CFO.

Benefits: The company offers a full benefits program.

Human Resources: Marian Wissman.

Application Procedures: The company accepts solicited and unsolicited resumes and advertises vacant positions through the classified ads. Interested candidates should direct submissions to the company.

▶ **Internships**

Type: The company offers an internship program.

U.S. Occupational Health Inc.

205 W. Randolph St.
Chicago, IL 60606
Phone: (312)641-1449

Human Resources: Dr. Fisher.

Universal Health Services Inc.

367 S. Gulph Rd.
King of Prussia, PA 19406
Phone: (215)768-3300

Business Description: A hospital management company for acute care and psychiatric hospitals. Operates 20 acute care hospitals and

13 psychiatric hospitals. Three hospitals are located in the United Kingdom.

Officers: Alan B. Miller, CEO & Pres.; Sidney Miller, Exec. VP.

Benefits: Benefits include medical insurance, dental insurance, 401(k), and short- and long-term disability insurance. Part-time employees must work at least 20 hours a week to receive benefits.

Human Resources: Eileen Dove.

Application Procedures: Send resume and cover letter to the attention of Eileen Dove.

▶ **Internships**

Type: The company offers an internship program.

University Hospital-Shaughnessy Site

4500 Oak St.
Vancouver, BC, Canada V6H 3N1
Phone: (604)875-2722
Fax: (604)875-2995

Employees: 4,500.

Average Entry-Level Hiring: Unknown.

Opportunities: RN—associate degree, diploma, or bachelor's degree. Physical therapist—bachelor's degree in physical therapy.

Application Procedures: Contact the Human Resources Department for more information.

Upjohn Co.

7000 Portage Rd.
Kalamazoo, MI 49001
Phone: (616)323-4000

Business Description: Develops, manufactures, and markets pharmaceuticals and other healthcare products for humans and animals. Also develops and markets agronomic seeds. Provides healthcare services.

Officers: Theodore Cooper, CEO & Chairman of the Board; Jack J. Jackson, VP of Sales; Robert C. Salisbury, VP & CFO.

Benefits: Benefits include child-care programs, child-care referrals, adoption aid, maternity leave, disability insurance, job sharing, flex time, a stock option plan, flexible spending accounts for medical and dependent care expenses, and a savings plan.

Application Procedures: Accepts unsolicited

resumes. Send resume and cover letter. Maintains a job hotline at (616)329-5550.

VA Medical Center
5500 Armstrong Rd.
Battle Creek, MI 49016
Phone: (616)966-5600
Fax: (616)966-5433

Employees: 1,600.

Average Entry-Level Hiring: 200.

Opportunities: Registered nurses, physicians, and physical therapists are needed in the areas of acute psychiatry, intermediate medicine, general medicine, and gerontology. Registered nurses—license required. Physicians—requires license and either Board eligible or certified. Physical therapist—requires appropriate degree and certification.

Human Resources: Mary Lightbody; Cynthia Sipp; Ronald Kelly.

VA Medical Center
Leestown Rd.
Lexington, KY 40511
Phone: (606)233-4511
Fax: (606)281-3994

Employees: 2,000.

Average Entry-Level Hiring: Unknown.

Opportunities: RN—two-, three- or four-year degree required. No other information available.

Human Resources: D.C. Schmonsky.

Application Procedures: Call for information.

VA Medical Center
113 Holland Ave.
Albany, NY 12208
Phone: (518)462-3311
Fax: (518)462-2519

Opportunities: Not hiring at this time.

Human Resources: Carol Ann Bedford RN, Nursing; Lawrence H. Flesh MD, Chief of Staff; Alice A. Flynn.

VA Medical Center
Fort Meade, SD 57741
Phone: (605)347-2511

Employees: 529.

Average Entry-Level Hiring: Unknown.

Opportunities: Registered nurse—associate or

bachelor's degree in nursing. LPN/LVN—completed vocational training. Physical therapist—bachelor's degree in physical therapy.

Human Resources: Sylvia Desjarlais, Registered Nurse; Ron Jacobs, Management Specialist; Mike Larson.

Application Procedures: Those dedicated to, and interested in, helping veterans in a quality work environment, are encouraged to apply.

Vari-Care Inc.
277 Alexander St.
Rochester, NY 14607
Phone: (716)325-6940

Business Description: Nursing homes.

Officers: Robert H. Hurlbut, President; William F. Doud, Exec. VP.

Opportunities: Hires entry-level accounts payable, accounts receivable, and reception staff. Previous experience required; college degree is mandatory for administrative positions.

Benefits: Benefits include medical insurance, life insurance, dental insurance, and vision insurance.

Human Resources: Patricia Gardner.

Application Procedures: Apply in person or send resume and cover letter to the attention of Patricia Gardner.

▶ Internships

Type: The company does not offer an internship program.

Vencor Inc.
Brown & Williamson Twr., Ste. 700
Louisville, KY 40202
Phone: (502)569-7300

Business Description: Specializes in providing long-term hospital care for patients suffering from catastrophic illness. The company's current operations include hospitals located in Arizona, Florida, Illinois, Indiana, Louisiana, Texas, Missouri, and Michigan.

Officers: Michael R. Barr, VP of Operations; W. Bruce Lunsford, CEO & Pres.; W. Earl Reed, III, VP of Finance.

Benefits: Offers a full benefits program including retirement plans.

Application Procedures: Places newspaper advertisements for certain openings and accepts unsolicited resumes. Send resume and cover letter to the attention of Human Resources.

▶ **Internships**

Type: Offers an internship program.

Villa Feliciana Chronic Disease Hospital and Rehabilitation Center

PO Box 438
Jackson, LA 70748
Phone: (504)634-4000

Opportunities: Hires nurses and civil service workers.

Benefits: Benefits include an HMO plan, life insurance, dental insurance, and a retirement plan.

Human Resources: Mary Banks.

Application Procedures: Contact the Civil Service Department in person or by phone to obtain a Civil Service application.

Warner-Lambert Co.

201 Tabor Rd.
Morris Plains, NJ 07950
Phone: (201)540-2000

Business Description: Develops, markets, and manufactures health care and consumer products, including ethical and non-prescription pharmaceuticals, chewing gum, breath mints, shaving products, and empty hard gelatin capsules. The company has focused its research on cognitive disorders, central nervous system conditions such as Alzheimer's disease, schizophrenia, and cardiovascular diseases such as congestive heart failure.

Officers: Ernest J. Lavini, Exec. VP & CFO; Lodewijk deVink, Pres. & COO; Melvin R. Goodes, CEO & Chairman of the Board.

Benefits: Benefits include family leave, vacation days, personal/sick days, overtime pay, child-care referrals, elder-care referrals, telecommuting, extended leave, part-time employment, job sharing, employee parking, 401(k), flex time, summer hours, on-site services such as a credit union, dry cleaners, sick pay, health insurance, and long-term disability.oil change and vehicle inspections and company store.

Human Resources: Raymond M. Fino.

Application Procedures: Interested candidates should forward resumes to the corporate human resources department. Raymond M. Fino.

▶ **Internships**

Contact: Robert Hoffman, Human Resources Dir.

Type: Provides paid internships during the summer (10 to 12 weeks). **Number Available Annually:** 12-15. **Applications Received:** 150-200.

Duties: Tasks vary depending on job. Most positions offer general project work.

Qualifications: Accepts candidates with masters degrees in Business Administration only.

Application Procedure: Campus recruiting only.

Washington Hospital Center

110 Irving St., NW
Washington, DC 20010
Phone: (202)877-6048
Toll-free: 800-432-3993
Fax: (202)877-7315

Business Description: Washington Hospital Center is an acute care, level one trauma center with 907 beds.

Employees: 5,100.

Average Entry-Level Hiring: 50-75.

Opportunities: Positions available in the following areas: nursing, PT, OT, medical technology, radiology, nuclear medicine, medical social work, respiratory therapy, pharmacy, surgical technology, cardiovascular technology, and as physician assistants. For the respective occupations, graduation from an accredited program, college, or university, and licensure is required.

Human Resources: Cynthia Wolfe, RN Nursing; Terra Cox, RN; Denise Stribling, RN.

Application Procedures: Contact Terra Cox for the following positions; PT, OT, medical technology, radiology, medical social work, nuclear medicine, and respiratory therapy. Contact Denise Stribling for the following positions; pharmacy, surgical technology, physician's assistant, and cardiovascular technology.

Wausau Hospital

333 Pine Ridge Blvd.
Wausau, WI 54401
Phone: (715)847-2800
Fax: (715)847-2017

Employees: 1,700.

Average Entry-Level Hiring: Varies with occupation.

Opportunities: RN—associate or bachelor's degree required. Also fills positions in PT, OT, medical technology, radiology, nuclear medicine, medical social work, respiratory therapy, pharmacy, surgical technology, and cardiovascular technology.

Human Resources: Cecilia R. Rudolph, RN.

Application Procedures: Call for more information.

Western Maryland Center

1500 Pennsylvania Ave.
Hagerstown, MD 21742
Phone: (301)791-4400

Opportunities: Requires at least a high school diploma. Hires physical therapists with master's degrees and patient care and direct care assistants with previous training.

Benefits: Benefits include medical insurance, life insurance, dental insurance, savings plan, and paid sick leave.

Human Resources: Pat Robinson.

Application Procedures: Send resume and cover letter to the attention of Pat Robinson, Personnel Department.

Wilderness Alternative School Inc.

200 Hubbart Dam Rd.
Marion, MT 59925
Phone: (406)854-2832

Business Description: Operator of specialized outpatient facilities.

Officers: Pete Anderson, Dir. of Mktg. & Sales; J. Brekke, President; Nancy Brekke, Dir. of Admin.

Benefits: Offers full benefits.

Human Resources: Cheryl Kirchner.

Application Procedures: Accepts unsolicited resumes. Send resume and cover letter to the attention of Human Resources.

▶ Internships

Contact: Loren Johnston.

Type: Offers non-paid internships. Meals and housing are provided.

Qualifications: Wilderness instructors with a background in guiding and a desire to become involved in wilderness expeditions.

Application Procedure: Send application to the attention of Loren Johnston.

Wilton Physical Therapy

396 Danbury Rd.
Wilton, CT 06897
Phone: (203)762-5623

Opportunities: Hires physical therapists with a college degree and previous experience.

Benefits: Benefits include medical insurance, dental insurance, tuition assistance, and sometimes profit sharing.

Human Resources: Gale Neilson.

Application Procedures: Send resume and cover letter to the attention of Gale Neilson.

The optimum time for follow-up calls after job interviews is from 9 to 11 am, Tuesday through Friday, according to Jeffrey G. Allen, author of *The Perfect Follow-Up Method to Get the Job*. The book provides a suggested script for follow-up calls or letters, gives tips on handling an interview while dining, and covers typical questions raised in a follow-up interview.

Source: *Career Opportunities News*

Women & Infants Hospital of Rhode Island

101 Dudley St.
Providence, RI 02905
Phone: (401)274-1100

Business Description: An obstetrical/gynecological teaching hospital that provides neonatal intensive care and gynecological oncology care.

Officers: Marke Crevier, Sr. VP & Finance Officer; Phyllis W. Jackowitz, VP of Mktg.; Thomas G. Parris, Jr., President; Bruce A. Reirden, Info. Systems Mgr.

Average Entry-Level Hiring: Hiring levels are expected to remain constant for the next few years.

Opportunities: Hires specialists such as genetic counselors, nurse practitioners, midwives, and pharmacists; and technicians such as diagnostic medical sonographers, medical technologists, cytotechnologists, and research assistants. Also hires medical transcriptionists, secretaries, clerical workers, electricians, and HVAC mechanics.

Benefits: Provides medical insurance, dental insurance, vision insurance, life insurance, long-term disability, and short-term disability. Also provides an employee pension plan. Other benefits include child-care programs, tuition assistance, a subsidized cafeteria, and a smoke-free environment.

Human Resources: Krista M. Sauvageau.

Application Procedures: Places newspaper advertisements for certain openings and accepts unsolicited resumes. Send resume and cover letter to the attention of Krista M. Sauvageau, Human Resources Department.

▶ **Internships**

Type: The company does not offer an internship program.

Woodhull Medical & Mental Health Center

760 Broadway
Brooklyn, NY 11206
Phone: (718)963-8000
Fax: (718)963-8169

Employees: 3,000.

Average Entry-Level Hiring: Unknown.

Opportunities: RN—associate or bachelor's degree required. Social workers—M.S.W. required. Occupational and physical therapist—bachelor's degree.

Application Procedures: Contact the Human Resources Department for more information.

Wound Care Resources Inc.

8320 W. Bluemound
Milwaukee, WI 53213
Phone: (414)476-5515

Human Resources: Gene Collins.

Application Procedures: Hires licensed physical therapists or assistant physical therapists with a college degree. Applications can be filled out on site or send resume and cover letter to the attention of Gene Collins.

▶ **Internships**

Type: The company does not offer an internship program.

Wyoming Medical Center

1233 E. 2nd St.
Casper, WY 82601
Phone: 800-526-5190

Business Description: As a teaching hospital for the University of Wyoming and Casper College, WMC is committed to education. In addition to 100% tuition reimbursement, WMC offers on-site, satellite, and national conferences and seminars; staff development and management programs; multiple certification classes; and OR and Critical Care Residency Programs. Orientation is unit-based and individualized and includes an extended program for new graduates.

Employees: 1,025.

Average Entry-Level Hiring: 15-30.

Opportunities: A wide variety of nursing specialities are available; pediatrics, cardiac surgery, rehabilitation, neurology, oncology, plastic surgery, emergency services, orthopedics, obstetrics and gynecology, and intensive and coronary care.

Human Resources: Mark Smith; Marilyn Thomas.

Additional Companies

Bellevue Hospital Center

1st Ave. & 27th St.
New York, NY 10016
Phone: (212)561-4141

Bryn Mawr Rehabilitation Hospital

414 Paoli Pike
Malvern, PA 19355
Phone: (215)251-5400

Burke Rehabilitation Hospital
785 Mamaroneck Ave.
White Plains, NY 10605
Phone: (914)948-0050

Charlotte Institute of Rehabilitation
1100 Blythe Blvd.
Charlotte, NC 28203
Phone: (704)355-4300

Dallas Rehabilitation Institute
9713 Harry Hines Blvd.
Dallas, TX 75220
Phone: (214)358-6000

Drake Center
151 W. Galbraith Rd.
Cincinnati, OH 45216
Phone: (513)948-2500

Edwin Shaw Hospital
1621 Flickinger Rd.
Akron, OH 44312
Phone: (216)784-1271

Frazier Rehab Center
220 Abraham Flexner Way
Louisville, KY 40202
Phone: (502)582-7400

Garden State Rehabilitation Hospital
14 Hospital Dr.
Toms River, NJ 08755
Phone: (908)244-3100

Great Lakes Rehabilitation Hospital
143 E. 2nd St.
Erie, PA 16507
Phone: (814)870-7070

Healthsouth Rehabilitation Hospital
2935 Colonial Dr.
Columbia, SC 29203
Phone: (803)254-7777

Healthsouth Rehabilitation Hospital
700 N.W. 7th St.
Oklahoma City, OK 73102
Phone: (405)236-3131

Helen Hayes Hospital
Rte. 9W
West Haverstraw, NY 10993
Phone: (914)947-3000

John Muir Medical Center
1601 Ygnacio Valley Rd.
Walnut Creek, CA 94598
Phone: (510)938-2400

Kessler Institute for Rehabilitation
1199 Pleasant Valley Way
West Orange, NJ 07052
Phone: (201)731-3600

Madonna Rehabilitation Hospital
5401 South St.
Lincoln, NE 68506
Phone: (402)489-7102

Main Line Health Inc.
259 Radnor-Chester Rd.
Radnor, PA 19087
Phone: (215)254-2908

Marshall Rehabilitation Center
PO Box 190
Marshall, MO 65340
Phone: (816)886-2202
Fax: (816)886-3047

Memorial Hospital of Rhode Island Notre Dame Ambulatory
1000 Broad St.
Central Falls, RI 02863
Phone: (401)726-1800

Methodist Health Systems Inc.
1211 Union Ave.
Memphis, TN 38104
Phone: (901)726-2300

Metrohealth Center for Rehabilitation
2500 Metrohealth Dr.
Cleveland, OH 44109
Phone: (216)459-5020

Mississippi Methodist Hospital and Rehabilitation Center
1350 Woodrow Wilson Dr.
Jackson, MS 39216
Phone: (601)981-2611

Missouri Rehabilitation Center
600 N. Main St.
Mt. Vernon, MO 65712
Phone: (417)466-3711

Moss Rehabilitation Hospital
1200 W. Tabor Rd.
Philadelphia, PA 19141
Phone: (215)456-9900

Northeast Rehabilitation Hospital
70 Butler St.
Salem, NH 03079
Phone: (603)893-2900

Oak Forest Hospital of Cook County
15900 S. Cicero Ave.
Oak Forest, IL 60452
Phone: (708)425-8000

Oak Hill Nursing Homes
34225 Grand River Ave.
Farmington Hills, MI 48335
Phone: (313)477-7373

Rehabclinics Inc.
1018 9th Dr.
King of Prussia, PA 19406
Phone: (215)992-7600

Rehabilitation Institute of San Antonio
9119 Cinnamon Hill
San Antonio, TX 78240
Phone: (512)691-0737

Reproductive Institute Inc.
3780 Holcomb Bridge Rd.
Norcross, GA 30092
Phone: (404)416-9781

Sacred Heart Rehabilitation Hospital
1545 S. Layton Blvd.
Milwaukee, WI 53215
Phone: (414)383-4490

St. David's Rehabilitation Center
PO Box 4270
Austin, TX 78765
Phone: (512)867-5100

St. John's Hospital, Inc.
12617 River Rd.
Richmond, VA 23233
Phone: (804)784-3501

St. Joseph Rehabilitation Hospital and Outpatient Center
505 Elm St., N.E.
Albuquerque, NM 87102
Phone: (505)766-4700

St. Lawrence Rehabilitation Center
2381 Lawrenceville Rd.
Lawrenceville, NJ 08648
Phone: (609)896-9500

Santa Fe Health Care Inc.
720 SW 2nd Ave.
Gainesville, FL 32601
Phone: (904)375-4321

Santa Rosa Health Care Corp.
PO Box 7330
San Antonio, TX 78207
Phone: (210)228-2011

Schwab Rehabilitation Center
1401 S. California Blvd.
Chicago, IL 60608
Phone: (312)522-2010

Spalding Rehabilitation Hospital
4500 E. Iliff Ave.
Denver, CO 80222
Phone: (303)782-5700

Stopwatch Inc.
341 Seaspray Ct.
Neptune, NJ 07753
Phone: (908)774-5959

**Sunnyview Hospital and
Rehabilitation Center**
1270 Belmont Ave.
Schenectady, NY 12308
Phone: (518)382-4523

Thoms Rehabilitation Hospital
PO Box 15025
Asheville, NC 28813
Phone: (704)274-2400

A Touch of Care
2231 S. Carmelina Ave.
Los Angeles, CA 90064
Phone: (310)473-6525
Fax: (310)479-1287

Western Rehabilitation Institute
8074 S. 1300 E.
Sandy, UT 84094
Phone: (801)572-2600

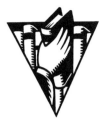

CAREER

RESOURCES

Career Resources

T he Career Resources chapter covers additional sources of job-related information that will aid you in your job search. It includes full, descriptive listings for sources of help wanted ads, professional associations, employment agencies and search firms, career guides, professional and trade periodicals, and basic reference guides and handbooks. Each of these sections is arranged alphabetically by organization, publication, or service name. For complete details on the information provided in this chapter, consult the introductory material at the front of this directory.

Sources of Help Wanted Ads

AACP News
American Association of Colleges of Pharmacy (AACP)
1426 Prince St.
Alexandria, VA 22314
Phone: (703)739-2330

Monthly. Free to members; $10.00/year for non-members. Newsletter; includes information on employment opportunities, association activities, and new members.

AAPA Newsletter
American Association of Pathologists' Assistants (AAPA)
c/o Leo J. Kelly
Dept. of Pathology

VA Medical Center
West Haven, CT 06516
Phone: (203)932-5711

Quarterly. Free to members. Includes employment and educational opportunity listings.

AARC Times: The Magazine for the Respiratory Care Professional
American Association for Respiratory Care (AARC)
11030 Ables Ln.
Dallas, TX 75229
Phone: (214)243-2272
Fax: (214)484-2720

Monthly. Free to members; $60.00/year for non-members. Includes employment opportunities, advertisers' index, calendar of events, and legislative update.

American Annals of the Deaf
800 Florida Ave., NE
Washington, DC 20002
Phone: (202)651-5340

Five times/year. $40.00/year.

The American Chiropractor
5005 Riviera Ct.
Ft. Wayne, IN 46825
Phone: (219)484-9600
Fax: (219)484-9604

Monthly.

F or some, breaking into a new career path is as simple as being in the right place at the right time; other positions are the result of calculated, progressive growth.

Source: *Journal of the American Dietetic Association*

American Druggist
Hearst Business Publishing Group
60 E. 42nd St.
New York, NY 10165
Phone: (212)297-9680

Magazine for pharmacists who practice in independent drug stores, chain drug stores, and hospitals. Sandra Riskin, editor-in-chief. Monthly. $36.00/year; $3.00/single issue.

The American Journal of Clinical Nutrition
428 E. Preston St.
Baltimore, MD 21202
Phone: (301)528-4000
Fax: (301)530-7038

Alice O'Donnell, editor. Monthly. $85.00/year. Medical and nutrition journal.

American Journal of Hospital Pharmacy
American Society of Hospital Pharmacists
4630 Montgomery Ave.
Bethesda, MD 20814
Phone: (301)657-3000

Monthly. $105.00/year. Journal for directors and staffs of pharmaceutical departments in hospitals and health-care institutions.

American Journal of Occupational Therapy
American Occupational Therapy Association, Inc.
1383 Piccard Dr.
PO Box 1725
Rockville, MD 20850-4375
Phone: (301)948-9626
Fax: (301)948-5512

Elaine Viseltear, editor. Monthly. $25.00/year; $55.00/year for nonmembers; $6.00/issue. Journal providing a forum for occupational therapy personnel to share research, case studies, and new theory.

American Journal of Physical Medicine and Rehabilitation
Williams and Wilkens, Inc.
428 E. Preston St.
Baltimore, MD 21202
Phone: (301)528-4068

Bimonthly. $55.00/year; $75.00/year for foreign subscribers; $87.00/year for institutions; $15.00/single issue.

American Journal of Public Health
American Public Health Association (APHA)
1015 15th St., NW
Washington, DC 20005
Phone: (202)789-5600
Fax: (202)789-5681

Monthly. Free to members; $80.00/year for nonmembers. Includes annual membership directory and news briefs.

American Pharmacy: The Journal of the American Pharmaceutical Association
American Pharmaceutical Association
2215 Constitution Ave., NW
Washington, DC 20037
Phone: (202)628-4410
Fax: (202)783-2381

Marlene Bloom, editor. Monthly. $50.00/year. Journal for pharmacy professionals.

American Review of Respiratory Diseases
American Lung Association
1740 Broadway
New York, NY 10019
Phone: (212)315-8700

Monthly. $110.00/year; $120.00/year for foreign subscribers excluding Canada and Mexico.

APAP Update
Association of Physician Assistant Programs
(APAP)
950 N. Washington St.
Alexandria, VA 22314
Phone: (703)836-2272

Monthly. Free to members. Includes employment listings and meeting announcements. Newsletter for physician assistant program faculty and others concerned with curricula and government/legislative developments affecting the profession.

Archives of Physical Medicine and Rehabilitation
78 E. Adams St.
Chicago, IL 60603-6103

Careers in Respiratory Therapy
Goldstein & Assoc., Inc.
1150 Yale St., No. 12
Santa Monica, CA 90403
Phone: (213)828-1309
Fax: (213)829-1169

Bimonthly.

Chef Institutional
Culinary Review, Inc.
134 Main St.
New Canaan, CT 06840
Phone: (203)972-3022
Fax: (203)972-3874

Quarterly. $20.00/year; $5.00/single issue.

Clinical Pharmacology & Therapeutics
Mosby-Year Book Inc.
11830 Westline Ind. Dr.
St. Louis, MO 63146
Phone: (314)872-8370
Fax: (314)432-1380

Monthly. $85.00/year; $7.50/single issue.

Clinical Pharmacy
American Society of Hospital Pharmacists
4630 Montgomery Ave.
Bethesda, MD 20814
Phone: (301)657-3000
Fax: (301)652-8278

Monthly. $45.00/year; $6.00/single issue.

Cognitive Rehabilitation
NeuroScience Publication
6555 Carrollton Ave.
Indianapolis, IN 46220
Phone: (317)257-9672

Bimonthly. $35.00/year; $7.00/issue.

As much as half of the impression you make on a prospective employer may have to do with your general knowledge of issues in your profession as well as issues in the industry in which you currently work or the industry in which you want to work. Subscribe to the journals in your field and industry, and don't forget to stay on top of the broader picture of the national and world economies.

Source: *Working Woman*

Dental Hygiene
American Dental Hygienists Association
444 N. Michigan Ave., Ste. 3400
Chicago, IL 60611
Phone: (312)440-8900

Monthly. $40.00/year; $5.00/issue.

DICP: The Annals of Pharmacotherapy
PO Box 42696
Cincinnati, OH 45242
Phone: (513)793-3555

Monthly. $100.00/year for institutions. Drug therapy clinical pharmacy magazine.

The Digest of Chiropractic Economics
Chiropractic News Publishing Corp.
29229 W. 6 Mile Rd.
Livonia, MI 48152
Phone: (313)427-5720

Bimonthly. $24.00/year; $4.00/single issue.

Drug Topics
Medical Economics Co.
5 Paragon Dr.
Montvale, NJ 07645-1742
Phone: (201)356-7200
Fax: (201)573-8979

23 times/year. $55.00/year; $5.00/single issue.

Employment Update

American Therapeutic Recreation Association (ATRA)
PO Box 15215
Hattiesburg, MS 39404-5215
Phone: 800-553-0304

Monthly. Free to members. Features employment and internship opportunities for therapeutic recreation professionals.

---

n a crowded job market, employers become more selective. With more applicants to choose from, they're not just looking for those who do what's expected. They look for those who take the initiative to exceed designated objectives or to improve the status quo in some way. Any instances you can point to in which you've reduced expenditures or staffing requirements, customer complaints, or product defects will tend to improve your chances. Examples of enhanced revenue, productivity, or customer satisfaction you've managed to produce will also tend to impress employers looking for ways to compete and survive.

Source: *Newark Star-Ledger*

Federal Career Opportunities

Federal Research Service, Inc.
243 Church St. NW
Vienna, VA 22183
Phone: (703)281-0200

Biweekly. $160.00/year; $75.00/six months; $38.00/three months; $7.50/copy. Provides information on more than 4,200 current federal job vacancies in the United States and overseas; includes permanent, part-time, and temporary positions. Entries include: Position title, location, series and grade, job requirements, special forms, announcement number, closing date, application address. Arrangement: Classified by federal agency and occupation.

Federal Jobs Digest

Federal Jobs Digest
325 Pennsylvania Ave., SE
Washington, DC 20003
Phone: (914)762-5111

Biweekly. $110.00/year; $29.00/three months; $4.50/issue. Covers over 20,000 specific job openings in the federal government in each issue. Entries include: Position name, title, General Schedule grade and Wage Grade, closing date for applications, announcement number, application address, phone, and name of contact. Arrangement: By federal department or agency, then geographical.

Food Industry News

Foodservice Publishing Co., Inc.
2702 W. Touhy Ave.
Chicago, IL 60645
Phone: (312)743-4200

Monthly. $9.50/year; $2.00/single issue.

Food Management

7500 Old Oak Blvd.
Cleveland, OH 44130
Phone: (216)243-8100

Monthly. $35.00/year; $5.00/single issue. Institutional foodservice magazine.

Food-Service East

The Newbury Street Group, Inc.
545 Boylston St.
No. 605
Boston, MA 02116
Phone: (617)267-9080

Seven times/year. $20.00/year; $3.00/single issue.

Food Technology

221 N. La Salle St.
Ste. 300
Chicago, IL 60601
Phone: (312)782-8424

Monthly. $72.00/year. Food technology and science magazine.

Foodservice Director

Restaurant Business, Inc.
633 3rd Ave.
New York, NY 10017
Phone: (212)986-4800
Fax: (212)983-3198

Monthly.

Hawaiian Dental Journal

1000 Bishop St.
Ste. 805
Honolulu, HI 96813

Hearing Instruments

Edgell Communications, Inc.
120 W. 2nd St.
Duluth, MN 55802
Phone: (218)723-9289

Monthly. $25.00/year.

Hearing Journal

Laux Co., Inc.
63 Great Rd.
Maynard, MA 07154
Phone: (508)897-5552
Fax: (508)897-6842

Monthly. $28.00/year; $3.00/single issue.

Heart and Lung—Journal of Critical Care

11830 Westline Industrial Dr.
St. Louis, MO 63146
Phone: (314)872-8370

Bimonthly. $24.50/year; $85.00/year for institutions; $16.00/year for students; $6.00/issue.

HMO Practice

Lippincott Healthcare Publications
130 Madison Ave., 3rd Fl.
New York, NY 10016
Phone: (212)679-9710
Fax: (212)679-9716

Bimonthly. $50.00/year; $13.00/single issue.

Hospital Pharmacist Report

Medical Economics Co.
5 Paragon Dr.
Montvale, NJ 07645-1742
Phone: (201)356-7200
Fax: (201)573-8979

Monthly. $35.00/year; $3.00/single issue.

Hospital Pharmacy

Lippincott Healthcare Publications
130 Madison Ave., 3rd Fl.
New York, NY 10016
Phone: (212)679-9710

Monthly. $60.00/year; $11.00/single issue.

Journal of Agricultural and Food Chemistry

American Chemical Society
1155 16th St., NW
Washington, DC 20036
Phone: (202)872-4600

Bimonthly. $24.00/year for members; $126.00/year for nonmembers.

Techniques for winning people over to your team when you're new on the job and change is in your program: make sure those who work for you see your vision as clearly as you do; listen to your critics—if you respect their work, they probably have good advice; make it clear that you're not on a power trip—be honest and don't promise what you can't deliver; get people involved in different aspects of the business so they know how everything works.

Source: *Working Woman*

Journal of Allied Health

1101 Connecticut Ave., NW
Ste. 700
Washington, DC 20036

Journal of Burn Care & Rehabilitation

Mosby Yearbook Inc.
11830 Westline Industrial Dr.
St. Louis, MO 63146
Phone: (314)872-8370
Fax: (314)432-1380

Bimonthly. Covers burn treatment and rehabilitation for the entire burn team and lists a variety of rehabilitation positions.

Journal of Cardiopulmonary Rehabilitation

J.b. Lippincott Co.
E. Washington Sq.
Philadelphia, PA 19105
Phone: (215)238-4200

Bimonthly. $55.00/year; $75.00/year for institutions; $9.00/single issue.

Journal of Chiropractic

American Chiropractic Association (ACA)
1701 Clarendon Blvd.
Arlington, VA 22209
Phone: (202)276-8800
Fax: (703)243-2593

Monthly. $24.00/year for members; $3.00/year for student members; $80.00/year for nonmembers. Contains employment listings, convention calendar, council reports on specific areas of chiropractic, and information on new members. Provides information on the progress of chiropractic procedures and research, and developments in other fields of interest to chiropractors; includes news of members, advertisers index, book reviews, and college calendar and news.

Some handy books to help you contemplate the job-change process: *Switching Gears: How to Master Career Change and Find the Work That's Right for You,* by Carole Hyatt; *Congratulations! You've Been Fired* , by Emily Knoltnow; and *How to Get the Job You Want,* by Melvin Danaho and John L. Meyer.

Source: *Better Homes and Gardens*

Journal of Dental Hygiene

American Dental Hygienists' Assn.
444 N. Michigan Ave., Ste. 3400
Chicago, IL 60611
Phone: (312)440-8900
Fax: (312)440-8929

Professional journal of dental hygiene.

Journal of Dental Research

American Association for Dental Research
1111 14th St., NW, Ste. 1000
Washington, DC 20005
Phone: (202)898-1050

Monthly. $220.00/year; $230.00 for foreign subscribers.

Journal of Learning Disabilities

5615 W. Cermak Rd.
Cicero, IL 60650

Journal of Nutrition Education

428 E. Preston
Baltimore, MD 21202-3993
Phone: (301)528-4068

Bimonthly. $70.00/year; $85.00/year for institutions; $15.00/ single issue.

The Journal of Orthopaedic and Sports Physical Therapy

Williams and Wilkins
428 E. Preston St.
Baltimore, MD 21202
Phone: (301)528-4068

Monthly. $60.00/year; $13.00/single issue.

Journal of Parenteral and Enteral Nutrition

Williams and Wilkins
428 E. Preston St.
Baltimore, MD 21202
Phone: (301)528-4000

Bimonthly. $60.00/year.

Journal of Rehabilitation

633 S. Washington St.
Alexandria, VA 22314
Phone: (703)836-0850

Quarterly. $35.00/year; $40.00/year for Canada; $50.00/year for foreign subscribers.

Journal of the American Dietetic Association

208 S. La Salle St., Ste. 1100
Chicago, IL 60604-1003
Phone: (312)899-0040

Monthly. $60.00/year; $6.00/issue. Magazine reporting original research on nutrition, diet therapy, education, and administration.

Journal of the California Dental Association

California Dental Association
818 'K' St. Mall
PO Box 13749
Sacramento, CA 95853
Phone: (916)443-0505

Monthly. $24.00/year; $6.00/issue.

McKnight's Long-Term Care News

McKnight Medical Communications, Inc.
1419 Lake Cook Rd., Ste. 110
Deerfield, IL 60015
Phone: (708)945-0345
Fax: (708)945-0532

Monthly. $41.00/year; $5.00/single issue.

Modern Food Service News

Grocers Publishing Co., Inc.
15 Emerald St.
Hackensack, NJ 07601
Phone: (201)488-1800

Monthly. $24.00/year; $2.00/single issue.

The Nation's Health

American Public Health Association (APHA)
1015 15th St., NW
Washington, DC 20005
Phone: (202)789-5600
Fax: (202)789-5681

Ten times/year. Free to members; $8.00/year for nonmembers. Includes employment opportunity listings and reports on current health issues, association actions, and legislative, regulatory, and policy issues affecting public health.

New York State Dental Journal

Dental Society of the State of New York
7 Elk St.
Albany, NY 12207
Phone: (518)465-0044

Ten times/year (monthly, except June/July and August/September combined). $40.00/year; $5.00/single issue.

Northwest Dentistry

2236 Marshall Ave.
St. Paul, MN 55104

NRA Newsletter: Committed to Enhancing the Lives of Persons with Disabilities

National Rehabilitation Association (NRA)
633 S. Washington St.
Alexandria, VA 22314
Phone: (703)836-0850
Fax: (703)836-2209

Eight times/year. Free to members. Includes

listing of employment opportunities, calendar of events, and chapter news.

NSCA Bulletin

National Strength and Conditioning Association (NSCA)
PO Box 81410
Lincoln, NE 68501
Phone: (402)472-3000
Fax: (402)476-6976

Monthly. Free to members. Newsletter; includes employment opportunity listings, book reviews, certification information, and symposia proceedings.

Optical Index

Professional Press Group
825 7th Ave.
New York, NY 10019
Phone: (212)887-1832

Monthly. $40.00/year.

Optical Management

5 N. Greenwich Rd.
Armonk, NY 10504

Optometric Monthly

101 E. Ontario St.
Chicago, IL 60611

Orthopaedic Review

301 Gibraltar Rd.
Box 528
Morris Plains, NJ 07950
Phone: (201)644-0802

Monthly. $55.00/year; $65.00/year for institutions; $82.00/year for foreign subscribers; $7.50/single issue.

PAJF Employment Magazine
American Academy of Physician Assistants
(AAPA)
950 N. Washington St.
Alexandria, VA 22314
Phone: (703)836-2272
Fax: (703)684-1924

Biweekly. $20.00/year for members;
$50.00/year for nonmembers. Provides nation-
wide listing of employment opportunities for
physician assistants.

Pharmaceutical Executive
859 Willamette St.
PO Box 10460
Eugene, OR 97440-1046
Phone: (503)343-1200

Monthly. $54.00/year; $8.00/issue.

Most Often-Cited Corporate Restructuring Goals

1. Reduce expenses
2. Increase profits
3. Improve cash flow
4. Increase productivity
5. Increase shareholder return on investment
6. Increase competitive advantage
7. Reduce bureaucracy
8. Improve decision making
8. Increase customer satisfaction
10. Increase sales

Source: *The Wall Street Journal*

Pharmaceutical Technology
859 Willamette St.
PO Box 10460
Eugene, OR 97440-1046
Phone: (503)343-1200

Monthly. $49.00/year.

Pharmacy Times
80 Shore Rd.
Port Washington, NY 11050
Phone: (516)883-6350

Monthly. $30.00/year. Magazine providing infor-
mation on health items to independent, chain,
and hospital pharmacists.

Physical Therapy
American Physical Therapy Association
(APTA)
1111 N. Fairfax St.
Alexandria, VA 22314
Phone: (703)684-2782

Monthly. Free to members; $50.00/year for non-
members. Journal featuring employment listings, continuing education course listings,
abstracts of current literature, book reviews, and
product and computer news. Contains advertisers' index and special features indexes each
issue; also contains annual index.

Physicians Assistant
American Academy of Physician Assistants
950 N. Washington St.
Alexandria, VA 22314-1534
Phone: (703)836-2272

1993. Eighteen-page booklet describing roles,
work settings, education, credentials, cost effectiveness, history, and organizations related to
physician assistants.

Pneumogram
California Society for Respiratory Care
24307 Magic Mountain Pkwy., Ste. 288
Valencia, CA 91355
Phone: (805)298-4010
Fax: (805)298-0235

Quarterly.

The Professional Medical Assistant
The American Association of Medical
Assistants
20 N. Wacker Dr., Ste. 1575
Chicago, IL 60606
Phone: (312)899-1500

Bimonthly. $20.00/year; $3.00/single issue.

PT Bulletin
American Physical Therapy Association
(APTA)
1111 N. Fairfax St.
Alexandria, VA 22314
Phone: (703)684-2782

Weekly. Free to members; $1.00/year for non-
member physical therapists; $80.00/year for all
others. Newsletter; includes employment listings and information on upcoming seminars.

RDH: The National Magazine for Dental Hygiene Professionals
Stevens Publishing Corp.
PO Box 2573
225 N. New Rd.
Waco, TX 76702-2573
Phone: (817)776-9000
Fax: (817)776-9018

Monthly.

Rehab Management
1849 Sawtelle, Ste. 770
Los Angeles, CA 90025
Phone: (213)479-1769
Fax: (213)479-6275

Six times/year.

Rehabilitation Today
Sportscape, Inc.
Framingham Corp. Ct.
492 Old Connecticut Path
3rd Fl.
Framingham, MA 01701
Phone: (508)872-2021
Fax: (508)872-2114

Nine times/year.

Respiratory Care
American Association for Respiratory Care
11030 Ables Ln.
PO Box 29686
Dallas, TX 75229
Phone: (214)243-2272
Fax: (214)484-2720

Monthly. $50.00/year; $5.00/single issue.
Describes the work of the respiratory therapist,
educational preparation, and employment outlook.

Respiratory Management
11742 Wilshire Blvd.
Los Angeles, CA 90025
Phone: (213)473-1354

Six times/year. $48.00/year.

The Respiratory Practitioner
Reliable Multi-Media Productions
5705 S. Sepulveda Blvd.
Culver City, CA 90230
Phone: (213)397-2229

Quarterly. $25.00/year.

Restaurant Exchange News
PO Box 2655
Greenwich, CT 06836
Phone: (203)661-9090

Monthly. $36.00/year; $3.00/single issue.

S trategies for "jump-starting" stalled job searches are
included in *Parting Company: How To Survive the
Loss of a Job and Find Another Successfully*, co-authored
by William J. Morin, chairman of Drake Beam Morin Inc.,
the world's largest career-management consulting firm.
Other chapters cover such timely topics as: assessing your
skills and interests, making career decisions, financial
planning, exploring different options such as early retirement, starting a business, consulting, targeting your job
search, resumes and references, marketing strategy, job
interviews, negotiating an offer, starting a new job.

Review of Optometry
Chilton Company
Chilton Way
Radnor, PA 19089
Phone: (215)946-4376

Monthly. $36.00/year. Journal for the optomet-
ric profession and optical industry.

RT: The Journal for Respiratory Care Practitioners
1849 Sawtelle Blvd., Ste. 770
Los Angeles, CA 90025
Phone: (213)476-1769
Fax: (213)479-6275

Quarterly. Free to qualified subscribers.

Rural Health Care
National Rural Health Association (NRHA)
301 E. Armour Blvd., Ste. 420
Kansas City, MO 64111
Phone: (816)756-3140
Fax: (816)756-3144

Bimonthly. Free to members. Association
newsletter; includes listing of employment
opportunties, listing of publications, book
reviews, information on new members, and legislative and state news.

Southeast Food Service News
Southeast Publishing Co.
PO Box 47719
Atlanta, GA 30362
Phone: (404)452-1807

Monthly. $25.00/year.

Southern Medical Journal
Southern Medical Association
35 Lakeshore Dr.
PO Box 19008
Birmingham, AL 35219-0088
Phone: (205)945-1840
Fax: (205)942-0642

Multispecialty medical journal that lists positions in various medical disciplines.

Some personal improvement guides: *Marketing Yourself*, by Dorothy Leeds; *The Perfect Interview: How To Get the Job You Really Want*, by John D. Drake; and *The Management Skills Builder: Self-Directed Learning Strategies for Career Development.*

Source: *Library Journal*

Southern Pharmacy Journal
3030 Peachtree Rd., Ste. 411
Atlanta, GA 30305
Phone: (404)231-1267

Monthly. $18.00/year; $2.00/single issue.

Southwest Medical Opportunities
6750 West Loop S., Ste. 500
Bellaire, TX 77401
Phone: (713)666-8976

Bimonthly. Healthcare recruitment journal.

Sunbelt Foodservice
Shelby Publishing Co., Inc.
517 Green St.
Gainesville, GA 30501
Phone: (404)534-8380

Monthly. $25.00/year; $3.50/single issue.

Teaching Exceptional Children
The Council for Exceptional Children
1920 Association Dr.
Reston, VA 22091-1589
Phone: (703)620-3660
Fax: (703)264-9494

Quarterly. Free to members; $25.00/year for nonmembers. Magazine including classroom-oriented information about instructional methods, materials, and techniques for students of all ages with special needs.

TeamRehab Report
Miramar Publishing
6133 Bristol Pkwy.
PO Box 3640
Culver City, CA 90231-3640
Phone: (213)337-9717

Bimonthly. $24.00/year.

Today's Chiropractic
Life Chiropractic College
1269 Barclay Circle
Marietta, GA 30060
Phone: (404)499-9824

Bimonthly. $24.00/year; $4.00/single issue.

Topics in Language Disorders
200 Orchard Ridge Dr.
Gaithersburg, MD 20878
Phone: (301)417-7500
Fax: (301)417-7550

Quarterly. $52.00/year; $62.00/year for foreign subscribers; $17.00/single issue.

The Volta Review
3417 Volta Pl., NW
Washington, DC 20007-2778
Phone: (202)337-5220

Seven times/year. $42.00/year.

Yankee Food Service
Griffin Publishing Co., Inc.
PO Box 190
549 Columbian St.
South Weymouth, MA 02190
Phone: (617)337-2900

Monthly. $32.00/year.

Professional Associations

Accreditation Review Committee on Education for Physicians Assistants (ARC-PA)

515 N. State St.
Chicago, IL 60610
Phone: (312)464-4623
Fax: (312)464-4184

Purpose: Serves as an accrediting review body for physician assistant education nationwide. Makes recommendations to Committee on Allied Health Education and Accreditation.

American Academy of Clinical Toxicology (AACT)

Kansas State University
Comparative Toxicology Laboratories
Manhattan, KS 66506-5606
Phone: (913)532-4334
Fax: (913)532-4481

Membership: Physicians, veterinarians, pharmacists, research scientists, and analytical chemists. Activities: Maintains placement services. Objectives are to: unite medical scientists and facilitate the exchange of information; encourage the development of therapeutic methods and technology; establish a mechanism for the certification of medical scientists in clinical toxicology. Conducts workshops and professional training in poison information and emergency service personnel. Maintains speakers' bureau. Bestows awards.

American Academy of Physician Assistants (AAPA)

950 N. Washington St.
Alexandria, VA 22314
Phone: (703)836-2272
Fax: (703)684-1924

Membership: Physician assistants who have graduated from an American Medical Association accredited program and/or are certified by the National Commission on Certification of Physician Assistants; individuals who are enrolled in an accredited PA educational program. **Purpose:** To educate the public about the physician assistant profession; represent physician assistants' interests before Congress, government agencies, and health-related organizations; assure the competence of physician assistants through development of educational curricula and accreditation programs; provide services for members. Organizes annual National PA Day. Develops research and education programs; maintains library. Awards scholarships; compiles statistics. **Publication(s):** *AAPA Bulletin*, monthly. • *AAPA News*, monthly. • *Journal of the American Academy of Physician Assistants*, 10/year. • *Legislative Watch*, monthly. • *Membership Directory*, annual. • *PA Career*, monthly.

Best Business Schools in Executive Education

1. Harvard University
2. Stanford University
3. Northwestern University
4. University of Michigan
5. University of Pennsylvania

Source: *US News & World Report*

American Association for Leisure and Recreation (AALR)

1900 Association Dr.
Reston, VA 22091
Phone: (703)476-3472
Fax: (703)476-9527

Membership: Teachers of recreation and park administration, leisure studies, and recreation programming in colleges and universities; professional recreation and park practitioners; people involved in other areas of health, physical education, and recreation with an interest in recreation. Activities: Maintains placement service. Goals of AALR are to: encourage professional involvement and exchange; monitor recreation legislation and render consultation at the request of legislators; disseminate information on topics of current interest in leisure and recreation; maintain liaison with organizations having allied interests in leisure and recreation; support, encourage, and provide guidance to members in the development of programs of leisure services; aid in the development of quality educational/recreational programs in the schools; facilitate communication between professionals and lay people and between the schools and the community; create opportunity for professional growth and development; sponsor programs at district and national conventions, workshops, and conferences; nurture the conceptualization of a philosophy of leisure through curriculum development and professional preparation. Bestows awards; maintains library.

> **M**anagers are turning to tried-and-true as well as innovative imperatives to boost staff performance. Among them: communicate, creatively and often, through electronic bulletin boards, multimedia presentations, videotapes, handwritten notes, and employee-generated mottoes; build role-playing into training efforts; bring problem-solving and decision-making down to as low an organizational level as possible, giving everyone the training, information, and tools they need to make the right choices; set up incentive programs that are linked to both team effort and individual performance.
>
> Source: *Working Woman*

American Association for Respiratory Care (AARC)

11030 Ables Ln.
Dallas, TX 75229
Phone: (214)243-2272
Fax: (214)484-2720

Membership: Allied health society of respiratory care technicians and therapists employed by hospitals, group practices, educational institutions, and municipal organizations. **Purpose:** To encourage, develop, and provide educational programs for persons interested in the profession of respiratory care; and to advance the science of respiratory care. **Publication(s):** *AARC Times: The Magazine for the Respiratory Care Professional*, monthly. • *Respiratory Care*, monthly.

American Association of Cardiovascular and Pulmonary Rehabilitation (AACVPR)

7611 Elmwood Ave., Ste. 201
Middleton, WI 53562
Phone: (608)831-6989
Fax: (608)831-5122

The AACVPR's membership includes allied health professionals involved in the field of car-

diovascualr and pulmonary rehabilitation. It fosters the improvement of clinical practice in CVPR; promotes scientific CVPR research; seeks the advancement of CVPR education for healthcare professional and the public. The group publishes an annual directory, several professional journals, and a quarterly newsletter.

American Association of Colleges of Pharmacy (AACP)

1426 Prince St.
Alexandria, VA 22314
Phone: (703)739-2330

Membership: College of pharmacy programs accredited by American Council on Pharmaceutical Education; corporations and individuals. **Purpose:** Sponsors competitions; bestows awards; compiles statistics. **Publication(s):** *AACP News*, monthly. • *American Association of Colleges of Pharmacy–Graduate Program Book*, annual. • *American Journal of Pharmaceutical Education*, quarterly. • *Pharmacy School Admission Requirements*, annual. • *Roster of Teaching Personnel in Colleges of Pharmacy*, annual. Electronic bulletin board, Pharmline.

American Association of Healthcare Consultants (AAHC)

11208 Waples Mill Rd., Ste. 109
Fairfax, VA 22030
Phone: (703)691-AAHC

AAHC is a professional association of individuals exclusively devoted to hospital and healthcare consultation. It serves as a resource for healthcare providers, offers continuing education to members, conducts institutes for individuals and groups intersted in topical subjects related to healthcare delivery systems. The group publishes an annual directory.

American Association of Medical Assistants (AAMA)

20 N. Wacker Dr., Ste. 1575
Chicago, IL 60606
Phone: (312)899-1500

Membership: Assistants, receptionists, secretaries, bookkeepers, nurses, and laboratory personnel employed in the offices of physicians and other medical facilities. **Purpose:** Activities include a certification program consisting of study and an examination, passage of which entitles the individual to a certificate as a Certified Medical Assistant. Conducts accreditation of one- and two-year programs in medical assisting in conjunction with the Committee on Allied Health Education and Accreditation and the American Medical Association. Provides assistance and information to institutions of higher learning desirous of initiating courses for medical assistants. Sponsors the Maxine Williams Scholarship program. Offers continuing education to assistants who cannot return to school and guided study courses in human relations and medical law. Awards continuing education units for selected educational programs. Maintains library of textbooks and a reference list. **Publication(s):** *Professional Medical Assistant*, bimonthly. • Also publishes brochures and pamphlets.

American Association of Nutritional Consultants (AANC)

1641 E Sunset Rd., B117
Las Vegas, NV 89119
Phone: (702)361-1132

Membership: Professional nutritional consultants. **Purpose:** Seeks to: develop a certification board; create a forum for exchange of nutritional information; establish state chapters. Offers benefits such as car rental and laboratory discounts. **Publication(s):** *Herald of Holistic Health Newsletter*, periodic. • *Membership Directory*, annual. • *Nutrition and Dietary Consultant*, monthly.

American Association of Pathologists' Assistants (AAPA)

c/o Leo J. Kelly
Dept. of Pathology
VA Medical Center
West Haven, CT 06516
Phone: (203)932-5711

Membership: Pathologists' assistants and individuals qualified by academic and practical training to provide service in anatomic pathology under the direction of a qualified pathologist who is responsible for the performance of the assistant. Activities: Offers placement services. Purposes of AAPA are to promote the mutual association of trained pathologists' assistants and to inform the public and the medical profession concerning the goals of this profession.

Presents Newsletter Contributor Award. Compiles statistics on salaries, geographic distribution, and duties of pathologists' assistants. Sponsors a continuing medical education program.

American Association of Pharmaceutical Scientists (AAPS)

1650 King St.
Alexandria, VA 22314-2747
Phone: (703)548-3000
Fax: (703)684-7349

Membership: Pharmaceutical scientists. Activities: Offers placement service. Provides a forum for exchange of scientific information; serves as a resource in forming public policies to regulate pharmaceutical sciences and related issues of public concern. Promotes pharmaceutical sciences and provides for recognition of individual achievement; works to foster career growth and the development of members. Bestows awards.

> **M**ore than any other profession, medicine is constantly evolving, changing quickly with every new piece of high-tech equipment or the latest published research.
>
> Source: *Glamour*

American Auditory Society (AAS)

1966 Inwood Rd.
Dallas, TX 75235
Phone: (214)905-3001
Fax: (214)905-3022

Membership: Audiologists, otolaryngologists, scientists, hearing aid industry professionals, and educators of hearing impaired people; individuals involved in industries serving hearing impaired people, including the amplification systems industry. **Purpose:** Seeks to increase knowledge about hearing; promotes conservation of hearing. Promotes self-sufficiency and rehabilitation for hearing impaired people. **Publication(s):** *Corti's Organ*, quarterly. • *Ear and Hearing*, bimonthly.

American Chiropractic Association (ACA)

1701 Clarendon Blvd.
Arlington, VA 22209
Phone: (703)276-8800
Fax: (703)243-2593

Purpose: Enhances the philosophy, science, and art of chiropractic, and the professional welfare of individuals in the field. Promotes legislation defining chiropractic health care and improves the public's awareness and utilization of chiropractic. Conducts chiropractic survey and statistical study. Sponsors Correct Posture Week in May and Spinal Health Month in October. Chiropractic colleges have student ACA groups. **Publication(s):** *ACA/FYI*, monthly. • *American Chiropractic Association Membership Directory*, annual. • *Journal of Chiropractic*, monthly.

By the year 2000, 41 percent of new jobs created will require average or above-average skills, compared with fewer than 24 percent in 1992.

Source: *The Futurist*

American College of Clinical Pharmacy (ACCP)

3101 Broadway, Ste. 380
Kansas City, MO 64111
Phone: (816)531-2177

Membership: Clinical pharmacists dedicated to: promoting rational use of drugs in society; advancing the practice of clinical pharmacy and interdisciplinary health care; assuring high quality clinical pharmacy by establishing and maintaining standards in education and training at advanced levels. Activities: Maintains placement service. Encourages research and recognizes excellence in clinical pharmacy. Offers educational programs, symposia, research forums, fellowship training, and college-funded grants through competitions; bestows Therapeutic Frontiers Lecture Award.

American College of Sports Medicine (ACSM)

PO Box 1440
Indianapolis, IN 46206-1440
Phone: (317)637-9200
Fax: (317)634-7817

The association advances and disseminates information on the benefits and effects of exercise, and the treatment and prevention of injuries incurred in sports, exercise, and fitness activities. The group certifies fitness instructors, exercise test technologists, exercise specialists, and exercise program directors. It grants continuing medical education and continuing education credits. ACSM publishes a monthly newsletter, an annual directory, and a monthly journal.

American Council on Pharmaceutical Education (ACPE)

311 W. Superior St., Ste. 512
Chicago, IL 60610
Phone: (312)664-3575
Fax: (312)664-4652

Membership: Accrediting agency for the professional programs of colleges and schools of pharmacy and approval of providers of continuing pharmaceutical education. **Publication(s):** *Accredited Professional Programs of Colleges of Schools of Pharmacy* and *Approved Providers of Continuing Pharmaceutical Education*.

American Dental Assistants Association (ADAA)

919 N. Michigan Ave., Ste. 3400
Chicago, IL 60611
Phone: (312)664-3327
Fax: (312)664-5288

Membership: Individuals employed as dental assistants in dental offices, clinics, hospitals, or institutions; instructors of dental assistants; dental students. **Purpose:** Sponsors workshops and seminars; maintains governmental liaison. Offers group insurance; maintains scholarship trust fund. **Publication(s):** *The Dental Assistant*, bimonthly. • Also publishes educational materials.

American Dental Association (ADA)

211 E. Chicago Ave.
Chicago, IL 60611
Phone: (312)440-2500

Membership: Professional society of dentists. **Purpose:** Encourages the improvement of the health of the public and promotes the art and science of dentistry in matters of legislation and regulations. Inspects and accredits dental schools and schools for dental hygienists, assistants, and laboratory technicians. Conducts research programs at ADA Health Foundation Research Institute. Produces most of the dental health education material used in the U.S. Sponsors National Children's Dental Health Month. Compiles statistics on personnel, practice, and dental care needs and attitudes of patients with regard to dental health. Operates library of 50,000 volumes. Maintains biographical records of U.S. dentists, past and present; and collection of published and original documentary material of historical interest to the profession. Sponsors 11 councils. **Publication(s):** *American Dental Directory*, annual. • *Index to Dental Literature*, quarterly. • *News*, biweekly.

American Dental Hygienists' Association (ADHA)

444 N. Michigan Ave., Ste. 3400
Chicago, IL 60611
Phone: (312)440-8900
Toll-free: 800-243-ADHA
Fax: (312)440-8929

Membership: Professional organization of licensed dental hygienists possessing a degree or certificate in dental hygiene granted by an accredited school of dental hygiene. **Purpose:** Administers Dental Hygiene Candidate Aptitude Testing Program and makes available scholarships, research grants, and continuing education programs. Maintains accrediting service through the American Dental Association's Commission on Dental Accreditation. Bestows awards; compiles statistics. **Publication(s):** *American Dental Hygienists' Association Access*, 10/year. • *Dental Hygiene*, 9/year.

American Dietetic Association (ADA)

216 W. Jackson Blvd., Ste. 800
Chicago, IL 60606
Phone: (312)899-0040
Fax: (312)899-1979

Membership: Professional organization of dietetic professionals and registered dietitians in hospitals, colleges, universities, school food services, day care centers, research, business, and industry; dietetic technicians who meet ADA requirements. **Purpose:** Seeks to provide direction and leadership for dietetic practice, educa-

tion, and research; promote optimal health and nutritional status of the population. Sets and approves standards of education and practice. Provides career guidance. Offers scholarships and awards through the American Dietetic Association Foundation. **Publication(s):** *Journal of the American Dietetic Association*, monthly.

American Group Practice Association (AGPA)

1422 Duke St.
Dayton, OH 45401-2307
Phone: (513)223-9630

A group representing more than 21,000 physicians, the AGPA fosters accredidation of medical clinics, compiles statistics on group practice, and sponsors research, patient education, and insurance programs. The group maintains a database, biographical archives, and publishes an annual directory, a bimonthly journal, and a periodic newsletter.

With big corporations no longer rewarding loyalty and performance with lifetime guarantees of employment, individuals are transforming themselves into itinerant professionals who sell their human capital on the open market. "Instead of climbing up the ladder, people now have to develop a portfolio of skills and products that they can sell directly to a series of customers," explains Charles Handy, visiting professor at the London Business School and author of *The Age of Unreason*, a book about the changing nature of work. "We are all becoming people with portfolio careers."

Source: *Business Week*

American Health Information Management Association (AHIMA)

919 N. Michigan Ave.
Chicago, IL 60611
Phone: (312)787-2672

The association publishes a journal containing job listings, a directory, runs a referral service, and conducts educational programs.

American Hospital Association (AHA)

840 N. Lake Shore Dr.
Chicago, IL 60611
Phone: (312)280-6000
Toll-free: 800-621-6712
Fax: (312)280-5979

Membership: Individuals and health care institutions including hospitals, health care systems, and pre- and postacute health care delivery organizations. **Purpose:** Is dedicated to promoting the welfare of the public through its leadership and assistance to its members in the provision of better health services for all people. Carries out research and education projects in such areas as health care administration, hospital economics, and community relations; represents hospitals in national legislation; offers programs for institutional effectiveness review, technology assessment, and hospital administrative services to hospitals; conducts educational programs furthering the in-service education of hospital personnel; collects and analyzes data; furnishes multimedia educational materials; maintains 44,000 volume health care administration library, and biographical archive. Bestows awards. **Publication(s):** *AHANews*, weekly. • *Guide to the Health Care Field*, annual. • *Hospital Statistics*, annual. • *Hospitals*, biweekly.

Best books for new bosses

1. *Servant Leadership*, Robert K. Greenleaf, 1977
2. *The Female Advantage*, Sally Helgesen, 1990
3. *The Grace of Great Things*, Robert Grudin, 1990
4. *301 Great Management Ideas from America's Most Innovative Small Companies*, from *Inc.* magazine, 1991

Source: Selected by Nancy K. Austin, co-author of *A Passion for Excellence*, *Working Woman*

American Kinesiotherapy Association (AKA)

c/o Ed Reiling
PO Box 611
Wright Brothers Sta.
Dayton, OH 45409
Phone: 800-326-0268

Membership: Professional society of kinesiotherapists and exercise therapists, and associate and student members with interest in physical and mental rehabilitation and adapted physical education. Activities: Maintains placement service. Promotes and sponsors medically-prescribed rehabilitation programs; encourages research and publication. Offers specialized education program. Operates library. Bestows awards; compiles statistics.

American Managed Care Pharmacy Association (AMCPA)

2300 9th St. S., Ste. 210
Arlington, VA 22204
Phone: (703)920-8480

Membership: Preferred provider organizations that specialize in maintainence drug therapy in managed care environments and make available home-delivery pharmacy services. **Purpose:** Promotes managed care prescription services as suppliers of medication to home-delivery pharmacy services. Seeks to assist health plan officers and consumers in obtaining maximum value from prescription services; inform consumers and health care organizations about members' efforts to improve prescription services through cost containment measures. Compiles statistics. **Publication(s):** Informational booklet.

American Massage Therapy Association (AMTA)

1130 W. North Shore Ave.
Chicago, IL 60626-4670
Phone: (312)761-AMTA
Fax: (312)761-0009

The AMTA is made up of massage therapists or technicians. It provides referrals to area therapists and certified schools, conducts community outreach programs and research and educational projects, and accredits massage training programs. The group publishes a quarterly newsletter, an annual registry, and informational brochures.

American Medical Association (AMA)

515 N. State St.
Chicago, IL 60610
Phone: (312)464-5000
Fax: (312)645-4184

Membership: County medical societies and physicians. **Purpose:** Disseminates scientific information to members and the public. Informs members on significant medical and health legislation on state and national levels and represents the profession before Congress and governmental agencies. Cooperates in setting standards for medical schools, hospitals, residency programs, and continuing medical education courses. Offers physician placement service and counseling on practice management problems. Operates library which lends material and provides specific medical information to physicians. Ad-hoc committees are formed for such topics as health care planning and principles of medical ethics. **Publication(s):** *American Journal of Diseases of Children*, monthly. • *American Medical News*, weekly. • *Archives of Dermatology*, monthly. • *Archives of General Psychiatry*, monthly. • *Archives of Internal Medicine*, monthly. • *Archives of Neurology*, periodic. • *Archives of Ophthalmology*, monthly. • *Archives of Otolaryngology--Head and Neck Surgery*, monthly. • *Archives of Pathology and Laboratory Medicine*, monthly. • *Archives of Surgery*, monthly. • *Journal of the American Medical Association*, weekly.

American Medical Technologists (AMT)

710 Higgins Rd.
Park Ridge, IL 60068
Phone: (708)823-5169
Fax: (708)823-0458

Membership: National professional registry of medical laboratory technologists, technicians, medical assistants, and dental assistants. Activities: Maintains placement service. Bestows awards in six categories: Distinguished Achievement; Exceptional Merit; Order of the Golden Microscope; Member and Student Writing; President's Award; Technologist of the Year. Sponsors AMT Institute for Education which has developed continuing education programs. Affiliated With: Accrediting Bureau of Health Education Schools.

American Nutritionists Association (ANA)

5530 Wisconsin Ave. NW, Ste. 1149
Washington, DC 20815
Fax: (301)656-0989

Membership: Nutritionists holding graduate degrees from accredited universities. **Purpose:** Seeks to represent nutritionists before federal and state policymakers; works to educate the public about nutrition; fosters nutrition science in research, public health, clinical, and educa-

tional settings. **Publication(s):** *ANA Highlights*, monthly. • *The Nutrition Report*, monthly. • Also publishes *Surgeon General's Reports on Nutrition and Health* (book).

> **G**ood negotiating skills are not just more important in times of social and economic change, they are also more difficult to master, according to Max H. Bazerman and Margaret A. Neale, authors of *Negotiating Rationally*. "Negotiation is used every day to resolve differences and allocate resources," they explain; negotiating rationally means making the best decisions to maximize your interests. It's especially important for the job seeker.
>
> Source: *Library Journal*

American Occupational Therapy Association (AOTA)

1383 Piccard Dr., Ste. 301
Rockville, MD 20850-4375
Phone: (301)948-9626
Toll-free: 800-THE-AOTA
Fax: (301)948-5512

Membership: Registered occupational therapists and certified occupational therapy assistants who provide services to people whose lives have been disrupted by physical injury or illness, developmental problems, the aging process, or social or psychological difficulties. **Purpose:** Occupational therapy focuses on the active involvement of the patient in specially designed therapeutic tasks and activities to improve function, performance capacity, and the ability to cope with demands of daily living. Conducts research program and compiles statistics. Bestows awards. Resources include a 3500 volume library and an occupational therapy archives. Supports the American Occupational Therapy Foundation, which administers a program of professional training and development in research and provides research information related to occupational therapy. **Publication(s):** *American Journal of Occupational Therapy*, monthly. • *Developmental Disabilities Specialty Section Newsletter*, quarterly. • *Occupational Therapy Week*. • *Physical Disabilities Special Interest Section Newsletter*, quarterly. • *Sensory Integration Special Interest Section Newsletter*, quarterly. • Also publishes monographs.

American Optometric Association (AOA)

243 Lindbergh Blvd.
St. Louis, MO 63141
Phone: (314)991-4100
Fax: (314)991-4101

AOA is a professional society of optometrists, students of optometry, and paraoptometic assistants and technicians. Its purposes are to improve the quality, availability, and accessibility of eye and vision care; to represent the optometric profession; to help members conduct their practices; and to promote the highest standards of patient care. The group presents annual awards, conducts specialized education programs, and operates a placement service. Several monthly journals are published by AOA.

American Pharmaceutical Association (APhA)

2215 Constitution Ave., NW
Washington, DC 20037
Phone: (202)628-4410
Toll-free: 800-237-APhA
Fax: (202)783-2351

APhA is a professional association that includes pharmacists, educators, students, researchers, editors and publishers of pharmaceutical literature, pharmaceutical chemists and scientists, food and drug officials, hospital pharmacists, and pharmacists in government service. The group promotes quality healthcare and rational drug therapy through the appropriate use of pharmacy services. It works to assure the quality of drug products, represent the interests of the profession before governmental bodies, and interpret and disseminate information on developments in healthcare. APhA fosters professional education and training of pharmacists.

American Physical Therapy Association (APTA)

1111 N. Fairfax St.
Alexandria, VA 22314
Phone: (703)684-2782

Membership: Professional organization of physical therapists and physical therapy assistants and students. Activities: Provides placement services at conference. Formed to foster the development and improvement of physical therapy service, education, and research; to evaluate the organization and administration of cur-

ricula; to direct the maintenance of standards and promote scientific research. Acts as an accrediting body for educational programs in physical therapy and is responsible for establishing standards. Offers advisory and consultation services to schools of physical therapy and facilities offering physical therapy. Maintains library, archives, speakers' bureau, and Information Central. Presents awards and scholarships.

American Physiological Society (APS)

9650 Rockville Pike
Bethesda, MD 20814
Phone: (301)530-7164
Fax: (301)571-1814

Membership: Professional society of physiologists. **Purpose:** Maintains biographical archives; bestows awards. **Publication(s):** *Advances in Physiology Education*, semiannual. • *American Journal of Physiology*, monthly. • *American Journal of Physiology: Cell Physiology*, monthly. • *American Journal of Physiology: Endocrinology and Metabolism*, monthly. • *American Journal of Physiology: Gastrointestinal and Liver Physiology*, monthly. • *American Journal of Physiology: Heart and Circulatory Physiology*, monthly. • *American Journal of Physiology: Lung Cellular and Molecular Physiology*, bimonthly. • *American Journal of Physiology: Regulatory, Integrative, and Comparative Physiology*, monthly. • *American Journal of Physiology: Renal, Fluid and Electrolyte Physiology*, monthly. • *FASEB Directory*, annual. • *Journal of Applied Physiology*, monthly. • *Journal of Neurophysiology*, monthly. • *News in Physiological Sciences*, bimonthly. • *Physiological Reviews*, quarterly. • *The Physiologist*, bimonthly. • Also publishes handbooks of physiology and clinical physiology.

American Public Health Association (APHA)

1015 15th St., NW
Washington, DC 20005
Phone: (202)789-5600
Fax: (202)789-5681

Membership: Professional organization of physicians, nurses, educators, academicians, environmentalists, epidemiologists, new professionals, social workers, health administrators, optometrists, podiatrists, pharmacists, pharmacy assistants, dentists, dental assistants, nutritionists, health planners, health care workers, other community and mental health specialists, and interested consumers. Activities: Sponsors job placement service. Seeks to protect and promote personal, mental, and environmental health. Services include: promulgation of standards; establishment of uniform practices and procedures; development of the etiology of communicable diseases; research in public health; exploration of medical care programs and their relationships to public health. Presents Award for Excellence to individuals for outstanding contributions to the improvement of public health; also bestows the Drotman Award to a young health professional who demonstrates potential in the health field and Sedgwick Memorial Medal to those who have advanced public health knowledge and practices. Maintains Action Board and Program Development Board.

American School Health Association (ASHA)

7263 State Rt. 43
PO Box 708
Kent, OH 44240
Phone: (216)678-1601
Fax: (216)678-4526

Membership: School physicians, dentists, nurses, nutritionists, health educators, dental hygienists, and public health workers. Activities: Maintains placement service. Formed to promote comprehensive and constructive school health programs including the teaching of health, health services, and promotion of a healthful school environment. Offers a professional referral service, classroom teaching aids, and professional reference materials. Conducts research programs; compiles statistics. Sponsors annual foreign travel study tour. Bestows William A. How Award annually for distinguished service in school health.

American Society of Allied Health Professions

1101 Connecticut Ave., NW, Ste. 700
Washington, DC 20036
Phone: (202)857-1150

The organization is made up of national allied health professional membership associations, clinical service programs, academic institutions, and other organizations whose interests include the advancement of allied health education, research, and service delivery. The group publishes an annual directory, a monthly journal, and a monthly newsletter.

American Society of Hand Therapists (ASHT)

1002 Vandora Springs Rd., Ste. 101
Garner, NC 27529
Phone: (919)779-ASHT
Fax: (919)779-5642

Membership: Registered and licensed occupational and physical therapists specializing in hand therapy and committed to excellence and professionalism in hand rehabilitation. Activities: Maintains placement service. Purposes are to promote research, publish information, improve treatment techniques, and standardize hand evaluation and care. Fosters education and communication between therapists in the U.S. and abroad. Compiles statistics; conducts research and education programs. Maintains speakers' bureau and resource library of materials and publications available for rental or purchase.

"**W**e need occupational therapists who are insightful, resourceful, able to solve complex problems rapidly and can interact with individuals from culturally diverse backgrounds," states researcher E.S. Cohn.

Source: *The American Journal of Occupational Therapy*

American Society of Hospital Pharmacists (ASHP)

4630 Montgomery Ave.
Bethesda, MD 20814
Phone: (301)657-3000
Fax: (301)652-8278

Membership: Professional society of pharmacists employed by hospitals and related institutions. Activities: Provides personnel placement service for members. Sponsors professional and personal liability program. Conducts educational and exhibit programs. Maintains library of medical and pharmacy journals. Presents Harvey A.K. Whitney Lecture Award. Has 25 practice interest areas, 11 specialty practice groups, and research and education foundation.

American Society of Podiatric Medical Assistants (ASPMA)

2124 S. Austin Blvd.
Cicero, IL 60650
Phone: (708)863-6303

Membership: Podiatric assistants. **Purpose:** Purposes are to hold educational seminars and to administer certification examinations. Maintains scholarship trust fund and biographical archives. Holds annual seminar. **Publication(s):** *Journal*, bimonthly. • *Newsletter*, quarterly. • *Podiatric Assistant*, quarterly.

American Speech-Language-Hearing Association (ASHA)

10801 Rockville Pike
Rockville, MD 20852
Phone: (301)897-5700
Fax: (301)571-0457

Membership: Speech-language pathologists and audiologists. **Purpose:** Acts as an accrediting agency for college and university graduate school programs and clinic and hospital programs and as a certifying body for professionals providing speech, language, and hearing therapy to the public. Offers career information, listing of university training programs, and certification requirements. Conducts research on communication disorders and community needs. Presents annual awards. **Publication(s):** *Asha*, monthly. • *ASHA Monographs*, periodic. • *ASHA Reports*, periodic. • *Guide to Graduate Education in Speech-Language Pathology and Audiology*, biennial. • *Journal of Speech and Hearing Research*, bimonthly. • *Language, Speech, and Hearing Services in Schools*, quarterly.

American Therapeutic Recreation Association (ATRA)

PO Box 15215
Hattiesburg, MS 39402-5215
Toll-free: 800-553-0304
Fax: (601)583-4024

Membership: Therapeutic recreation professionals and students; interested others. **Purpose:** (Therapeutic recreation involves the use of sports, handicrafts, and other recreational activities to improve the physical, mental, and emotional functions of persons with illnesses or disabling conditions.) Promotes the use of therapeutic recreation in hospitals, mental rehabilitation centers, physical rehabilitation centers, senior citizen treatment centers, and other public health facilities. Conducts discussions on certification and legislative and regulatory concerns that affect the industry. Sponsors seminars and workshops; conducts research; bestows awards. **Publication(s):** *Employment Update*, monthly. • *Newsletter*, bimonthly. • *The Therapeutic Recreation Journal*, annual (in conjunction with American Association for Leisure and Recreation). • Also publishes *Risk Management in Therapeutic Recreation* and *Evaluation of Therapeutic Recreation Through Quality Assurance*.

Association for Holistic Health (AHH)

PO Box 1122
Del Mar, CA 92014
Phone: (619)535-0101

Membership: Registered nurses, medical doctors, osteopathic physicians, chiropractors, dentists, social workers, psychologists, therapists, ministers, and healers. Activities: Maintains placement service. Formed to promote and support holistic health and to build a bridge between traditional and alternative health care methods. Informs holistic health operations of successful methods of traditional and alternative healing and health programs; provides a forum for individuals and organizations dedicated to promotion of holistic health; attempts to set standards for responsible practitioners and centers. Conducts workshops, seminars, and correspondence courses. Bestows awards; maintains speakers' bureau.

Association for Practitioners in Infection Control (APIC)

505 E. Hawley St.
Mundelein, IL 60060
Phone: (708)949-6052
Fax: (312)566-7282

Membership: Physicians, microbiologists, nurses, epidemiologists, medical technicians, sanitarians, and pharmacists. **Purpose:** To improve patient care by improving the profession of infection control through the development of educational programs and standards. Promotes quality research and standardization of practices and procedures. Develops communications among members, and assesses and influ-ences legislation related to the field. Conducts seminars at local level. **Publication(s):** *American Journal of Infection Control*, bimonth-ly. • *Newsletter*, quarterly.

Association of Physician Assistant Programs (APAP)

950 N. Washington St.
Alexandria, VA 22314
Phone: (703)836-2272

Membership: Educational institutions with training programs for assistants to primary care and surgical physicians. Activities: Coordinates program logistics such as career placements. Assists in the development and organization of educational curricula for physician assistant (PA) programs to assure the public of compe-tent PAs; contributes to defining the roles of PAs in the field of medicine to maximize their benefit to the public; serves as a public information cen-ter on the profession. Sponsors Annual Survey of Physician Assistant Educational Programs in the United States. Maintains library of 200 vol-umes on books and articles. Conducts research projects; compiles statistics. Affiliated With: American Academy of Physician Assistants.

Association of Physician's Assistants in Cardio-Vascular Surgery (APACVS)

2000 Tate Springs Rd.
PO Box 2242
Lynchburg, VA 24501-2242
Phone: 800-528-1506

Membership: Physician's assistants who work with cardiovascular surgeons. Activities: Offers placement service. Objective is to assist in defin-ing the role of physician's assistants in the field of cardiovascular surgery through educational forums. Compiles statistics.

Association on Handicapped Student Service Programs in Postsecondary Education (AHSSPPE)

PO Box 21192
Columbus, OH 43221
Phone: (614)488-4972

Membership: Individuals interested in promot-ing the equal rights and opportunities of handi-capped postsecondary students and graduates.

Activities: Offers employment exchange for posi-tions in handicapped student services, and resource referral system. Facilitates communica-tion among those professionally involved with handicapped students; encourages and supports legislation for the benefit of handicapped stu-dents. Conducts surveys and research pro-grams; bestows awards; compiles statistics.

Child Life Council (CLC)

7910 Woodmont Ave., Ste. 300
Bethesda, MD 20895

Membership: Professional organization repre-senting child life personnel, patient activities specialists, recreational therapists, and students in the field. Activities: Offers a job bank service listing employment openings. Promotes psycho-logical well-being and optimum development of children, adolescents, and their families in health care settings. Works to minimize the stress and anxiety of illness and hospitalization. Addresses professional issues such as program standards, competencies, and core curriculum. Provides resources and conducts research and educational programs. Bestows awards.

When training is unavailable free on the job, the next cheapest way to acquire new skills may be right in the back yard. The majority of Americans live with-in 30 miles of one of the nation's nearly 1,200 community and technical colleges, which are rapidly gaining impor-tance as centers of retraining.

Source: *U.S. News & World Report*

Christian Chiropractors Association (CCA)

3200 S. LeMay Ave.
Ft. Collins, CO 80525
Phone: (303)482-1404
Fax: (303)482-1538

Membership: Christian chiropractors orga-nized to spread the gospel of Christ throughout the U.S. and abroad. Activities: Aids in place-ment of Christian chiropractors as missionaries. Works to unify Christian chiropractors around the essentials of Christianity, "leaving lesser points of doctrine to the conscience of the indi-vidual believers." Focus is on world missions;

seeks to expand the variety of mission fields. Sponsors missions in Ecuador, Ethiopia, France, Kenya, Monaco, Peru, Philippines, the U.S., and Canada. Maintains speakers' bureau; bestows awards.

Committee on Allied Health Education and Accreditation (CAHEA)
515 N. State St.
Chicago, IL 60610
Phone: (312)464-4660
Fax: (312)464-5830

Purpose: Serves as an accrediting agency for 2885 allied health programs in 28 occupational areas. Sponsored by the American Medical Association. Compiles statistics on enrollment and graduates of CAHEA-accredited allied health education programs. **Publication(s):** *Allied Health Education Directory*, annual.

If an ad requests salary information, provide it or you'll find your resume in the wrong pile. The reason firms want the information is to ensure they're interviewing candidates they can afford. Interviews take time and cost money.

Source: *Business Monday/Detroit Free Press*

Convention of American Instructors of the Deaf (CAID)
c/o Dr. Stephanie Polowe
Office of the President
PO Box 9887
LBJ 2264
Rochester, NY 14623-0887
Phone: (716)475-6201
Fax: (716)475-6500

Membership: Professional organization of teachers, administrators, and professionals in allied fields related to education of the deaf. Activities: Offers placement services. Facilitates communication and publication of information on educating the deaf, and develops more effective methods of teaching hearing impaired children. Bestows awards; maintains speakers' bureau.

Council on Chiropractic Education (CCE)
4401 Westown Pkwy., Ste. 120
West Des Moines, IA 50266
Phone: (515)226-9001
Fax: (515)226-9031

Membership: Representatives of member colleges. **Purpose:** Advocates high standards in chiropractic education; establishes criteria of institutional excellence for educating chiropractic physicians; acts as national accrediting agency for chiropractic colleges. Conducts workshops for college teams, consultants, and chiropractic college staffs. **Publication(s):** *CCE Board of Directors*, annual. • *Educational Standards for Chiropractic Colleges*, semiannual. • *Newsletter*, periodic. • Also publishes pamphlets, news releases, and lists of institutions conforming to its standards and policies.

Council on Medical Education of the American Medical Association (CME-AMA)
515 N. State St.
Chicago, IL 60610
Phone: (312)464-5000

Purpose: Participates in the accreditation of and provides consultation to medical school programs, graduate medical educational programs, and educational programs for several allied health occupations. Provides information on medical and allied health education at all levels. Bestows Physicians Recognition Award. **Publication(s):** *Allied Health Education Directory*, annual. • *Annual Report of Medical Education in the Journal of the AMA*. • *Continuing Education Courses for Physicians Supplement to the Journal of the AMA*, semiannual. • *Directory of Graduate Medical Education Programs*, annual.

Council on Professional Standards in Speech-Language Pathology and Audiology
Amer. Speech-Language-Hearing Assn.
10801 Rockville Pike
Rockville, MD 20852
Phone: (301)897-5700

Purpose: Defines standards for clinical certification and for the accreditation of graduate education and professional services. Monitors the interpretation and application of these standards to individuals, institutions, and organizations.

Arbitrates appeals regarding certification and accreditation. **Publication(s):** *Annual Report.* • Also publishes *Appeals Procedure.*

Dental Assisting National Board (DANB)

216 E. Ontario St.
Chicago, IL 60611
Phone: (312)642-3368

Purpose: Certifying agency that administers examinations to dental assistants.

International Chiropractors Association (ICA)

1110 N. Glebe Rd., Ste. 1000
Arlington, VA 22201
Phone: (703)528-5000

Membership: Professional society of chiropractors, chiropractic educators, students, and laypersons. **Purpose:** Sponsors professional development programs and practice management seminars. Presents annual Chiropractor of the Year Award. **Publication(s):** *ICA Today*, bimonthly. • *International Chiropractors Association Membership Directory*, annual. • *International Review of Chiropractic*, bimonthly. • Also publishes materials on patient education.

International Society of Phonetic Sciences (ISPhS)

IASP
50 Dauer Hall
University of Florida
Gainesville, FL 32611
Phone: (904)392-2046

Membership: Phoneticians, phonologists, linguists, engineers, communication scientists, language teachers, speech pathologists, phoniatrists, logopedists, and national phonetic sciences organizations. Activities: Maintains placement service. Purposes are: to promote phonetic sciences on a worldwide basis; to serve as a clearinghouse for issues on phonetics; to become a communication link among the world's phoneticians and affiliated groups; to promote research in phonetics. Bestows awards; compiles statistics.

National Association of Activity Professionals (NAAP)

1225 I St., NW, Ste. 300
Washington, DC 20005
Phone: (202)289-0722
Fax: (202)842-0621

Membership: Those who are or have been therapists, activity directors, and activity consultants in nursing homes, senior centers, retirement housing, or adult day care programs; other interested individuals. Activities: Offers placement service. Purposes of NAAP are to: promote quality care and services for elderly and/or handicapped persons; assist in the delivery of activity services; foster research and the production of relevant literature; upgrade educational programs. Sets standards and has established a certification process. Bestows awards; compiles statistics; maintains speakers' bureau and resource review; sponsors National Activity Professional Day. Offers correspondence courses. Publishes *NAAP News: News of the Activity Profession*, monthly newsletter including educational opportunities, and information on new members and upcoming events (free to members).

National Association of Chain Drug Stores (NACDS)

PO Box 1417-D49
Alexandria, VA 22313-1417
Phone: (703)549-3001

The group is made up of manufacturers, suppliers, manufacturers' representatives, publishers, and advertising agencies. It sponsors meetings and pharmacy student recruitment programs. NACGS publishes an annual calendar and several periodic newsletters.

National Board for Respiratory Care (NBRC)

8310 Nieman Rd.
Lenexa, KS 66214
Phone: (913)599-4200
Fax: (913)541-0156

Purpose: Offers credentialing examinations for respiratory therapists, respiratory therapy technicians, and pulmonary technologists. **Publication(s):** *Annual Directory.* • *Newsletter*, bimonthly.

National Commission on Certification of Physician Assistants (NCCPA)

2845 Henderson Mill Rd. NE
Atlanta, GA 30341
Phone: (404)493-9100

Purpose: Certifies physicians' assistants at the entry level and for continued competence. Has certified 19,000 physicians' assistants. **Publication(s):** *Directory of Physician's Assistants - Certified*, annual.

National Council for Therapeutic Recreation Certification (NCTRC)

PO Box 479
Thiells, NY 10984-0479
Phone: (914)947-4346

Purpose: To establish national evaluative standards for certification and recertification of individuals who work in the therapeutic recreation field; grant recognition to individuals who voluntarily apply and meet established standards; monitor adherence to standards by certified personnel. **Publication(s):** *NCTRC Newsletter*, semiannual.

People assume that they get better within their careers over time, that growth is a step-by-step improvement. Studies have shown that growth occurs in episodic movement, often triggered by a small event. People tend to remain at a uniform level until some change propels them toward a new level of performance.

Source: *The Canadian Nurse*

National Health Council (NHC)

1730 M St., NW, Ste. 500
Washington, DC 20036
Phone: (202)785-3910

Membership: National membership association of voluntary and professional societies in the health field; federal government agencies concerned with health; national organizations and business groups with strong health interests. **Publication(s):** *Standards of Accounting and Reporting for Voluntary Health and Welfare Organizations (The Black Book)*, *Directory of Health Groups in Washington*, *Congress and Health*, *Long-Term Care: Economic Impacts & Financing Dilemmas*, and other books.

National Hospice Organization (NHO)

1901 N. Moore St., Ste. 901
Arlington, VA 22209
Phone: (703)243-5900

The organization is made up of hospices and individuals interested in the promotion of the hospice concept and program of care. It promotes standards of care in program planning and implementation, monitors healthcare legislation and regulation relevant to hospice care. The group publishes an annual guide, a quarterly journal, and monthly newsletter.

National Rehabilitation Association (NRA)

633 S. Washington St.
Alexandria, VA 22314
Phone: (703)836-0850
Fax: (703)836-2209

Membership: Physicians, counselors, therapists, disability examiners, vocational evaluators, and others interested in rehabilitation of persons with disabilities. Activities: Maintains Job Placement Division. Sponsors Graduate Literary Awards Contest. Conducts legislative activities; develops accessibility guidelines; offers specialized education.

National Rehabilitation Counseling Association (NRCA)

1910 Association Dr., Ste. 206
Reston, VA 22091
Phone: (703)620-4404

Membership: A division of the National Rehabilitation Association. Professional and student rehabilitation counselors. **Purpose:** Works to expand the role of counselors in the rehabilitation process and seeks to advance members' professional development. Supports legislation favoring the profession. **Publication(s):** *Journal of Applied Rehabilitation Counseling*, quarterly. • *Professional Report of the National Rehabilitation Counseling Association*, bimonthly.

National Rural Health Association (NRHA)

301 E. Armour Blvd.
Ste. 420
Kansas City, MO 64111
Phone: (816)756-3140
Fax: (816)756-3144

Membership: Administrators, physicians, dentists, nurses, physician assistants, health planners, academicians, and others interested or involved in rural health care. Activities: Provides placement services. Purpose is to: create a better understanding of health care problems unique to rural areas; utilize a collective approach in finding positive solutions; articulate and represent the health care needs of rural America; supply current information to rural health care providers; serve as a liaison between rural health care programs throughout the country. Offers continuing education credits for medical, dental, nursing, and management courses. Bestows awards.

National Strength and Conditioning Association (NSCA)

PO Box 81410
Lincoln, NE 68501
Phone: (402)472-3000
Fax: (402)476-6976

Membership: Professional coaches, athletic trainers, physical therapists, sports medicine physicians, and sports science researchers. Activities: Provides job update service hot line and maintains Job Placement Committee. Promotes the total conditioning of athletes to a level of optimum performance, with the belief that a better conditioned athlete not only performs better but is less prone to injury. Sanctions national, regional, state, and local clinics and workshops. Funds private research projects; provides professional liability insurance; offers scholarships. Operates professional certification program.

National Therapeutic Recreation Society (NTRS)

2775 S. Quincy St., Ste. 300
Arlington, VA 22206
Phone: (703)820-4940
Fax: (703)671-6772

Membership: Professional personnel whose full-time employment is directly related to the therapeutic application of recreation in clinical, residential, or community programs for people with disabilities. **Purpose:** Encourages professional growth that will directly benefit the ill and handicapped through studies, workshops, seminars, institutes, and staff training programs in cooperation with specialists, educators, and other interdisciplinary groups; supports the

application of the principles of other allied groups in total treatment programs; encourages scientifically designed research; advocates undergraduate and graduate college curricula to provide recreational therapists the opportunity to apply for national professional registration. Bestows awards. A branch of the National Recreation and Park Association. **Publication(s):** *NTRS Newsletter*, quarterly. • *Parks and Recreation*, monthly. • *Therapeutic Recreation Journal*, quarterly.

Opticians Association of America (OAA)

10341 Democracy Ln.
PO Box 10110
Fairfax, VA 22030
Phone: (703)691-8355
Fax: (703)691-3929

Membership: Retail dispensing opticians who fill prescriptions for glasses or contact lenses written by a vision care specialist. **Purpose:** To advance the science of ophthalmic optics. **Publication(s):** *OAA News*, 8/year.

T o economize on headhunters' fees and classified advertising, a growing number of companies are now filing the resumes that snow in each year where they might actually do job seekers some good: in an electronic database.

Source: *U.S. News & World Report*

Private Practice Section/American Physical Therapy Association (PPS)

1101 17th St. NW, Ste. 1000
Washington, DC 20036
Phone: (202)457-1115
Fax: (202)457-9191

Membership: Physical therapists who are members of the American Physical Therapy Association and who are in private practice. **Purpose:** Purposes are: to provide physical therapists with information on establishing and managing a private practice; to promote high standards of private practice physical therapy; to represent private practitioners before governmental and professional agencies; to disseminate information relating to private practice. Monitors federal and state legislation. Holds forums and seminars. Bestows Robert G. Dicus Award to recognize individuals for achievement in and commitment to the private practice of physical therapy. **Publication(s):** Operates telephone referral service. *Private Practice Section Membership Directory*, annual. • *Physical Therapy Today*, quarterly. • Also publishes *An Employers Guide to Obtaining Physical Therapy Services.*

In a survey of allied health students, all students agreed that the labor shortages so widely reported are indeed existent. Because of these shortages, career prospects are excellent for all of the allied health professions. In many cases students reported being called by "headhunters" to discuss jobs available immediately after graduation.

Source: *Healthcare Careers*

Special Recreation, Inc. (SRI)

362 Koser Ave.
Iowa City, IA 52246-3038
Phone: (319)337-7578
Fax: (319)338-3320

Membership: Disabled consumers, rehabilitation professionals, parents of the disabled, and volunteers. Activities: Offers career guidance and placement service. Formed to support, encourage, and promote self-determination, equal opportunity, consumerism, and normalization in recreation and leisure for disabled individuals; to launch the formation and advancement of national policy and philosophy for special recreation; to provide national information services on federal, state, and local laws, regulations, and public programs for special recreation. Conducts research and demonstrations; prepares and disseminates information; cooperates with and assists voluntary associations and public agencies in initiating, expanding, and improving special recreation programs and services and provides personnel training. Maintains Pioneers in Special Recreation Hall of Fame and biographical archives. Maintains 2000 volume library and speakers' bureau; presents awards; compiles statistics.

U.S. Physical Therapy Association (USPTA)

1803 Avon Lane
Arlington Heights, IL 60004

Membership: Professional physical therapists and assistants. Activities: Maintains placement service. Maintains U.S. Physical Therapy Academy which: conducts continuing education programs for members; sponsors workshops to acquaint personnel from other medical fields with physical therapy; accredits hospital and nursing home physical therapy departments, universities, and colleges of physical therapy; certifies physical therapists through board examinations. Promotes ethical standards; maintains charitable program; bestows awards; compiles statistics; conducts children's services.

Employment Agencies and Search Firms

A.C. Personnel Consultants

1175 S. Fairplay
Circle D
Aurora, CO 80012
Phone: (303)751-9208

Academy Medical Personnel Services

571 High St.
Worthington, OH 43085
Phone: (614)848-6011

Employment agency. Fills openings on a regular or temporary basis.

Alpine Consultants

10300 SW Greenburg Rd., Ste. 290
Portland, OR 97223
Phone: (503)244-3393

Employment agency.

Bryant Bureau

3030 NW Expressway, 400
Oklahoma City, OK 73112
Phone: (405)946-3001

Employment agency.

Davis-Smith Medical Employment Service, Inc.

24725 W. 12 Mile Rd.
No. 2302 Lockdale Office Plaza
Southfield, MI 48034
Phone: (313)354-4100

Employment agency. Executive search firm.

Dent-Assist Personnel Service

2020 29th St., Ste. 202
Sacramento, CA 94817
Phone: (916)456-1111

Employment agency. Provides placement on regular or temporary basis.

DentaPro, Inc.

3930 Knowles Ave., Ste. 301
Kensington, MD 20985
Phone: (301)942-3366

Employment agency.

Durham Medical Search, Inc.

6300 Transit
Depew, NY 14043
Phone: (716)681-7402

Employment agency.

Dynamic Dental Services, Inc.

863 Holcolm Bridge Rd., Ste. 230
Roswell, GA 30076
Phone: (404)998-7779
Fax: (404)552-0176

Employment agency.

Eden Personnel, Inc.

280 Madison Rd., Rm. 202
New York, NY 10016
Phone: (212)685-8600

Employment agency. Places individuals in regular or temporary positions.

Harper Associates-Detroit, Inc.

29870 Middlebelt
Farmington Hills, MI 48334
Phone: (313)932-1170

Employment agency.

Health and Science Center

PO Box 213
Lima, PA 19037
Phone: (215)891-0794

Employment agency. Executive search firm.

Massachusetts Medical Bureau

101 Tremont St.
Boston, MA 02108
Phone: (617)842-2400
Fax: (617)482-7290

Employment agency. Executive search firm.

Medical Personnel Pool

Ala Moana Bldg., Ste. 1320
1441 Kapiolani Bldg.
Honolulu, HI 96814
Phone: (808)955-1102

Offices throughout the continental U.S. as well. Provides temporary staffing assistance.

Networking isn't talking about yourself. You can get information only if the other party is talking about himself or herself, his or her company and associates. If you find networking is your-sided, you'd better rethink your approach.

Source: *Business Monday/Detroit Free Press*

Medical Personnel Service

4801 Woodway, No. 333 West
Houston, TX 77056
Phone: (713)623-2200

Employment agency.

Midwest Medical Consultants

8910 Purdue Rd., Ste. 200
Indianapolis, IN 46268-1155
Phone: (317)872-1053

Employment agency. Executive search firm.

Ocean Personnel Agency

PO Box 698
Malibu, CA 90265
Phone: (213)451-8183

Employment agency.

Opportunities Unlimited of N.E., Inc.

40 Speer St.
PO Box 9106
Framingham, MA 01701
Phone: (508)872-3517

Employment agency.

Professional Placement Associates, Inc.
11 Rye Ridge Plaza
Port Chester, NY 10573
Phone: (914)939-1195
Fax: (914)939-1959

Employment agency.

Ranier Home Health Care
1530 S. Union, Ste. 10
Tacoma, WA 98405
Phone: (206)759-8060

Employment agency.

Retail Recruiters/Spectra Professional Search
1 Bala Cynwyd Plaza, Ste. 217
Bala Cynwyd, PA 19004
Phone: (215)667-6565
Fax: (215)667-5323

Employment agency. Affiliate offices in many locations across the country.

One thousand unsolicited resumes typically arrive in the daily mail at Fortune 50 companies. Four out of five are tossed after a quick perusal.

Source: *U.S. News & World Report*

Ritt-Ritt and Associates
1400 E. Touhy Ave.
Des Plaines, IL 60018
Phone: (708)298-2510

Employment agency.

Staley/Adams and Associates Personnel Services Inc.
4615 Post Oak Pl., Ste. 140
Houston, TX 77027
Phone: (713)965-0402

Employment agency.

Travcorps, Inc.
40 Eastern Ave.
Malden, MA 02148
Phone: (617)322-2600

Places staff in temporary assignments.

Career Guides

The 100 Best Companies to Work for in America
Signet/NAL Penguin
1633 Broadway
New York, NY 10019

Levering, Robert, Moskowitz, Milton, and Katz, Michael. 1985. $5.95. 477 pages. Describes the best companies to work for in America, based on such factors as salary, benefits, job security, and ambience. The authors base their 'top 100' rating on surveys and personal visits to hundreds of firms.

120 Careers in the Health Care Field
U.S. Directory Service, Publishers
PO Box 13
New Providence, NJ 07974
Phone: (305)769-1700
Toll-free: 800-521-8110
Fax: (908)665-6688

Stanley Alperin. Second edition, 1989.

300 New Ways to Get a Better Job
Bob Adams, Inc.
260 Center St.
Holbrook, MA 02343
Phone: (617)767-8100

Advocates a job search approach designed to meet the changing nature of the job market.

850 Leading USA Companies
Jamenair Ltd.
PO Box 241957
Los Angeles, CA 90024
Phone: (213)470-6688

Studner, Peter K. $49.95. Compatible with IBM and IBM-compatibles.

About Therapeutic Recreation
National Therapeutic Recreation Society
2775 S. Quincy St., Ste. 300
Arlington, VA 22206
Phone: (703)820-4940

1989. This 15-page booklet discusses the importance of therapeutic recreation and its role as part of the client treatment team; describes educational preparation, certification, and licensure.

Allied Health Education Directory
American Medical Association (AMA)
515 N. State St.
Chicago, IL 60610
Phone: (312)464-5000
Toll-free: 800-621-8335

William R. Burrow, editor. Sixteenth edition, 1991. Describes 26 allied health occupations and lists educational programs accredited by the Committee on Allied Health Education and Accreditation of the American Medical Association.

The American Almanac of Jobs and Salaries
Avon Books
1350 Avenue of the Americas
New York, NY 10019
Phone: (212)261-6800
Toll-free: 800-238-0658

John Wright, editor. Revised and updated, 1990. A comprehensive guide to the wages of hundreds of occupations in a wide variety of industries and organizations.

Being a Long-Term Care Nursing Assistant
Prentice Hall
Rte. 9W
Englewood Cliffs, NJ 07632
Phone: (201)592-2000

Connie A. Will. 1991.

The Berkeley Guide to Employment for New College Graduates
Ten Speed Press
PO Box 7123
Berkeley, CA 94707
Phone: (415)845-8414

Briggs, James I. $7.95. 256 pages. Basic job-hunting advice for the college student.

The Best Companies for Women
Simon and Schuster
Simon and Schuster Bldg.
1230 Avenue of the Americas
New York, NY 10020
Phone: (212)698-7000

1989. $8.95.

Best of the National Business Employment Weekly
Consultants Bookstore
Templeton Rd.
Fitzwilliam, NJ 03447
Phone: (603)585-2200
Fax: (603)585-9555

$5.00/booklet. Booklets summarizing the best articles from the *National Business Employment Weekly* on a variety of job hunting topics.

Career Directions for Dental Hygienists
Career Directions Press
171 Hwy. 34
Holmdel, NJ 07733
Phone: (908)946-8457

Regina A. Dreyer-Thomas. Revised edition, 1992. Describes the personal characteristics needed to be a dental hygienist. Explores career opportunities in public health, the federal government, long-term care facilities, education, dental centers, health maintenance organizations, industry, working abroad, and private practice. Gives job hunting advice including how to write the resume and preparing for the interview.

A recent study by Northwestern National Life Insurance Company found that 46 percent of American workers worry about their jobs and feel more pressured to prove their value because of the recession. . . Unfortunately, the more you worry about whether you are doing a good enough job, the more likely you are to erode your efficiency, creativity and morale—and damage your health.

Source: *Business Monday/Detroit Free Press*

The Career Fitness Program: Exercising Your Options
Gorsuch Scarisbrick, Publishers
8233 Via Paseo del Norte, Ste. F-400
Scottsdale, AZ 85258

Sukiennik et al. 1989. $16.00. 227 pages. Textbook, with second half devoted to the job search process.

Career for the Future: Chiropractic Health Care

International Chiropractors Association
1110 N. Glebe Rd., Ste. 1000
Arlington, VA 22201
Phone: (703)528-5000

1991. This six-panel pamphlet describes personal qualifications, nature of the job, educational preparation, professional practice, licensure, income, and financial aid.

What makes one job better than another? High pay? Prestige? Pleasant working conditions? Or, these days, might the clincher be job security? The answer is that there is no single deciding factor. Truly great jobs offer all of the above and more . . . . Jobs, after all, are a complicated mix of pluses and minuses.

Source: *Money*

The Career Guide—Dun's Employment Opportunities Directory

Dun's Marketing Services
Dun and Bradstreet Corp.
3 Sylvan Way
Parsippany, NJ 07054-3896
Phone: (201)605-6000

Annual, December. $450.00; $385.00 for public libraries (lease basis). Covers: More than 5,000 companies that have a thousand or more employees and that provide career opportunities in sales, marketing, management, engineering, life and physical sciences, computer science, mathematics, statistics planning, accounting and finance, liberal arts fields, and other technical and professional areas; based on data supplied on questionnaires and through personal interviews. Also covers personnel consultants; includes some public sector employers (governments, schools, etc.) usually not found in similar lists. Entries include: Company name, location of headquarters, and other offices of plants; entries may also include name, title, address, and phone of employment contact; disciplines or occupational groups hired; brief overview of company; discussion of types of positions that may be available; training and career development programs; benefits offered. Arrangement: Companies are alphabetical; consultants are geo-

graphical. Indexes: Geographical, Standard Industrial Classification code.

A Career in Pharmacy

National Association of Retail Druggists
205 Daingerfield Rd.
Alexandria, VA 22314
Phone: (703)683-8200

1992. This one-page information sheet outlines high school courses, pre-pharmacy courses, and pharmacy school courses. Briefly describes professional opportunities in different work settings, working hours per week, salary, and employment outlook.

Career Information Systems (CIS)

National Career Information System
1787 Agate St.
Eugene, OR 97403
Phone: (503)686-3872

Includes information on job search techniques and self-employment options. Also provides extensive career planning information.

Career Opportunities

Quanta Press, Inc.
1313 5th St. SE, Ste. 223A
Minneapolis, MN 55414
Phone: (612)379-3956

CD-ROM (Compact Disc-Read Only Memory) database that provides job titles and job descriptions and information on education levels, chances for advancement, average salaries, and working conditions.

Career Placement Registry (CPR)

Career Placement Registry, Inc.
302 Swann Ave.
Alexandria, VA 22301
Phone: (703)683-1085
Fax: (703)683-0246

Contains brief resumes of job candidates currently seeking employment. Comprises two files, covering college and university seniors and recent graduates, and alumni, executives, and others who have already acquired substantial work experience. Entries typically include applicant name, address, telephone number, degree level, function, language skills, name of school, major field of study, minor field of study, occupational preference, date available, city/area preference, special skills, citizenship status, employer name, employer address, description of duties, position/title, level of education, civil service register, security clearance type/availability, willingness to relocate, willingness to travel, salary expectation, and overall work experience. Available online through DIALOG Information Services, Inc.

Career Strategies—From Job Hunting to Moving Up

Association for Management Success
2360 Maryland Rd.
Willow Grove, PA 19090

Six video cassettes. Kennedy, Marilyn Moats. $36.95/each. $203.70/set. 30 minutes each. Covers the following topics: planning the job hunt, networking, resumes, interviewing, negotiating salaries and benefits, and moving up on the job.

Careering and Re-Careering for the 1990's

Consultants Bookstore
Templeton Rd.
Fitzwilliam, NH 03447
Phone: (603)585-6544
Fax: (603)585-9555

Krannich, Ronald. 1989. $13.95. 314 pages. Details trends in the marketplace, how to identify opportunities, how to retrain for them, and how to land jobs. Includes a chapter on starting a business. Contains index, bibliography, and illustrations.

Careers

National Textbook Co.
4255 W. Touhy Ave.
Lincolnwood, IL 60646
Phone: (312)679-5500
Toll-free: 800-323-4900

1990. Includes a bibliography and an index.

Careers and the College Grad

Bob Adams, Inc.
260 Center St.
Holbrook, MA 02343
Phone: (617)767-8100
Fax: (617)767-0994

Ranno, Gigi. 1992. $12.95. 64 pages. An annual resource guide addressing the career and job-hunting interests of undergraduates. Provides company profiles and leads.

Careers in Health Care

Chelsea House Publishers
1974 Sproul Rd., Ste. 400
Broomall, PA 19008
Phone: (215)353-5166
Fax: (215)359-1439

Rachel S. Epstein. 1989.

Careers in Occupational Therapy

American Occupational Therapy Association
1383 Piccard Dr., Ste. 301
PO Box 1725
Rockville, MD 20849-1725
Phone: (301)948-9626

1990. This sheet describes employment outlook for occupational therapists, as well as education, places of employment, and earnings.

> In the next decade, diet treatment alone or combined with drugs may be recommended for over 25 percent of Americans; administration of dietary treatment on this scale is a major challenge for the dietetics profession.
>
> Source: *Journal of the American Dietetic Association*

Careers in Physiology

American Physiological Society
9650 Rockville Pike
Bethesda, MD 20814-3991
Phone: (301)530-7164

1990. Briefly describes physiology careers and the education required.

Careers in Speech-Language Pathology and Audiology

American Speech-Language-Hearing Association (ASHA)
10801 Rockville Pike
Rockville, MD 20852
Phone: (301)897-5700

1993. Packet containing four information sheets describing what speech-language pathologists and audiologists do, as well as certification, educational preparation, and financial aid.

Careers in the Dental Profession: Dental Assisting

SELECT
211 E. Chicago Ave., Ste. 1804
Chicago, IL 60611-2678
Phone: (312)440-2500

1991. This eight-page booklet describes what dental assistants do, where they work, educational preparation and certification.

The Certified Occupational Therapy Assistant: Roles and Responsibilities

Slack, Inc.
6900 Grove Rd.
Thorofare, NJ 08086
Phone: (609)848-1000
Toll-free: 800-257-8290

Sally E. Ryan, editor. 1992. Includes a bibliography. Illustrated.

There are two types of ads: open (the company identified) and blind. Open ads are great for job-hunters. They give you the opportunity to do some investigation on the firm. Be sure to tailor your cover letter with your knowledge of the company. If you're lucky, you may uncover a contact.

Source: *Business Monday/Detroit Free Press*

Certified Occupational Therapy Assistants: Opportunities and Challenges

Haworth Press, Inc.
10 Alice St.
Binghamton, NY 13904-1580
Phone: (607)722-2493
Toll-free: 800-342-9678

Jerry A. Johnson, editor. 1989. Includes bibliographical references. Illustrated.

Chiropractic State of the Art

American Chiropractic Association (ACA)
1701 Clarendon Blvd.
Arlington, VA 22209
Phone: (703)276-8800
Toll-free: 800-368-3083

1992. This 57-page booklet gives history, occu-pational information, educational information, licensure, and employment outlook. Lists accredited chiropractic colleges.

Chronicle Career Index

Chronicle Guidance Publications
PO Box 1190
Moravia, NY 13118-1190
Phone: (315)497-0330

Annual. $14.25. Provides bibliographic listings of career and vocational guidance publications and other resources. Arrangement: Alphabetical by source. Indexes: Occupation; vocational and professional information.

College Majors and Careers: A Resource Guide to Effective Life Planning

Garrett Park Press
PO Box 190E
Garrett Park, MD 20896
Phone: (301)946-2553

Paul Pfifer. 1993. Includes chapters titled "Biology", "Botany", "Physiology", and "Zoology". Lists 61 college majors, with definitions; related occupations and leisure activities; skills, values, and personal attributes needed; suggested readings; and a list of associations.

The Complete Job Search Book

John Wiley and Sons
605 3rd Ave.
New York, NY 10158

Beatty, Richard H. 1988. $12.95. 256 pages.

The Complete Job-Search Handbook

Consultants Bookstore
Templeton Rd.
Fitzwilliam, NH 03447
Phone: (603)585-6544
Fax: (603)585-9555

Figler, Howard. 1988. $12.95. 366 pages. Contains information on how to look for career opportunities every day. Focuses on 20 life skills in self-assessment, detective work, communication skills, and selling oneself. Includes skill-building exercises.

Comprehensive Review of Dental Assisting

Krieger Publishing Co., Inc.
PO Box 9542
Melbourne, FL 32902
Phone: (407)724-9542
Fax: (407)951-3671

Jacqueline W. Sapp. 1981.

The Corporate Directory of U.S. Public Companies

Gale Research Inc.
835 Penobscot Bldg.
Detroit, MI 48226
Phone: (313)961-2242
Fax: (313)961-6241

1991. $325.00. Provides information on more than 9,500 publicly-traded firms having at least $5,000,000 in assets. Entries include: General background, including name, address and phone, number of employees; stock date; description of areas of business; major subsidiaries; officers; directors; owners; and financial data. Indexes: Officers and directors, owners, subsidiary/parent, geographic, SIC, stock exchange, company rankings, and newly registered corporations.

CSI National Career Network

Computer Search International Corporation (CSI)
7926 Jones Branch Dr., Ste. 120
McLean, VA 22102
Phone: (302)749-1635

Contains job listings from potential employers and candidate resumes from executive recruiting firms. Covers more than 40 technical and managerial job categories.

Dental Assistant

National Learning Corp.
212 Michael Dr.
Syosset, NY 11791
Phone: (516)921-8888

Jack Rudman. 1989. Part of Career Examination Series.

The Dental Assistant

Lea & Febiger
200 Chester Field Pkwy.
Malvern, PA 19355
Phone: (215)251-2230
Fax: (215)251-2229

Roger E. Barton, editor. Sixth edition, 1988.

Dental Assisting

National Learning Corp.
212 Michael Dr.
Syosset, NY 11791
Phone: (516)921-8888

Jack Rudman. 1989. Part of Occupational Competency Examination Series.

Dental Assisting: Basic & Dental Sciences

Mosby Year Book, Inc.
11830 Westline Industrial Dr.
St. Louis, MO 63146
Phone: (314)872-8370

Leimone. 1987.

The United States economy is projected to provide 24 million more jobs in 2005 than it did in 1990, an increase of 20 percent.

Source: *Occupational Outlook Quarterly*

Directory of Employment Opportunities in the Federal Government

Arco Publishing Company
Simon and Schuster, Inc.
15 Columbus Circle
Order Dept., 16th Fl.
New York, NY 10023
Phone: (212)373-8931
Fax: (212)767-5852

1985. $24.95. Covers: Federal agencies offering employment opportunities in the U.S. government. Entries include: Agency name and address, geographical area served, subsidiary and branch names and locations, eligibility requirements, application and testing procedures, and job descriptions. Arrangement: Alphabetical. Indexes: Department name, position title, subject (occupational categories).

Dun and Bradstreet Million Dollar Directory

Dun's Marketing Services
Dun and Bradstreet Corp.
3 Sylvan Way
Parsippany, NJ 07054-3896
Phone: (201)605-6000
Fax: (201)605-6911

An annual directory covering 160,000 businesses with a net worth of $500,00 or more, including industrial corporations, utilities, transportation companies, bank and trust companies, stock brokers, mutual and stock insurance companies, wholesalers, retailers, and domestic subsidiaries of foreign corporations.

Encyclopedia of Career Choices for the 1990s: A Guide to Entry Level Jobs

Walker and Co.
720 5th Ave.
New York, NY 10019
Phone: (212)265-3632
Toll-free: 800-289-2553

1991. Describes entry-level careers in a variety of industries. Presents qualifications required, working conditions, salary, internships, and professional associations.

In all cases, the people with an edge will be those who know how to use a computer to do their jobs more efficiently, who can present ideas cogently and who work well in teams.

Source: *U.S. News & World Report*

The Encyclopedia of Careers and Vocational Guidance

J.G. Ferguson Publishing Co.
200 W. Monroe, Ste. 250
Chicago, IL 60606
Phone: (312)580-5480

William E. Hopke, editor-in-chief. Eighth edition, 1990. Four-volume set that profiles 900 occupations and describes job trends in 71 industries.

The Encyclopedia of Careers and Vocational Guidance

J. G. Ferguson Publishing Co.
200 W. Monroe, Ste. 250
Chicago, IL 60606
Phone: (312)580-5480

William E. Hopke, editor-in-chief. ninth edition, 1993. Four-volume set that profiles 900 occupations and describes job trends in 71 industries. Volume 2–*Professional Careers*–chapters on biological scientists include "Biochemists" (p. 60) and "Biologists" (p. 63). Includes career descrip-

tion, educational requirements, history of the job, methods of entry, advancement, employment outlook, earnings, conditions of work, social and psychological factors, and sources of further information.

Exciting Opportunities Ahead for Speech, Language and Hearing Scientists

American Speech-Language-Hearing Association
10801 Rockville Pike
Rockville, MD 20852
Phone: (301)897-5700

1990. Eight-panel brochure describing research careers in communication sciences and disorders; also explains educational preparation required.

The Experienced Hand: A Student Manual for Making the Most of an Internship

Carroll Press
43 Squantum St.
Cranston, RI 02920
Phone: (401)942-1587

Stanton, Timothy, and Ali, Kamil. 1987. $6.95. 88 pages. Guidance for deriving the most satisfaction and future benefit from an internship.

Exploring Nontraditional Jobs for Women

Rosen Publishing Group, Inc.
29 E. 21st St.
New York, NY 10010
Phone: (212)777-3017
Toll-free: 800-237-9932
Fax: (212)777-0277

Rose Neufeld. Revised edition. 1989. $13.95 per volume; $139.50 per set. Part of a 10 volume set that describes occupations where few women are found. Covers job duties, training routes, where to apply for jobs, tools used, salary, and advantages and disadvantages of the job.

Fact Sheet on Chiropractic

American Chiropractic Association
1701 Clarendon Blvd.
Arlington, VA 22209
Phone: (703)276-8800
Toll-free: 800-368-3083
Fax: (703)243-2593

1990. Describes the position of chiropractors in the health care system.

Facts About Chiropractic Education: Patient Information

American Chiropractic Association
1701 Clarendon Blvd.
Arlington, VA 22209
Phone: (703)276-8800
Toll-free: 800-368-3083
Fax: (703)243-2593

1990. This pamphlet describes the educational preparation and licensure of chiropractors and gives a profile of a typical chiropractic student.

Facts . . . About Dental Hygienists

American Dental Hygienists' Association (ADHA)
444 N. Michigan Ave., Ste. 3400
Chicago, IL 60611
Phone: (312)440-8900
Fax: (312)440-8929

1982. This two-panel brochure describes what dental hygienists do, necessary educational preparation, and places of employment.

Financial World—500 Fastest Growing Companies

Financial World Partners
1328 Broadway
New York, NY 10001
Phone: (212)594-5030

An annual directory listing 500 U.S. firms showing greatest growth in net earnings for the year.

Financial World America's Top Growth Companies Directory Issue

Financial World Partners
1328 Broadway
New York, NY 10001
Phone: (212)594-5030

An annual listing of companies selected on the basis of earnings per share growth rate over a 10-year period ending with the current year.

Forbes Up-and-Comers 200: Best Small Companies in America

Forbes, Inc.
60 5th Ave.
New York, NY 10011
Phone: (212)620-2200
Fax: (212)620-1863

An annual directory that lists 200 small companies judged to be exceptionally fast-growing on the basis of 5-year return on equity and other qualititative measurements.

Fortune Directory

Time, Inc.
Time and Life Bldg.
Rockefeller Center
New York, NY 10020
Phone: (212)586-1212

An annual directory that covers 500 of the largest U.S. industrial corporations and 500 largest U.S. non-industrial corporations.

A Future in Physical Therapy

American Physical Therapy Association
1111 N. Fairfax St.
Alexandria, VA 22314
Phone: (703)684-2782

Annual. Sixteen-page booklet including a description of the field, what physical therapists do, education, licensure, and salaries. Gives a state-by-state listing of accredited programs. List sources of financial aid.

> "**M**edicine is changing faster than ever and changing in more significant ways," says Lowell S. Levin, Ed.D., professor of public health at Yale University School of Medicine. Dr. Levin points not only to the millions of pages of research published in medical journals each year, but also to recent breakthroughs in fields such as genetics that are changing some of our basic notions about health.
>
> Source: *Glamour*

Get a Better Job!

Peterson's
PO Box 2123
Princeton, NJ 08543-2123
Phone: (609)243-9111

Rushlow, Ed. 1990. $11.95. 255 pages. Counsels the reader on job search techniques. Discusses how to win the job by bypassing the Personnel Department and how to understand the employer's system for screening and selecting candidates. Written in an irreverent and humorous style.

277

Get That Job!

Consultants Bookstore
Templeton Rd.
Fitzwilliam, NH 03447
Phone: (603)585-6544
Fax: (603)585-9555

Camden, Thomas. 1981. $24.95. Two 30-minute cassettes supplemented by a 45-page booklet that include dramatizations of interviews, cover what questions to expect, and how to respond to them. Provides sample resumes and letters.

Getting a Job in the Computer Age

Peterson's Guides, Inc.
PO Box 2123
Princeton, NJ 08543-2123
Phone: (609)395-0676
Toll-free: 800-338-3282

Harold Goldstein and Bryna S. Fraser. 1986. Includes about 75 occupations, based on a study of all occupations in which computers are used. Contains chapters titled "Writers" (p. 80) and "Technical Writers" (p. 79-80). Describes the type of equipment used; discusses types of computer training (most computer skills needed are learned on the job).

> **O**ne way to improve your chances in the job hunt is to define "you" as broadly as possible . . . . Defining yourself in terms of your skills rather than your job history is the key.
>
> Source: *Business Monday/Detroit Free Press*

Guide to Federal Jobs

Resource Directories
3361 Executive Pkwy.
Toledo, OH 43606
Phone: (419)536-5353
Toll-free: 800-274-8515
Fax: (419)536-7056

Rod W. Durgin, editor. Third edition, 1992. Contains information on finding and applying for federal jobs. Describes more than 200 professional and technical jobs for college graduates. Includes chapters titled "Geologist" (p. 221), "Geophysicist" (p. 215), and "Hydrologist" (p. 211). Covers the nature of the work, salary, and geographic location. Lists college majors preferred for that occupation. Section one describes the function and work of government agencies that hire the most significant number of college graduates.

Have You Considered Dental Hygiene?

American Dental Association (ADA)
211 E. Chicago Ave.
Chicago, IL 60611
Phone: (312)440-2500
Toll-free: 800-947-4746

1990. This nine-page booklet describes what dental hygienists do and where they work, earnings, accreditation, licensure, and education.

The Health Care Worker: An Introduction to Health Occupations

Prentice-Hall, Inc.
Route 9W
Englewood Cliffs, NJ 07632
Phone: (201)592-2000

Shirley A. Badasch, and Doreen S. Chesebro. Second edition, 1988. Includes a bibliography and an index.

Health Career Planning: A Realistic Guide

Human Sciences Press
233 Spring St.
New York, NY 10013
Phone: (212)620-8000

Ellen F. Lederman. 1988.

Health Careers Today

C.V. Mosby Co.
11830 Westline Industrial Dr.
St. Louis, MO 63146
Phone: (314)872-8370

Judith A. Gerdin. 1991. Surveys health occupations. Includes information on basic health care skills and careers.

The Hidden Job Market

Peterson's
PO Box 2123
Princeton, NJ 08543-2123
Phone: (609)243-9111

1991. $16.95. Subtitled *A Job Seeker's Guide to America's 2,000 Little-Known but Fastest-*

Growing High-Tech Companies. Listing of high technology companies in such fields as environmental consulting, genetic engineering, home health care, telecommunications, alternative energy systems, and others.

Hospital Salary Survey Report

Hospital Compensation Service
John R. Zabka Associates, Inc.
69 Minnehaha Blvd.
PO Box 376
Oakland, NJ 07436
Phone: (201)405-0075
Fax: (201)405-1258

Annual. Reports salaries for management employees, registered nurses, and licensed practical nurses by hospital bed size, by profit and nonprofit status for governmental hospitals, and by geographic area.

How to Get a Good Job and Keep It

VGM Career Horizons
4255 W. Touhy Ave.
Lincolnwood, IL 60646-1975
Phone: (708)679-5500

Bloch, Deborah Perlmutter. 1993. $7.95. Aimed at the recent high school or college graduate, this guide provides advice on finding out about jobs, completing applications and resumes, and managing successful interviews.

Inc.—The Inc. 100 Issue

The Goldhirsh Group
38 Commercial Wharf
Boston, MA 02110
Phone: (617)248-8000
Fax: (617)248-8090

An annual directory listing the 100 fastest-growing publicly held companies in manufacturing and service industries that had revenues greater than $100,000 but less than $25 million five years prior to compilation.

Inc.—The Inc. 500 Issue

The Goldhirsh Group
38 Commercial Wharf
Boston, MA 02110
Phone: (617)248-8000
Fax: (617)248-8090

An annual directory that lists 500 fastest-growing privately held companies in service, manufacturing, retail, distribution, and construction industries, based on percentage increase in sales over the five-year period prior to compilation.

The Internship Experience—A Manual for Pharmacy Preceptors and Interns

National Association of Boards of Pharmacy (NABP)
700 Bussey Hwy.
Park Ridge, IL 60068
Phone: (708)698-6227

Paul Grussing, editor. 1991.

Four out of five companies say their employees can't write well. But only 21 percent of corporate training aims at writing skills.

Source: *U.S. News & World Report*

Internships: On-the-Job Training Opportunities for All Types of Careers

Peterson's Guides, Inc.
20 Carnegie Center
PO Box 2123
Princeton, NJ 08543-2123
Phone: (609)243-9111
Fax: (609)243-9150

Annual, December. $27.95., plus $3.00 shipping. Covers: 850 corporations, social service organizations, government agencies, recreational facilities (including parts and forests), entertainment industries, and science and research facilities which offer about 50,000 apprenticeships and internships in 23 different career areas. Entries include: Organization name, address, name of contact; description of internship offered, including duties, stipend, length of service; eligibility requirements; deadline for application and application procedures. Arrangement: Classified by subject (arts, communications, business, etc.). Indexes: Subject/organization name, geographical.

Introduction to the Health Professions

Jones and Bartlett Publishers, Inc.
1 Exeter Plaza
Boston, MA 02116
Phone: (617)859-3900

Peggy Stanfield. 1990.

> **A** career path should not be restrictive—there should be forks in the path, allowing you to adapt as changes occur within professional and personal lifestyles. The best intentions can go astray, leading to discouragement and disillusionment if alternative paths have not been prepared.
>
> Source: *The Canadian Nurse*

The Job Bank Series

Bob Adams, Inc.
260 Center St.
Holbrook, MA 02343
Phone: (617)767-8100
Fax: (617)767-0994

$12.95/volume. There are 18 volumes in the Job Bank Series, each covering a different job market. Volumes exist for the following areas: Atlanta, Boston, Chicago, Dallas/Fort Worth, Denver, Detroit, Florida, Houston, Los Angeles, Minneapolis, New York, Ohio, Pennsylvania, Phoenix, San Francisco, Seattle, St. Louis, and Washington D.C. Each directory lists employers and provides name, address, telephone number, and contact information. Many entries include common positions, educational backgrounds sought, and fringe benefits provided. Cross-indexed by industry and alphabetically by company name. Profiles of professional associations, a section on the region's economic outlook, and listings of executive search and job placement agencies are included. Features sections on conducting a successful job search campaign and writing resumes and cover letters.

Jobs Rated Almanac: Ranks the Best and Worst Jobs by More Than a Dozen Vital Criteria

World Almanac
200 Park Ave.
New York, NY 10166
Phone: (212)692-3830

Les Krantz. 1988. Ranks 250 jobs by environment, salary, outlook, physical demands, stress, security, travel opportunities, and geographic location. Includes jobs the editor feels are the most common, most interesting, and the most rapidly growing.

Joyce Lain Kennedy's Career Book

VGM Career Horizons
4255 W. Touhy Ave.
Lincolnwood, IL 60646-1975
Phone: (708)679-5500

Kennedy, Joyce Lain. Co-authored by Dr. Darryl Laramore. 1992. $17.95 paperback. $29.95 hardcover. 448 pages. Guides the reader through the entire career planning and job hunting process.

Medical Assisting—A Career for Today and Tomorrow (RMA)

Registered Medical Assistants (RMA)
710 Higgins Rd.
Park Ridge, IL 60068-5765
Phone: (708)823-5169

Moody's Corporate Profiles

Moody's Investors Service, Inc.
Dun and Bradstreet Co.
99 Church St.
New York, NY 10007
Phone: (212)553-0300
Fax: (212)553-4700

Provides data on more than 5,000 publicly held companies listed on the New York Stock Exchange or the American Stock Exchange or NMS companies traded on the National Association of Securities Dealers Automated Quotations. Available through DIALOG Information Services, Inc.

National Directory of Internships

National Society for Internships and
Experiential Education
3509 Haworth Dr., Ste. 207
Raleigh, NC 27609
Phone: (919)787-3263

Biennial. $22.00. Covers over 30,000 educational

internship opportunities in 75 fields with over 2,650 organizations in the United States for youth and adults.

Nursing Assistants & the Long-Term Health Care Facility

J. B. Lippincott Co.
227 E. Washington Square
Philadelphia, PA 19106
Phone: (215)238-4200

Lorna Hanebuth. 1977.

Occupational Outlook Handbook

Bureau of Labor Statistics
441 G St., NW
Washington, DC 20212
Phone: (202)523-1327

A biennial directory containing profiles of various occupations, including description of occupation, educational requirements, market demand, and expected earnings.It also lists over 100 state employment agencies.

Occupational Therapy: Principles & Practice

Williams and Wilkins
428 E. Preston St.
Baltimore, MD 21202
Phone: (410)528-4000
Toll-free: 800-638-0672

Alice J. Punwar. 1988. Includes bibliographies and an index. Illustrated.

Opportunities in Chiropractic Health Careers

National Textbook Co.
NTC Publishing Group
4255 W. Touhy Ave.
Lincolnwood, IL 60646-1975
Phone: (708)679-5500
Toll-free: 800-323-4900

R.C. Schafer. 1987. Presents an overview of the profession, its history and development, the science and philosophy of chiropractic therapy. Describes the basic role of the chiropractic physician, career opportunities educational requirements, licensure, and the future of the profession.

Opportunities in Eye Care Careers

VGM Career Horizons
4255 W. Touhy Ave.
Lincolnwood, IL 60646-1975
Phone: (312)679-5500
Toll-free: 800-323-4900

Kathleen M. Ahrens. 1991.

Opportunities in Fitness Careers

National Textbook Co.
NTC Publishing Group
4255 W. Touhy Ave.
Lincolnwood, IL 60646
Phone: (312)679-5500
Toll-free: 800-323-4900

Jean Rosenbaum. 1991. Surveys fitness related careers, including the career of occupational therapist. Describes career opportunities, education and experience needed, how to get into entry-level jobs and what income to expect. Schools are listed in the appendix.

Opportunities in Nutrition Careers

National Textbook Co.
NTC Publishing Group
4255 W. Touhy Ave.
Lincolnwood, IL 60646-1975
Phone: (708)679-5500
Toll-free: 800-323-4900

Carol C. Caldwell. 1992. Describes how to become a registered dietitian and discusses different educational programs. Suggests many different work environments and overviews new career opportunities.

Opportunities in Occupational Therapy Careers

National Textbook Co.
NTC Publishing Group
4255 W. Touhy Ave.
Lincolnwood, IL 60646-1975
Phone: (708)679-5500
Toll-free: 800-323-4900

Marguerite Abbott. 1988. Discusses history, educational and licensure requirements, and the working conditions. Describes the occupational therapist in clinical work, in administration, and in education. Covers salaries, educational programs, and where to write for more information.

Opportunities in Pharmacy Careers

National Textbook Co.
NTC Publishing Group
4255 W. Touhy Ave.
Lincolnwood, IL 60646-1975
Phone: (708)679-5500
Toll-free: 800-323-4900

Gable, Fred B. 1990.

Opportunities in Physical Therapy Careers

National Textbook Co.
NTC Publishing Group
4255 W. Touhy Ave.
Lincolnwood, IL 60646-1975
Phone: (708)679-5500
Toll-free: 800-323-4900

Bernice Krumhansl. 1993. Gives the history and an overview of physical therapy as a career. Discusses the many different settings where physical therapists work. Describes training requirements and lists colleges and universities offering programs in physical therapy.

Growth in employment is only one source of job openings. In fact, most openings arise because of the need to replace workers who transfer to other occupations or leave the labor force.

Source: *Occupational Outlook Quarterly*

Opportunities in Speech-Language Pathology Careers

National Textbook Co.
NTC Publishing Group
4255 W. Touhy Ave.
Lincolnwood, IL 60646-1975
Phone: (708)679-5500
Toll-free: 800-323-4900

Patricia G. Larkins. 1988.

Optician

Careers, Inc.
PO Box 135
Largo, FL 34649-0135
Phone: (813)584-7333

1990. Eight-page brief offering the definition, history, duties, working conditions, personal qualifications, educational requirements, earn-

ings, hours, employment outlook, advancement, and careers related to this position.

Passbooks for Career Opportunities: Physical Therapist

National Learning Corporation
212 Michael Dr.
Syosset, NY 11791
Phone: (516)921-8888
Toll-free: 800-645-6337
Fax: (516)921-8743

1984.

Peterson's Job Opportunities for Business and Liberal Arts Graduates

Peterson's
PO Box 2123
Princeton, NJ 08543-2123
Phone: (609)243-9111

1993. $20.95. 300 pages. Lists hundreds of organizations that are hiring new business, humanities, and social science graduates in the areas of business and management.

Pharmacist

Careers, Inc.
PO Box 135
Largo, FL 34649-0135
Phone: (813)584-7333

1989. Eight-page brief offering the definition, history, duties, working conditions, personal qualifications, educational requirements, earnings, hours, employment outlook, advancement, and careers related to this position.

Pharmacy: A Caring Profession

American Association of Colleges of Pharmacy
1426 Prince St.
Alexandria, VA 22314-2841
Phone: (703)739-2330

1992. This six-panel brochure describes the profession and educational preparation required and lists schools of pharmacy.

Pharmacy Education and Careers: The APhA Resource Book

American Pharmaceutical Association (APhA)
2215 Constitution Ave., NW
Washington, DC 20037
Phone: (202)628-4410

Vicki L. Meade, editor. 1991-92.

Pharmacy. Is It the Career for You?

National Association of Chain Drug Stores
PO Box 1417-D49
Alexandria, VA 22313
Phone: (703)549-3001

1987. This eight-panel pamphlet describes the need for pharmacists; lists colleges and universities with pharmacy programs.

Physical Therapist

Careers, Inc.
PO Box 135
Largo, FL 34649-0135
Phone: (813)584-7333

1991. Eight-page brief offering the definition, history, duties, working conditions, personal qualifications, educational requirements, earnings, hours, employment outlook, advancement, and careers related to this position.

Physical Therapists

Chronicle Guidance Publications, Inc.
66 Aurora St.
PO Box 1190
Moravia, NY 13118-1190
Phone: (315)497-0330
Toll-free: 800-622-7284

1991. Career brief describing the nature of the job, working conditions, hours and earnings, education and training, licensure, certification, unions, personal qualifications, social and psychological factors, location, employment outlook, entry methods, advancement, and related occupations.

Physician Assistant

Careers, Inc.
PO Box 135
Largo, FL 34649-0135
Phone: (813)584-7333

1992. Two-page occupational summary card describing duties, working conditions, personal qualifications, training, earnings and hours, employment outlook, places of employment, related careers, and where to write for more information.

Physician Assistant Programs

American Academy of Physician Assistants
950 N. Washington St.
Alexandria, VA 22314-1552
Phone: (703)836-2272

1988. This information packet describes accreditation of physician assistant programs, curriculum, and degrees awarded to physician assistants.

The Physician Assistant Up Close

Pennsylvania Society of Physician Assistants
PO Box 8988
Pittsburgh, PA 15221-8988
Phone: (412)836-6411

1989. Eight-panel brochure explaining education, credentials, and roles of physician assistants.

---

ften the skill that distinguishes a person the most is her or his ability for self-promotion because, in the nontraditional job arena, communication links are less formal and structured. People learn about qualified practitioners through resumes, personal interviews, mutual friends, and acquaintances; through membership in organizations and on committees; through networking, publishing, and speaking. Dietitians find jobs by looking around, talking to people, becoming known, and marketing their particular area of expertise.

Source: *Journal of the American Dietetic Association*

Planning a Career in Chiropractic

American Chiropractic Association
1701 Clarendon Blvd.
Arlington, VA 22209
Phone: (703)276-8800
Toll-free: 800-368-3083

1992. This 15-page booklet provides general information on the history, growth, and goals of chiropractic as well as the educational requirements necessary for a doctor's degree, licensure information, and scholarship opportunities.

Professional's Job Finder

Planning/Communications
7215 Oak Ave.
River Forest, IL 60305-1935
Phone: (708)366-5297

$15.95. Discusses how to use sources of private sector job vacancies in a number of specialties and state by state, including job-matching services, job hotlines, directories, and more.

Recreation Therapist

Careers, Inc.
PO Box 135
Largo, FL 34649-0135
Phone: (813)584-7333
Toll-free: 800-726-0441

1992. Two-page occupational summary card describing duties, working conditions, personal qualifications, training, earnings and hours, employment outlook, places of employment, related careers, and where to write for more information.

Rehabilitation Counselors

Chronicle Guidance Publications, Inc.
66 Aurora St.
PO Box 1190
Moravia, NY 13118-1190
Phone: (315)497-0330
Toll-free: 800-622-7284

1991. Career brief describing the nature of the job, working conditions, hours and earnings, education and training, licensure, certification, unions, personal qualifications, social and psychological factors, location, employment outlook, entry methods, advancement, and related occupations.

By the end of this decade, 85 percent of all new entrants into the workforce will be women, minorities and immigrants, and they will bring with them very different cultures and values.

Source: *Television Quarterly*

Relief Pharmacist

Vocational Biographies, Inc.
PO Box 31
Sauk Centre, MN 56378-0031
Phone: (612)352-6516

1988. Four-page pamphlet containing a personal narrative about a worker's job, work likes and dislikes, career path from high school to the present, education and training, the rewards and frustrations, and the effects of the job on the rest of the worker's life. The data file portion of this pamphlet gives a concise occupational summary, including work description, working conditions, places of employment, personal characteristics, education and training, job outlook, and salary range.

Respiratory Care Practitioner

Careers, Inc.
PO Box 135
Largo, FL 34649-0135
Phone: (813)584-7333
Toll-free: 800-726-0441

1991. Two-page occupational summary card describing duties, working conditions, personal qualifications, training, earnings and hours, employment outlook, places of employment, related careers, and where to write for more information.

Respiratory Care Workers

Chronicle Guidance Publications, Inc.
66 Aurora St.
PO Box 1190
Moravia, NY 13118-1190
Phone: (315)497-0330
Toll-free: 800-622-7284

1990. Career brief describing the nature of the job, working conditions, hours and earnings, education and training, licensure, certification, unions, personal qualifications, social and psychological factors, location, employment outlook, entry methods, advancement, and related occupations.

Set Your Sights: Your Future in Dietetics—Educational Pathways

American Dietetic Association (ADA)
216 W. Jackson Blvd., Ste. 800
Chicago, IL 60606-6995
Phone: (312)899-0040
Toll-free: 800-877-1600

Three-page pamphlet describing different types of dietitians in different work settings, education, salary, financial aid, and job outlook.

Shall I Study Pharmacy?

American Association of Colleges of Pharmacy
1426 Prince St.
Alexandria, VA 22314-2841
Phone: (703)739-2330

Tenth edition, 1992. This 31-page booklet explains career opportunities in community and hospital pharmacy and the pharmaceutical industry; describes personal qualifications, educational preparation, professional courses, working conditions, and financial aid. Lists colleges and schools of pharmacy in the United States.

Speech-Language Pathologist

Careers, Inc.
PO Box 135
Largo, FL 34649-0135
Phone: (813)584-7333
Toll-free: 800-726-0441

1991. Eight-page brief offering the definition, history, duties, working conditions, personal qualifications, educational requirements, earnings, hours, employment outlook, advancement, and careers related to this position.

Speech Language Pathologists and Audiologists

Chronicle Guidance Publications, Inc.
Aurora St. Extension
PO Box 1190
Moravia, NY 13118-1190
Phone: (315)497-0330
Toll-free: 800-622-7284

1987. Career brief describing the nature of the job, working conditions, hours and earnings, education and training, licensure, certification, unions, personal qualifications, social and psychological factors, location, employment outlook, entry methods, advancement, and related occupations.

Standard and Poor's Register of Corporations, Directors, and Executives

Standard and Poor's Corp.
25 Broadway
New York, NY 10004
Phone: (212)208-8283

An annual directory that covers over 55,000 corporations in the United States, including names and titles of over 500,000 officials and 70,000 biographies of directors and executives.

Therapeutic Recreation Specialists

Chronicle Guidance Publications, Inc.
66 Aurora St. Extension
PO Box 1190
Moravia, NY 13118-1190
Phone: (315)497-0330
Toll-free: 800-622-7284

1988. Career brief describing the nature of the job, working conditions, hours and earnings, education and training, licensure, certification, unions, personal qualifications, social and psychological factors, location, employment out-

look, entry methods, advancement, and related occupations.

VGM's Careers Encyclopedia

National Textbook Co.
4255 W. Touhy Ave.
Lincolnwood, IL 60646-1975
Phone: (708)679-5500

Norback, Craig T., editor. Third edition, 1991. Profiles 180 occupations. Describes job duties, places of employment, working conditions, qualifications, education and training, advancement potential, and salary for each occupation. Chapters include "Geologist" (pp. 171-172), "Geophysicist" (pp. 173-175), and "Oceanographer" (pp. 280-282).

---

nterview proactively. Make a list of questions you'd like answered. Target the company's current and future plans, the job and where it could lead. You'll have the chance to ask most of them if you tie them into the answers you give on similar topics.

Source: Business Monday/Detroit Free Press

Ward's Business Directory of U.S. Private and Public Companies

Gale Research Inc.
835 Penobscot Bldg.
Detroit, MI 48226
Phone: (313)961-2242
Fax: (313)961-6241

1993. Four volumes. Contains information on over 85,000 U.S. businesses, over 90% of which are privately held. Entries include company name, address, and phone; sales; employees; description; names of officers; fiscal year end information; etc.

What Color Is Your Parachute?

Ten Speed Press
PO Box 7123
Berkeley, CA 94707
Phone: (415)845-8414

Bolles, Richard N. 1993. $12.95 paperback; $18.95 hardcover. Provides detailed and strategic advice on all aspects of the job search.

Where the Jobs Are: A Comprehensive Directory of 1200 Journals Listing Career Opportunities
Garrett Park Press
PO BOx 190
Garrett Park, MD 20896
Phone: (301)946-2553

1989. $15.00. Contains list of approximately 1,200 journals that publish advertisements announcing job opportunities.

W hen we consciously choose to do the work that we enjoy, not only can we get things done, but we can get them done well and be intrinsically rewarded for our effort, according to organizational psychologist Marsha Sinetar.

Source: *The Detroit News*

Where the Jobs Are: The Hottest Careers for the '90s
The Career Press
180 5th Ave.
PO Box 34
Hawthorne, NJ 07507

Satterfield, Mark. 1992. $9.95. Provides a look at current trends in the job market and the industries that offer the greatest opportunity for those entering the work force or making a career change.

Where to Start Career Planning
Peterson's
PO Box 2123
Princeton, NJ 08543-2123
Phone: (609)243-9111

Lindquist, Carolyn Lloyd and Miller, Diane June. 1991. $17.95 315 pages. Lists and describes the career planning publications used by Cornell University's Career Center, one of the largest career libraries in the country. It covers more than 2,000 books, periodicals, and audiovisual resources.

Professional and Trade Periodicals

ADA News
American Dental Assn.
211 E. Chicago Ave.
Chicago, IL 60611
Phone: (312)440-2786

James Berry, Editor. Every other week. Dental magazine.

Advance
Foundation for Chiropractic Education and Research
1701 Clarendon Blvd.
Arlington, VA 22209-2712
Phone: (703)276-7445

Editor(s): Patti Frattarola. Bimonthly. Provides information on programs and projects related to the Foundation, including research sponsored by the Foundation.

AHANews (AHA)
American Hospital Association (AHA)
840 N. Lake Shore Dr.
Chicago, IL 60611
Phone: (312)280-6000

Weekly.

American College of Apothecaries—Newsletter
American College of Apothecaries
205 Daingerfield Rd.
Alexandria, VA 22314
Phone: (703)684-8603

Editor(s): D.C. Huffman, Jr. Monthly. Presents national pharmacy news designed to assist association members in their professional practices.

American Hospital Association— Outreach
American Hospital Association
840 N. Lake Shore Dr.
Chicago, IL 60611
Phone: (312)280-5921

Editor(s): Marilyn Canna. Bimonthly. Analyzes the factors influencing market supply, demand, and competition.

American Occupational Therapy Association—Federal Report

American Occupational Therapy Association
1383 Piccard Dr.
PO Box 1725
Rockville, MD 20850
Phone: (301)948-9626

Frederick P. Somers, editor. Bimonthly. Analyzes legislative and regulatory issues related to occupational therapy, primarily Medicare and Medicaid. Carries information on health care inflation, cost reimbursement for hospitals, the prospective payment system, taxes, physician competition, rehabilitation services, hospitals, home health agencies, skilled nursing facilities, and health planning.

American Rehabilitation

U.S. Government Printing Office
Superintendent of Documents
Washington, DC 20402
Phone: (202)783-3238
Fax: (202)512-2233

Magazine on rehabilitation of the handicapped.

American Society of Allied Health Professions—Trends

American Society of Allied Health Professions
1101 Connecticut Ave., NW, Ste. 700
Washington, DC 20036
Phone: (202)857-1150
Toll-free: 800-879-2724
Fax: (202)223-4579

Editor(s): Thomas W. Elwood. Monthly. Discusses the educational programs, grants and funding, and employment opportunities available to those employed in allied health professions. Examines the achievements of allied health professionals as well as the effects and implications of their work.

ASHA

American Speech-Language-Hearing Association
10801 Rockville Pike
Rockville, MD 20852
Phone: (301)897-5700
Fax: (301)571-0457

Monthly magazine on hearing, language, and speech.

ASPMA Journal (ASPMA)

American Society of Podiatric Medical Assistants (ASPMA)
2124 S. Austin Blvd.
Cicero, IL 60650
Phone: (708)863-6303

Quarterly.

ASPMA Newsletter (ASPMA)

American Society of Podiatric Medical Assistants (ASPMA)
2124 S. Austin Blvd.
Cicero, IL 60650
Phone: (708)863-6303

Bimonthly.

Audiology: Official Organ of the International Society of Audiology

S. Karger Publishers, Inc.
26 W. Avon Rd.
PO Box 529
Farmington, CT 06085
Phone: (203)675-7834

J. N. Aran, editor. Bimonthly. Scientific medical journal.

Communication Outlook

Artificial Language Laboratory
405 Computer Center
Michigan State University
East Lansing, MI 48824-1042
Phone: (517)353-0870

Editor(s): Tammi Watt, Leann Tonn, and Tracy Birkenhauer. Quarterly. Provides information on modern techniques and aids for persons who experience communication handicaps due to neurological or neuromuscular conditions. Reports on current research, centers, programs, and projects in the field.

Contact Lens Spectrum

Viscom Publications, Inc.
50 Washington St.
Norwalk, CT 06854
Phone: (203)838-9100
Fax: (203)838-2550

Dr. Joseph T. Barr, Editor. Monthly. Magazine for eye care professionals providing contact lens care and contact lens products.

Current Opinion in Dentistry

Current Science
20 N. 3rd St.
Philadelphia, PA 19106-2113
Phone: (215)574-2266
Fax: (215)574-2270

S.T. Sonis, Editor. 3x/yr. Journal for dental professionals.

Employment for chiropractors is expected to rise because of the rapidly growing older population, with its greater likelihood of physiological problems, and as the awareness of chiropractic services grows.

Source: *Occupational Outlook Quarterly*

Dental Abstracts

C.E. Moseby
11830 Westline Industrial Dr.
St. Louis, MO 63146
Phone: (314)872-8370
Fax: (314)432-1158

Lawrence H. Meskin, Editor. Bimonthly. Dentistry professional magazine.

The Dental Assistant

American Dental Assistants Assn.
919 N. Michigan, Ste. 3400
Chicago, IL 60611
Phone: (312)664-3327
Fax: (312)664-5288

Mike Shaneyfelt, Editor. Quarterly.

Dental Clinics of North America

W.B. Saunders Co.
The Curtis Center
Independence Sq. W.
Philadelphia, PA 19106-3399
Phone: (215)238-7800
Fax: (215)238-7883

Susan C. Short, Editor. Quarterly. Journal reviewing current techniques in dentistry.

Dentistry Today

26 Park St.
Montclair, NJ 07042
Phone: (201)783-3935
Fax: (201)783-7112

Ted Fetner, Jr., Editor. 10x/yr. Dental magazine (tabloid).

Diet Center—the Update

Diet Center, Inc.
921 Penn Ave., 9th Fl.
Pittsburgh, PA 15222
Phone: 800-333-2581

Melissa Harrell, editor. Monthly. Promotes better health through sound nutrition. Contains articles on dietary goals and guidelines, anorexia, the cholesterol controversy, and other diet-related concerns.

Ear and Hearing

Williams & Wilkins
428 E. Preston St.
Baltimore, MD 21202
Phone: (410)528-4068
Fax: (410)528-4452

Susan Jerger, editor. Six issues/year. Original articles on auditory disorders.

Environmental Nutrition

Environmental Nutrition, Inc.
52 Riverside Dr.
New York, NY 10024
Phone: (212)362-0424

Densie Webb, editor. Monthly. Keeps readers abreast of new findings and breakthroughs in nutrition and diet. Discusses nutrition in connection with food additives, food fads and diets, pharmaceuticals and vitamins, and disease prevention.

The Explorer

National Association of Dental Assistants
900 S Washington St., No. G13
Falls Church, VA 22046-4020
Phone: (703)237-8616

Editor(s): Sue Young. Monthly. Reflects the Association's goal of improving the professional and personal lives of dental assistants and other staff. Provides information relating to the field of dentistry.

Health Business

Faulkner & Gray, Inc.
1133 15th St., NW
Washington, DC 20005
Phone: (202)828-4148

Editor(s): John Reichard. Weekly.

Health Labor Relations Reports

Interwood Publications
PO Box 20241
Cincinnati, OH 45220
Phone: (513)221-3715

Editor(s): Frank J. Bardack. Bimonthly. Focuses on employee and labor relations in the health care field. Reports on court and National Labor Relations Board (NLRB) decisions in the areas of wrongful discharge, employment-at-will, discrimination, and union organizing. Also notifies readers of arbitration awards and contract settlements.

Health Professions Report

Whitaker Newsletters, Inc.
313 South Ave.
Fanwood, NJ 07023-0340
Phone: (908)889-6336
Fax: (201)889-6339

Editor(s): Arne C. Bittner. Twenty-six issues/year. Tracks statistics on enrollment and educational costs, reports on relevant legislative and regulatory changes, and announces conferences, workshops, and other educational opportunities.

Healthwire

Federation of Nurses and Health Professionals
American Federation of Teachers
555 New Jersey Ave. NW
Washington, DC 20001
Phone: (202)879-4430

Editor(s): Priscilla M. Nemeth. 6/yr. Explores national news and issues affecting health care workers. Discusses general union developments as well as labor and union concerns specific to the health care field. Recurring features include local member news, book reviews, news of research, and columns titled Clipboard, Pulse Points, Stethescope, Second Opinion, and Making Rounds.

Hospital Practice

HP Publishing Co.
55 5th Ave., 14th Fl.
New York, NY 10003
Phone: (212)989-2100

Samuel C. Bukantz, M.D., editor. Eighteen issues/year. Magazine providing information on developments and problem areas in medicine and clinical research. Emphasizes application of medical knowledge to the direct care of patients.

JADA

ADA Publishing Company
211 E. Chicago Ave.
Chicago, IL 60611
Phone: (312)440-2740
Fax: (312)440-2550

James Berry, Editor. Monthly. Dental magazine.

At the same time that whale-size firms are whacking away the blubber, a net of 1.9 million new jobs will be created this year 1992, estimates Dun & Bradstreet, and 80 percent of them will be at companies with fewer than 100 employees.

Source: *U.S. News & World Report*

Natural Health Outreach

Nutripathic Formulas, Inc.
13402 N. Scottsdale Rd., B150
Scottsdale, AZ 85254
Phone: (602)948-5100
Toll-free: 800-654-3734
Fax: (602)948-8150

Gary A. Martin, editor. Ten issues/year. Discusses the merits of various "natural health products" (mainly dietary supplements) available through Nutripathic Formulas, Inc. Also provides information on studies and research relating to health problems brought on by vitamin deficiencies. Recurring features include letters from students of the company's nutripathic program.

Network-AAMA (AAMA)

American Association of Medical Assistants
(AAMA)
20 N. Wacker Dr., Ste. 1575
Chicago, IL 60606
Phone: (312)899-1500

Quarterly. Newsletter including calendar of events.

NNFA Today

National Nutritional Foods Association
150 Paularino Ave., Ste. 285
Costa Mesa, CA 92626
Phone: (714)966-6632
Fax: (714)641-7005

Burton Kallman, Ph.D., editor. Monthly. Supplies professionals in the health foods industry with analysis of business, social, technological, scientific, and economic developments affecting the industry. Provides information and suggestions about marketing, merchandising, public relations, and business management.

I n today's competitive marketplace, people who have not thought about their future may not have one, or at least not a very bright one. Job seekers must be able to match their skills to the jobs available. You'll stand a better chance of having the right skills if you know which ones will be in demand.

Source: *Occupational Outlook Quarterly*

NOHA News

Nutrition for Optimal Health Association
(NOHA)
PO Box 380
Winnetka, IL 60093
Phone: (708)835-5030

Marjorie Fisher and Lynn Lawson, editors. Quarterly. Examines the links between good nutrition and health. Reports nutritional information and research findings from scientific and medical sources.

Nutrition Action Healthletter

Center for Science in the Public Interest
1875 Connecticut Ave., NW, Ste. 300
Washington, DC 20009-5728
Phone: (202)332-9110
Fax: (202)265-4954

Stephen B. Schmidt, editor. Ten issues/year. Covers food and nutrition, the food industry, and relevant government regulations and legislation. Focuses upon the connections among diet, lifestyle, and disease. Includes nutritional comparisons of food products, reader questions and answers, and health-promoting recipies.

Nutrition and Health

Institute of Human Nutrition
Columbia University College of Physicians
and Surgeons
100 Haven Ave., No. 4F
Tower 3
New York, NY 10032
Phone: (212)305-6991

Monthly. Geared towards treating and preventing diseases. Covers a single topic each month.

Nutrition & the M.D.

PM, Inc.
7100 Hayvenhurst, Ste. 107
PO Box 10172
Van Nuys, CA 91410
Phone: (818)997-8011
Toll-free: 800-365-2468

Mary Stein, editor. Monthly. Covers such topics as foodborne illness, the effects of infection on nutrient metabolism, environmental contamination, food allergies, and amino acid therapy. Reports on specific food coloring dyes, preservatives, and other additives, and examines various health and nutrition studies conducted by major health institutions.

Nutrition Health Review

Vegetus Publications
Vegetus Foundation
171 Madison Ave.
New York, NY 10016
Phone: (212)679-3590

Frank Ray Rifkin, editor. Quarterly. Aims to educate the public about nutrition and health. Covers developments in areas including medical care, psychology, childraising, and geriatrics.

Nutrition News

Gurumantra S. Khalsa
4108 Watkins Dr.
Riverside, CA 92507
Phone: (714)784-7500

Siri Khalsa, editor. Monthly. Disseminates current research on nutrition and wellness in nontechnical, in-depth articles.

Nutrition Research Newsletter

Lyda Associates
PO Box 700
Palisades, NY 10964
Phone: (914)359-8282

Lillian Langseth, editor. 10/year. Summarizes over 400 biomedical journals to provide abstracts and citations to literature in nutrition research and clinical nutrition research.

Physical & Occupational Therapy in Geriatrics

The Haworth Press, Inc.
10 Alice St.
Binghamton, NY 13904
Phone: (607)722-2493
Toll-free: (607)722-5857

Ellen D. Taira, editor. Quarterly. Journal for allied health professionals focusing on current practice and emerging issues in the health care of the older client.

Physical Disabilities Special Interest Section—Newsletter

Physical Disabilities Special Interest Section
American Occupational Therapy Association
1383 Piccard Dr.
Rockville, MD 20850
Phone: (301)948-9626
Fax: (301)948-5512

Editor(s): Katherine Post. Quarterly. Focuses on the clinical management of people with physical disabilities. Publishes articles relevant to occupational therapy practice, including such topics as assessment protocols, treatment approaches, and program administration.

Professional Medical Assistant (AAMA)

American Association of Medical Assistants (AAMA)
20 N. Wacker Dr., Ste. 1575
Chicago, IL 60606
Phone: (312)899-1500

Bimonthly. Journal; includes association news, index of advertisers, book reviews, and calendar of events. Also contains annual directory.

Quintessence International

Quintessence Publishing Co., Inc.
551 N. Kimberly Dr.
Carol Stream, IL 60188-1881
Phone: (708)682-3223
Toll-free: 800-621-0387
Fax: (708)682-3288

Richard J. Simonsen, D.D.S., M.S., Editor-in-Chief. Monthly. Dental journal.

Special Care in Dentistry

Federation of Special Care Organizations in Dentistry
211 E. Chicago Ave., 17th Fl.
Chicago, IL 60611
Phone: (312)440-2660
Fax: (312)440-7494

Dr. Roseann Mulligan, Editor. 6x/yr. Dental journal.

Staying Well Newsletter

Foundation for Chiropractic Education and Research
c/o Acme Printing Company
66 Washington Blvd.
Des Moines, IA 50314
Phone: 800-622-6309

Editor(s): Tom Wolff. Bimonthly. Promotes health and fitness. Carries a feature article and news briefs on such topics as living a better life after age 65, the effect of fitness on life insurance premiums, milk intolerance, and other health-related issues.

Technology for Health Care Series

ECRI
5200 Butler Pike
Plymouth Meeting, PA 19462
Phone: (215)825-6000

Monthly. Concerned with the safety, performance, reliability, and cost effectiveness of health care technology. Covers areas of anesthesia, cardiology, emergengy medicine, imaging and radiology, laboratory medicine, materials management, nursing, respiratory therapy, and surgery. Reviews device test results and warns of hazards and deficiencies.

Selecting a boss who is a good match for your work style can be critical to your job success. The mismatched, or wrong boss, can make your work life miserable, as well as significantly damage your career.

Source: *The Detroit News*

Technology for Respiratory Therapy

ECRI
5200 Butler Pike
Plymouth Meeting, PA 19462
Phone: (215)825-6000
Fax: (215)834-1275

Editor(s): Elizabeth A. Richardson. Monthly. Reviews medical device technology and summarizes reported problems, hazards, and recalls.

Technology for Surgery

ECRI
5200 Butler Pike
Plymouth Meeting, PA 19462
Phone: (215)825-6000

Editor(s): Elizabeth Richardson. Monthly. Concerned with problems relating to surgical medical devices. Offers ECRI comparative product evaluations and summarizes reported problems, hazards, and recalls involving medical devices.

Therapeutic Recreation Journal

National Recreation and Park Assn.
3101 Park Center Dr., Ste. 1200
Alexandria, VA 22302-1593
Phone: (703)820-4940
Fax: (703)671-6772

Rikki S. Epstein, C.T.R.S., managing editor. Quarterly. Journal providing forum for research and discussion of therapeutic recreation for persons with disabilities.

Voice of the Pharmacist— Newsletter

Voice of the Pharmacist, Inc.
American College of Apothecaries
205 Daingerfield Rd.
Alexandria, VA 22314
Phone: (703)684-8603
Fax: (703)684-8603

Editor(s): D.C. Huffman, Jr., Ph.D. Quarterly. Examines current issues and opportunities affecting the retail, hospital, and consultant practices of pharmacy. Discusses controversial issues, often with commentary by pharmacists.

Work Programs Special Interest Section—Newsletter

Work Programs Special Interest Section
American Occupational Therapy Association
1383 Piccard Dr.
PO Box 1725
Rockville, MD 20850
Phone: (301)948-9626
Fax: (301)948-5512

Quarterly. Focuses on habilitation and rehabilitation of the worker in areas of physical disabilities, developmental disabilities, and mental health.

Basic Reference Guides

AANC Membership Directory

American Association of Nutritional Consultants (AANC)
1641 E. Sunset Rd., Ste. B117
Las Vegas, NV 89119
Phone: (702)361-1132

Annual.

AAPA Membership Directory

American Association of Pathologists' Assistants (AAPA)
c/o Leo J. Kelly
Dept. of Pathology
VA Medical Center
West Haven, CT 06516
Phone: (203)932-5711

Biennial.

AAPA Membership Directory

American Academy of Physician Assistants (AAPA)
950 N. Washington St.
Alexandria, VA 22314
Phone: (703)836-2272
Fax: (703)684-1924

Annual.

ACA Membership Directory

American Chiropractic Association (ACA)
1701 Clarendon Blvd.
Arlington, VA 22209
Phone: (202)276-8800
Fax: (703)243-2593

Annual.

ACCP Membership Directory

American College of Clinical Pharmacy (ACCP)
3101 Broadway, Ste. 380
Kansas City, MO 64111
Phone: (816)531-2177

Annual. Free to members; $30.00/copy for non-members.

Adapting Activities for Therapeutic Recreation Service: Concepts and Application

Campanile Press
San Diego State University
San Diego, CA 92182
Phone: (619)594-6724

Jesse T. Dixon. 1981. Includes a bibliography.

AGPA Directory

American Group Practice Association (AGPA)
1422 Duke St.
Alexandria, VA 22314
Phone: (703)838-0033

Annual, January. $125.00. Covers: About 300 pri-vate group medical practices and their professional staffs, totalling about 23,000 physicians. Entries include: Group member name, address, phone, names of administrator and other executives, names of physicians listed by medical specialties. Arrangement: Alphabetical. Indexes: Group location, personal name.

AHA Directory of Health Care Professionals

American Hospital Association
840 N. Lake Shore Dr.
Chicago, IL 60611
Phone: (312)280-5957

Annual, May. Covers over 161,000 hospital professionals and 4,000 health care system professionals.

A s the number of settings in which physical therapists' work increases, so do their roles. Community health, industry, sports medicine, and research are particular areas of recent expansion.

AHA Guide to the Health Care Field

Data Services Business Group
American Hospital Association
840 N. Lake Shore Dr.
Chicago, IL 60611
Phone: (312)280-5957

Annual, July. Covers hospitals, multi-health care systems, freestanding ambulatory surgery centers, psychiatric facilities, long-term care facilities, substance abuse programs, hospices, Health Maintenance Organizations (HMOs), and other health-related organizations.

AHSSPPE Membership Directory

Association on Handicapped Student Service Programs in Postsecondary Education (AHSSPPE)
PO Box 21192
Columbus, OH 43221
Phone: (614)488-4972

Annual.

American Academy of Implant Dentistry Directory

American Academy of Implant Dentistry
6900 Grove Rd.
Thorofare, NJ 08086
Phone: (609)848-7027
Fax: (609)853-5991

Annual, December. $1.00. Covers: 2,200 dentists and others engaged in the study of buried metals in the jaw and dental procedures involving implantation. Entries include: Name, address, phone. Arrangement: Geographical. Indexes: Alphabetical (with first year of membership).

American Academy of Pediatric Dentistry Membership Roster

American Academy of Pediatric Dentistry
211 E. Chicago Ave., Ste. 1036
Chicago, IL 60611
Phone: (312)337-2169

Annual, September. $200.00. Covers: 3,100 pediatric dentists in practice, teaching, and research. Entries include: Name, address, phone. Arrangement: Alphabetical. Indexes: Geographical.

Average starting salary for an M.B.A. with a liberal arts bachelor's degree: $35,734. A technical bachelor's degree adds $5,579.

Source: *U.S. News & World Report*

American Dental Directory

American Dental Association
211 E. Chicago Ave.
Chicago, IL 60611
Phone: (312)440-2500
Fax: (312)440-7494

Annual, January. $140.00. Covers: Over 180,000 dentists. Also includes list of active and historic dental schools, dental organizations, dental consultants, and state dental examining boards. Entries include: Name, address, year of birth, educational data, specialty, membership status. Arrangement: Geographical. Indexes: Alphabetical.

American Group Practice Association—Directory

American Group Practice Association
1422 Duke St.
Alexandria, VA 22314
Phone: (703)838-0033
Fax: (703)548-1890

Annual, January. Covers about 300 private group medical practices and their professional staffs, totalling about 23,000 physicians.

American Hospital Association— Guide to the Health Care Field

American Hospital Association (AHA)
840 N. Lakeshore Dr.
Chicago, IL 60611
Phone: (312)280-5957

Annual, July. $195.00; payment with order. Covers: 7,000 hospitals, long-term care facilities, and multihospital systems; individual members; and 1,800 health-related organizations. Entries include: For hospitals - Facility name, address, phone, administrator's name, number of beds, facilities and services, other statistics. For multihospital systems -Headquarters name, address, phone, chief executive. Arrangement: Hospitals are geographical; members are alphabetical. Indexes: Subject.

American Osteopathic Hospital Association Directory

American Osteopathic Hospital Association
5301 Wisconsin Ave. NW, Ste. 630
Washington, DC 20015-2015
Phone: (202)686-1700

Annual, April. $125.00; payment must accompany order. Covers: About 150 osteopathic hospitals. Includes list of individuals and institutional members; also lists osteopathic colleges and state osteopathic hospital associations. Entries include: For hospitals - Name of hospital, name of chief executive officer, address, phone, number of beds and other hospital data, including multi-hospital systems. Similar data given for other lists. Arrangement: Geographical.

APACVS Membership Directory

Association of Physician's Assistants in Cardio-Vascular Surgery (APACVS)
2000 Tate Springs Rd.
PO Box 2242
Lynchburg, VA 24501-2242
Phone: 800-528-1506

Annual.

ASHT Membership Directory

American Society of Hand Therapists (ASHT)
1002 Vandora Springs Rd., Ste. 101
Garner, NC 27529
Phone: (919)779-ASHT
Fax: (919)779-5642

Periodic. Free to members; $125.00/copy for nonmembers.

Billian's Hospital Blue Book

Billian Publishing Co.
2100 Powers Ferry Rd., Ste. 300
Atlanta, GA 30339
Phone: (404)955-5656

Annual, spring. $95.00, plus $4.50 shipping. Covers more than 7,100 hospitals. Entries include name of hospital, accreditation, mailing address, phone, number of beds, type of facility (nonprofit, general, state, etc.); list of administrative personnel and chiefs of medical services, with titles.

CCA Membership Register

Christian Chiropractors Association (CCA)
3200 S. LeMay Ave.
Ft. Collins, CO 80525
Phone: (303)482-1404
Fax: (303)482-1538

Annual.

Chiropractors Directory

American Business Directories, Inc.
American Business Information, Inc.
5711 S. 86th Circle
Omaha, NE 68127
Phone: (402)593-4600
Fax: (402)331-1505

Annual. $1730.00, payment with order. Number of listings: 52,456. Entries include: Name, address, phone (including area code), year first in 'Yellow Pages.' Regional editions available. Arrangement: Geographical.

CLC Directory

Child Life Council (CLC)
7910 Woodmont Ave., Ste. 300
Bethesda, MD 20895

Periodic.

A Clinical Manual for Nursing Assistants

Jones & Bartlett Publishers, Inc.
1 Exeter Plaza
Boston, MA 02116
Phone: (617)859-3900

Sharon McClelland. 1985.

> **C**iticorp is changing the way it uses interns, as are other companies. Instead of providing opportunities for students to examine various career paths, employers are taking a closer look at them as potential full-time employees. This means giving interns more responsibility.
>
> Source: *Fortune*

Clinical Practice of the Dental Hygienist

Lea and Febiger
200 Chesterfield Pkwy.
Malvern, PA 19355
Phone: (215)251-2230
Toll-free: 800-638-0672

Esther M. Wilkins. Sixth edition, 1989. Includes bibliographies and an index.

Complete Handbook for Dental Auxiliaries

Quintessence Publishing Company, Inc.
551 N. Kimberly Dr.
Carol Stream, IL 60188-1881
Phone: (708)682-3223
Toll-free: 800-621-0387
Fax: (708)682-3288

Charles A. Reap, Jr. 1981.

A Comprehensive Dictionary of Audiology

Hearing Aid Journal
63 Great Rd.
Maynard, MA 01754-2025
Phone: (508)897-5552

James H. Delk. 1983.

Comprehensive Respiratory Care

C. V. Mosby Co.
11830 Westline Industrial Dr.
St. Louis, MO 63146
Phone: (314)872-8370
Toll-free: 800-325-4177

1990.

A Comprehensive Review in Respiratory Care

Appleton and Lange
25 Van Zant St.
East Norwalk, CT 06855
Phone: (203)838-4400

Vijay Deshpande, Susan P. Pilbeam, and Robin J. Dixon. 1988. Includes bibliographies and an index.

Nothing can be more frustrating than getting typecast at work. You can get typecast in a certain job or image. Then, when you're ready to move up or into a different area of expertise, you can't get anyone to see you in a different way . . . . One technique to change your image is to dress in a more professional manner. You must also position yourself with people who can help you. One good way is to become active in a professional group, which also can provide you with good contacts and news of opportunities throughout your industry.

Source: *Business Monday/Detroit Free Press*

Contact Lenses Retail Directory

American Business Directories, Inc.
American Business Information, Inc.
5711 S. 86th Circle
Omaha, NE 68127
Phone: (402)593-4600
Fax: (402)331-1505

Annual. $520.00, payment with order. Number of listings: 14,908. Entries include: Name, address, phone (including area code), year first in 'Yellow Pages.' Arrangement: Geographical.

Dental Assisting Manuals

University of North Carolina Chapel Hill
University of North Carolina Press
116 S. Boundary St.
PO Box 2288
Chapel Hill, NC 27515-2288
Phone: (919)966-3561
Toll-free: 800-848-6224
Fax: 800-272-6817

Ethel M. Earl. Third edition.

Dentists Directory

American Business Directories, Inc.
American Business Information, Inc.
5711 S. 86th Circle
Omaha, NE 68127
Phone: (402)593-4600
Fax: (402)331-1505

Annual. $4,945.00. Number of listings: 163,527. Entries include: Name, address, phone (including area code), year first in 'Yellow Pages.' Regional editions available. Arrangement: Geographical.

Dictionary of Rehabilitation Medicine

Springer Publishing Co.
536 Broadway
New York, NY 10012
Phone: (212)431-4370

Herman L. Kamenetz. 1982.

A Dictionary of Speech Therapy

Singular Publishing Group
4284 41st St.
San Diego, CA 92105
Phone: 800-521-8545
Fax: (619)563-9008

David W. H. Morris. Second edition, 1992. Terms are grouped under such subjects as speech pathology, linguistics, phonetics/phonology, psychology/psychiatry, medicine, hearing, electronic devices, and microcomputers. Includes a bibliography and appendixes.

Directory of Drug Stores & HBA Chains

Chain Store Guide Information Services
3922 Coconut Palm Dr.
Tampa, FL 33619
Phone: (813)664-6700

Annual, December. $260.00, plus $5.00 shipping. Covers: Approximately 1,850 drug store chains operating over 31,000 drug and HBA (health and beauty aid) stores, 120 drug wholesalers and their 257 divisions. Also covers over 10,500 key personnel in the industry. Entries include: For drug store chains—Company name, address, phone, fax, product lines, annual sales volume, computerized RX indicator, distribution center, percentage of sales that are prescription sales, store names, number of prescriptions filled daily, number of pharmacies, and names and titles of key personnel. For drug wholesalers—Company name, address, phone, fax, product line, sales history, percentage of sales from prescription sales, number of stores served, and names and titles of key personnel. Arrangement: Separate geographical sections for chains and wholesalers; shows are chronological. Indexes: Top 100 drug store chains ranked by sales (with number of stores); chain headquarters. Regional editions available.

Directory of Hospital Personnel

Medical Device Register
5 Paragon Dr.
Montvale, NJ 07645-1725

Annual. $279.00, plus $5.00 shipping. Covers: 50,000 executives at hospitals with more than 200 beds. Entries include: Name of hospital, address, phone, number of beds, type of hospital, names and titles of key department heads and staff. Arrangement: Geographical. Indexes: Hospital name, personnel, hospital size.

Directory of Nursing Homes

Oryx Press
4041 N. Central, No. 700
Phoenix, AZ 85012
Phone: (602)265-2651
Fax: (602)253-2741

Reported as triennial; latest edition August 1991. $225.00. Covers: 16,259 state-licensed long-term care facilities. Entries include: Name of facility, address, phone, licensure status, number of beds; many listings also include name of administrator and health services supervisor; number of nursing, dietary, and auxiliary staff members; availability of social, recreational, and religious programs; and medicaid/medicare certification status. Arrangement: Geographical. Indexes: Facility name.

Directory of Physicians Assistants-Certified

National Commission on Certification of Physician Assistants (NCCPA)
2845 Henderson Mill Rd., NE
Atlanta, GA 30341
Phone: (404)493-9100

Annual.

Directory of Services for the Deaf in the U.S.

Convention of American Instructors of the Deaf (CAID)
c/o Dr. Stephanie Polowe
Office of the President
PO Box 9887
LBJ 2264
Rochester, NY 14623-0887
Phone: (716)475-6201
Fax: (716)475-6500

Annual.

Effective Dental Assisting

William C. Brown Group
2460 Kerper Blvd.
Dubuque, IA 52001
Phone: (319)588-1451
Fax: 800-346-2377

Shirley Schwarzrock. 1991.

Encyclopedia and Dictionary of Medicine, Nursing, and Allied Health

W. B. Saunders Co.
Curtis Center
Independence Sq., W.
Philadelphia, PA 19106
Phone: (215)238-7800
Toll-free: 800-545-2522

Benjamin F. Miller and Claire B. Keane. Fifth edition, 1992.

Encyclopedia of Medical Organizations and Agencies

Gale Research Inc.
835 Penobscot Bldg.
Detroit, MI 48226-4094
Phone: (313)961-2242
Toll-free: 800-877-GALE
Fax: (313)961-6083

Biennial, October. Covers over 12,000 state, national, and international medical associations, foundations, research institutes, federal and state agencies, and medical and allied health schools.

Essentials of Clinical Dental Assisting

Mosby Co.
11830 Westline Industrial Dr.
St. Louis, MO 63146
Phone: (314)872-8370

Joseph E. Chasteen. Fourth edition, 1989. Includes bibliographies and an index. Illustrated.

Federal Personnel Office Directory

Federal Reports, Inc.
1010 Vermont Ave., NW, Ste. 408
Washington, DC 20005
Phone: (202)393-3311
Fax: (202)393-1553

Biennial, March of even years. $27.00. Covers: Over 1,500 federal government personnel offices that hire people for federal jobs; limited international coverage. Entries include: Government agency name, address, phone, description of services, restrictions for employment eligibility, branch office names and locations. Includes information on federal recruitment programs for disabled persons, women and minorities, veterans, students, and summer employment. Arrangement: Geographical, classified by department or agency.

Some people will find the training they need right at the office. American companies desperate to produce more with fewer, better-skilled workers now are pumping $30 billion annually into employee-training programs that run the gamut from basic computer courses to company-sponsored M.B.A. degrees.

Source: *U.S. News & World Report*

Federal Staff Directory

Staff Directories Ltd.
Box 62
Mount Vernon, VA 22121-0062
Phone: (703)739-0900
Fax: (703)765-1300

Semiannual, December and July. $59.00. Covers: 30,000 persons in federal government offices

and independent agencies, with biographies of 2,500 key executives; includes officials at policy level in agencies of the Office of the President, Cabinet-level departments, independent and regulatory agencies, military commands, federal information centers, and libraries, and United States attorneys, marshals, and ambassadors. Entries include: Name, title, location (indicating building, address, and room), phone. Arrangement: By department or agency. Indexes: Personal name, subject.

Fundamentals of Private Practice in Physical Therapy

Charles C. Thomas, Publisher
2600 S. First St.
Springfield, IL 62794-9265
Phone: (217)789-8980

Mark A. Brimer. 1988. Covers starting a private practice, insurance, hiring personnel, managing the office, and marketing.

Geriatric Nursing Assistants: An Annotated Bibliography with Models to Enhance Practice

Greenwood Publishing Group, Inc.
88 Post Rd., W.
PO Box 5007
Westport, CT 06881
Phone: (203)226-3571
Fax: (203)222-1502

George H. Weber. 1991. Part of Bibliographies & Indexes in Gerontology Series.

Guide to Professional Services in Speech, Language Pathology and Audiology

American Speech-Language-Hearing Association (ASHA)
10801 Rockville Pike
Rockville, MD 20852
Phone: (301)897-5700
Fax: (301)571-0457

Irregular; latest edition April 1987. $28.00, payment with order. Covers: ASHA members in full-time private practice; accredited and nonaccredited clinical speech and hearing programs in the United States and Canada; and personnel of government agencies. Entries include: For accredited clinics - Clinic name, address, phone, director, size and certification of staff, type of clinic, referrals, and services offered. For members - Name, address, phone, specialty, and certification status. For nonaccredited clinics - Name, address, phone, specialty, director, referrals, languages, size and certification of staff. Arrangement: Geographical.

Guild of Prescription Opticians of America Guild Reference Directory

Guild of Prescription Opticians of America,
Division
Opticians Association of America
10341 Democracy Lane
Fairfax, VA 22030
Phone: (703)691-8355
Fax: (703)691-3929

Annual, January. $60.00, postpaid, payment with order. Covers: 250 member firms with a total of 300 retail locations. Entries include: Company name, address, name of manager, services. Arrangement: Geographical.

Handbook Of Clinical Nutrition: Clinician's Manual for the Diagnosis and Management of Nutritional Problems

C. V. Mosby Co.
11830 Westline Industrial Dr.
St. Louis, MO 63146
Phone: (314)872-8370
Fax: (314)432-1380

Roland L. Weinsier and C. E. Butterworth, Jr. 1989. Includes bibliographical references and an index. Illustrated.

Home Health Service Directory

American Business Directories, Inc.
American Business Information, Inc.
5711 S. 86th Circle
Omaha, NE 68127
Phone: (402)593-4600
Fax: (402)331-1505

Annual. $450.00, payment with order. Number of listings: 12,267. Entries include: Name, address, phone (including area code), year first in 'Yellow Pages.' Arrangement: Geographical.

Hospital Market Atlas

SMG Marketing Group, Inc.
1342 N. LaSalle Dr.
Chicago, IL 60610
Phone: (312)642-3026
Fax: (312)642-9729

Biennial. $595.00, postpaid; payment with order.

Covers: Over 8,200 hospitals, clinical laboratories, hospital systems, group purchasing organizations, health maintenance organizations, outpatient surgery centers, and diagnostic imaging centers. Entries include: Hospital or organization name, address, phone, management, type of hospital service, number of beds, admissions, surgical operations, and emergency room visits. Arrangement: Geographical.

Hospital Phone Book

U.S. Directory Service
655 NW 128th St.
Miami, FL 33168
Phone: (305)769-1700

Irregular; previous edition 1988; latest edition 1991/92. Covers about 7,975 hospitals, including military and other federal facilities.

A computer can make it easier to customize your resume. If you store your resume on a computer disk, you can copy it and rearrange it by skills, job chronology or almost any other method, customizing it for each job you apply for.

Source: *Business Monday/Detroit Free Press*

Hospital Phone Book

Reed Reference Publishing
121 Chanlon Rd.
New Providence, RI 07974
Toll-free: 800-521-8110

Contains thousands of numbers and basic information on hospitals around the country.

Hospitals Directory

American Business Directories, Inc.
American Business Information, Inc.
5711 S. 86th Circle
Omaha, NE 68127
Phone: (402)593-4600
Fax: (402)331-1505

Annual. $415.00, payment with order. Number of listings: 10,020. Entries include: Name, address, phone (including area code), year first in 'Yellow Pages.' Arrangement: Geographical.

ICA Membership Directory

International Chiropractors Association (ICA)
1110 N. Glebe Rd., Ste. 1000
Arlington, VA 22201
Phone: (703)528-5000

Annual.

International Association for Orthodontics Membership Directory

International Association for Orthodontics
211 E. Chicago Ave., Ste. 915
Chicago, IL 60611
Phone: (312)642-2602
Fax: (312)642-4191

Annual, June. $15.00. Covers: 1,700 general and children's dentists specializing in prevention or correction of facial and jaw irregularities. Entries include: Name, office address and phone, orthodontic techniques practiced. Arrangement: Geographical. Indexes: Personal name.

International Association of Oral Pathologists Membership List

International Association of Oral Pathologists
c/o Dr. William H. Binnie
3302 Gaston Ave.
Dallas, TX 75246
Phone: (214)828-8110

Annual. Free. Covers: 325 dentists who have had postgraduate instruction in oral pathology. Entries include: Personal name, address. Arrangement: Geographical.

ISPhS Directory

International Society of Phonetic Sciences (ISPhS)
IASP
50 Dauer Hall
University of Florida
Gainesville, FL 32611
Phone: (904)392-2046

Biennial. Free to members.

Life Sciences Organizations and Agencies Directory

Gale Research Inc.
835 Penobscot Bldg.
Detroit, MI 48226
Phone: (313)961-2242
Fax: (313)961-6241

First edition 1988. $155.00. Covers: About 7,500 associations, government agencies, research centers, educational institutions, libraries and information centers, museums, consultants, electronic information services, and other organizations and agencies active in agriculture, biology, ecology, forestry, marine science, nutrition, wildlife and animal sciences, and other natural and life sciences. Entries include: Organization or agency name, address, phone, name and title of contact, description. Arrangement: Classified by type of organization. Indexes: Organization/agency name and keyword.

Medical and Health Information Directory

Gale Research Inc.
835 Penobscot Bldg.
Detroit, MI 48226
Phone: (313)961-2242
Fax: (313)961-6241

Three volumes. Each volume published separately on a biennial basis; volume 1, latest edition 1991; volume 2, latest edition 1992; volume 3, latest edition 1992. $195.00 per volume; $480.00 for the three-volume set. Covers: In volume 1, medical and health oriented associations, organizations, institutions, and government agencies, including health maintenance organizations (HMOs), preferred provider organizations (PPOs), insurance companies, pharmaceutical companies, research centers, and medical and allied health schools. In volume 2, medical book publishers; medical periodicals, review serials, etc.; audiovisual producers and services, medical libraries and information centers, and computerized information systems and services. In volume 3, clinics, treatment centers, care programs, and counseling/diagnostic services for 30 subject areas (drawn from specialized lists published by governments and associations). Entries include: Institution, service, or firm name, address, phone; many include names of key personnel and, when pertinent, descriptive annotation. Arrangement: Classified by activity, service, etc. Indexes: Each volume has a complete master name and keyword index.

Medical Research Centres

Gale Research Inc.
835 Penobscot Bldg.
Detroit, MI 48226
Phone: (313)961-2242
Fax: (313)961-6241

Ninth edition, 1990. Two volumes; $470.00/set.

Covers medical and biochemical research conducted in over 100 countries. Entries include information on industrial enterprises, research laboratories, universities, societies, and professional associations engaged in research in medicine and related subjects like dentistry, nursing, pharmacy, psychiatry, and surgery.

Modern Dental Assisting

W. B. Saunders, Co.
Curtis Center
Independence Sq. W.
Philadelphia, PA 19106
Phone: (215)238-7800
Toll-free: 800-545-2522

Hazel O. Torres. Fourth edition, 1990.

Mosby's Textbook for Nursing Assistants

Mosby Year Book, Inc.
11830 Westline Industrial Dr.
St. Louis, MO 63146
Phone: (314)872-8370

Sorrentino. Third edition, 1991.

NACDS Membership Directory

National Association of Chain Drug Stores (NACDS)
PO Box 1417-D49
Alexandria, VA 22313-1480
Phone: (703)549-3001

Annual.

NAO Membership Directory

National Academy of Opticianry (NAO)
10111 Martin Luther King, Jr. Hwy., Ste. 112
Bowie, MD 20720
Phone: (301)577-4828
Fax: (301)577-3880

National Directory of Internships

National Society for Internships and Experiential Education
3509 Haworth Dr., Ste. 207
Raleigh, NC 27609-7229
Phone: (919)787-3263

Covers more than 30,000 educational internship opportunities in 75 fields with over 650 organizations in the United States. Includes information on deadlines, application procedures, contact names, and eligibility requirements.

National Wholesale Druggists' Association Membership & Executive Directory

National Wholesale Druggists' Association
Box 238
Alexandria, VA 22313
Phone: (703)684-6400
Fax: (703)548-2184

Annual, January. $295.00. Covers: Wholesalers, manufacturers, national drug-trade associations, and colleges of pharmacy. Entries include: For industry—Company name, address, phone, fax, names of principal executives. Arrangement: Classified by type of membership.

Jeffrey A. Sonnenfeld, an Emory University management professor, divides U.S. corporations into 4 categories: the Baseball Team—advertising, entertainment, investment banking, software, biotech research, and other industries based on fad, fashion, new technologies, and novelty; the Club—utilities, government agencies, airlines, banks, and other organizations that tend to produce strong generalists; the Academy—manufacturers in electronics, pharmaceuticals, office products, autos, and consumer products; and the Fortress—companies in fields such as publishing, hotels, retailing, textiles, and natural resources.

NBRC Annual Directory

National Board for Respiratory Care (NBRC)
8310 Nieman Rd.
Lenexa, KS 66214
Phone: (913)599-4200

NCTRC Registry

National Council for Therapeutic Recreation Certification (NCTRC)
49 S. Main St., Ste. 001
Spring Valley, NY 10977
Phone: (914)356-9660

Annual.

Nutrition and Diagnosis-Related Care

Lea and Febiger
200 Chesterfield Pkwy.
Malvern, PA 19355
Phone: (215)251-2230

Sylvia Escott-Stump. Third edition, 1992. Includes a bibliography and an index.

The Nutrition Desk Reference

Keats Publishing, Inc.
27 Pine St., Box 876
New Canaan, CT 06840
Phone: (203)966-8721

Robert H. Garrison and Elizabeth Somer. Second edition, 1990. Includes bibliographies and an index. Illustrated.

Nutritional Influences on Illness: A Sourcebook of Clinical Research

Third Line Press, Inc.
4751 Viviana Dr.
Tarzana, CA 91356
Phone: (818)996-0076

Melvyn R. Werbach. 1992. Discusses the effects of nutrients, toxins, and the environment on many common diseases.

Opticians Directory

American Business Directories, Inc.
American Business Information, Inc.
5711 S. 86th Circle
Omaha, NE 68127
Phone: (402)593-4600
Fax: (402)331-1505

Annual. $560.00, payment with order. Number of listings: 16,396. Entries include: Name, address, phone (including area code), year first in 'Yellow Pages.' Arrangement: Geographical.

The Penguin Encyclopaedia of Nutrition

Viking Penguin, Inc.
375 Hudson St.
New York, NY 10014
Phone: (212)366-2000
Toll-free: 800-631-3577

John Yudkin. 1986. This volume discusses food supplies, food preservation, and the use of food by the body.

Pharmaceutical Dosage Forms, Parenteral Medications

Marcel Dekker, Inc.
270 Madison Ave.
New York, NY 10016
Phone: (212)696-9000

Kenneth E. Avis, Leon Lachman, and Herbert A. Lieberman, editors. Volume 1 and 2, 1992; Volume 3, 1993. Includes bibliographies and an index.

Pharmaceutical Products-Wholesalers & Manufacturers

American Business Directories, Inc.
American Business Information, Inc.
5711 S. 86th Circle
Omaha, NE 68127
Phone: (402)593-4600
Fax: (402)331-1505

Annual. $125.00, payment with order. Number of listing: 2,679. Entries include: Name, address, phone (including area code), year first in 'Yellow Pages.' Arrangement: Geographical.

Physical and Occupational Therapy: Drug Implications for Practice

J. B. Lippincott Co.
227 E. Washington Sq.
Philadelphia, PA 19106
Phone: (215)238-4200
Toll-free: 800-638-3030

Terry Malone, editor. 1989. Includes bibliographies and an index.

Physical Therapists Directory

American Business Directories, Inc.
American Business Information, Inc.
5711 S. 86th Circle
Omaha, NE 68127
Phone: (402)593-4600
Fax: (402)331-1505

Annual. $630.00, payment with order. Number of listings: 18,213. Entries include: Name, address, phone (including area code), year first in 'Yellow Pages.' Arrangement: Geographical.

Physical Therapy Procedures: Selected Techniques

Charles C. Thomas, Publisher
2600 S. First St.
Springfield, IL 62794-9265
Phone: (217)789-8980

Ann H. Downer. Fourth edition, 1988.

Procedural Manual for the Utilization of Physician Extenders

Geisinger Medical Center
Kenneth Harbert, Physician Extender Services
Danville, PA 17822
Phone: (717)271-6094

1991. Manual providing general guidelines, job descriptions, and clinical privileges for physician assistants.

Recommended Dietary Allowances

National Academy Press
2101 Constitution Ave., NW
PO Box 285
Washington, DC 20055
Phone: (202)334-3318
Toll-free: 800-624-6242

Compiled by the National Research Council, Food and Nutrition Board. Tenth edition, 1989.

Rehabilitation Caseload Management: Concepts and Practice

PRO-ED
8700 Shoal Creek Blvd.
Austin, TX 78757-6897
Phone: (512)451-3246

Jack L. Cassell and S. Wayne Mulkey. 1985.

Rehabilitation Counseling and Services: Profession and Process

Charles C. Thomas, Publisher
2600 S. First St.
Springfield, IL 62794-9265
Phone: (217)789-8980

Gerald L. Gandy, et al., editors. 1987.

Remington's Pharmaceutical Sciences

Mack Publishing Co.
1991 Northhampton St.
Easton, PA 18042
Phone: (215)250-7241

Eighteenth edition, 1990. Textbook and reference work for pharmacists.

Respiratory Care of the Newborn: A Clinical Manual

J. B. Lippincott Co.
227 E. Washington Sq.
Philadelphia, PA 19106
Phone: (215)238-4200

Claire A. Aloan. 1993. Includes bibliographies and an index.

Respiratory Facts

F. A. Davis Co.
1915 Arch St.
Philadelphia, PA 19103
Phone: (215)568-2270

John H. Riggs. 1989. Includes bibliographies and an index.

Spinal Cord Injury: A Guide to Functional Outcomes in Occupational Therapy

Aspen Publishers, Inc.
1600 Research Blvd.
Rockville, MD 20850
Phone: (301)417-7500

Judy P. Hill. 1986. Includes a bibliography and an index. Illustrated.

Stroke/Head Injury: A Guide to Functional Outcomes in Physical Therapy Management

Aspen Publishers, Inc.
1600 Research Blvd.
Rockville, MD 20850
Phone: (301)251-5000

Ann Charness and Frederick Schneider, editors. 1986. Includes bibliographies and an index.

Successful Nurse Aide Management in Nursing Homes

Oryx Press
4041 N. Central at Indian School Rd., Ste. 700
Phoenix, AZ 85012-3397
Phone: (602)265-2651
Toll-free: 800-279-6799
Fax: 800-279-4663

Joann M. Day, editor. 1989.

Textbook for Nursing Assistants

Mosby Year Book, Inc.
11830 Westline Industrial Dr.
St. Louis, MO 63146
Phone: (314)872-8370

Sorretino. Second edition, 1988.

Therapeutic Recreation for Long-Term Care Facilities

Human Sciences Press
233 Spring St.
New York, NY 10013
Phone: (212)620-8000

Fred S. Greenblatt. 1988. Includes a bibliography and an index.

Therapeutic Recreation Intervention: An Ecological Perspective

Prentice-Hall, Inc.
Route 9W
Englewood Cliffs, NJ 07632
Phone: (201)592-2000

Roxanne Howe-Murphy and Becky G. Charboneau. Includes bibliographies and an index.

Therapeutic Recreation Program Design: Principles and Procedures

Prentice-Hall, Inc.
Route 9W
Englewood Cliffs, NJ 07632
Phone: (201)592-2000

Scout L. Gunn and Carol A. Peterson. Second edition, 1984. Includes bibliographies and an index.

U.S. Hospitals: The Future of Health Care

Deloitte & Touche
125 Summer St.
Boston, MA 02110
Phone: (617)261-8000

1990. Survey of 25 percent of all acute care hospitals in the United States. The report describes financial losses, low occupancy rates, and nursing shortages.

U.S. Medical Directory

U.S. Directory Service, Publishers
655 NW 128th St.
PO Box 68-1700
Miami, FL 33168
Phone: (305)769-1700
Fax: (305)769-0548

Latest edition 1989. $150.00, plus $5.00 shipping. Covers: Medical doctors, hospitals, nursing facilities, medical research laboratories, poison control centers, medical schools and libraries, and other medical services, organizations, facilities, and institutes.

The United States Pharmacopeia Twenty-Second Revision: The National Formulary, Sixteeth Edition

United States Pharmacopeial Convention, Inc.
PO Box 2248
Rockville, MD 20852
Phone: (301)881-0666
Toll-free: 800-227-8772

1990. Lists standards for drug identification, purity, strength, and formulas.

Veterinary and Human Toxicology

American Academy of Clinical Toxicology (AACT)
Kansas State University
Comparative Toxicology Laboratories
Manhattan, KS 66506-5606
Phone: (913)532-4334
Fax: (913)532-4481

Bimonthly. $50.00/year. Includes annual directory.

Who's Who among Human Services Professionals

National Reference Institute
3004 Glenview Rd.
Wilmette, IL 60091
Phone: (708)441-2387

Biennial, February of even years. $69.95. Covers: Nearly 20,000 human service professionals, in such fields as nursing, counseling, social work, psychology, audiology, and speech pathology. Entries include: Name, address, education, work experience, professional association memberships. Arrangement: Alphabetical. Indexes: Geographical, field of specialization.

Women's Auxiliary of the International Chiropractors Association Membership Roster

Women's Auxiliary of the International
Chiropractors Association
1925 Apple Ave.
Muskegon, MI 49442
Phone: (616)777-2622

Biennial. Covers: About 500 women who are chiropractic assistants, chiropractors, or related to members of the ICA.

MASTER
INDEX

Master Index

The Master Index provides comprehensive access to all four sections of the Directory by citing all subjects, organizations, publications, and services listed throughout in a single alphabetic sequence. The index also includes inversions on significant words appearing in cited organization, publication, and service names. For example, "Ward's Business Directory of U.S. Private and Public Companies" could also be listed in the index under "Companies; Ward's Business Directory of U.S. Private and Public."